People's Mission to the Ottoman Empire

People's Mission to the Ottoman Empire

M. A. Ansari and the Indian Medical Mission, 1912–13

BURAK AKÇAPAR

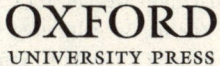

OXFORD
UNIVERSITY PRESS

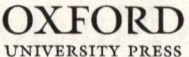

OXFORD
UNIVERSITY PRESS

Oxford University Press is a department of the University of Oxford.
It furthers the University's objective of excellence in research, scholarship,
and education by publishing worldwide. Oxford is a registered trademark of
Oxford University Press in the UK and in certain other countries

Published in India by
Oxford University Press
YMCA Library Building, 1 Jai Singh Road, New Delhi 110001, India

© Oxford University Press 2014

The moral rights of the authors have been asserted

First Edition published in 2014

ISBN-13: 978-0-19-809957-4
ISBN-10: 0-19-809957-6

Typeset in Trump Mediaeval LT Std 9.5/13
by MAP Systems, Bengaluru 560 082, India
Printed in India at Repro India Ltd., Mumbai

To My Beloved Mother,
Gürten Akçapar
(1937–2014)

Contents

Contents

Foreword

A century is a long time in individual memory, much less on the canvas of history. The task of the historian, as Ibn Khaldun said, is to 'lift the veil from conditions as they arose' in earlier generations. Ambassador Burak Akçapar has undertaken one such exercise to shed light on a happening in 1912–13 that highlighted and underlined the emotional bonds between the Muslims of India and the people of Turkey.

The story of the Indian Medical Mission to Turkey has been told in snippets as part of the larger discourse on the evolution of perceptions in India's Muslim community in the early decades of the twentieth century. They have to be understood in the context of the trauma emanating from the events of 1857—partly anti-Western and partly riveted on a vague sense of Islamic solidarity with the sole surviving Muslim political entity of any consequence. A 'memorandum on Indian Muslims' prepared by the then Government of India in 1915 opined that 'Orthodox (Sunni) Muslims regard the Sultan of Turkey as the rightful Caliph of Islam and owe him *spiritual* allegiance'. This, evidently, was time and situation specific since the evidence of earlier history is less emphatic. The memorandum added that 'most Muslims fear that the destruction of the Turkish Government will involve also the destruction of Mohammedan principles'.

The Medical Mission was motivated by a sentiment, a desire to help Turkey in a war against Christian powers. The decision to send it was a gesture of solidarity. There was also an amorphous element of internationalism in it, as is evident from Maulana Mohammad Ali's and Abul Kalam Azad's fiery writings of that period. In the course of the next few years, it took a firmer shape in the articulation of a demand for the independence of India from the British rule and merged into mainstream nationalist discourse shown in the convergence of the Khilafat and Non-Cooperation movements of 1911–22.

The work done by the Medical Mission in its two field hospitals, along with the financial assistance to the Turkish Red Crescent sent from India, was greatly appreciated then and is remembered to this day. The venue of one of these field hospitals, a village by the name Ömerli, was renamed Hindia Köy at the time. The most important result of the Mission, as Dr Ansari said on his return, was the forging of a bond between the Turkish nation and India. This was renewed some years later when Halide Edib visited India on his invitation and wrote her perceptive book *Inside India*.

Ambassador Akçapar's book is a timely reminder of a relevant chapter in India–Turkey relationship. I commend him on his effort.

New Delhi
18 October 2013

M. Hamid Ansari
Vice President of India and
Chairman of the Rajya Sabha

Acknowledgements

My greatest debt of gratitude is to those who have taken the challenge of writing earlier accounts of the 1912–13 Indian Medical Mission to Turkey. Their writings have been a blessing that did not allow the Medical Mission to fall into obscurity.

I wholeheartedly thank all those who made copies of the *Comrade* journal accessible. These include Radhey Shyam, Head Librarian of the Nehru Memorial Museum and Library (NMML), New Delhi, who helped locate and photocopy issues of the journal; Rebecca Cornelius, who went through copies of the *Comrade* to identify the relevant pages; and Pooja Palta and Albert Gibbs, who proofread the typed letters.

I thank the Turkish Red Crescent for providing records of the Red Crescent archives.

My thanks also go to Mushirul Hasan, Mohammad Sadiq, and Naimur Rahman Farooqi for providing corrections and valuable comments.

I owe special thanks to the honourable Vice President of the Republic of India, His Excellency M. Hamid Ansari, whose proud uncle led the Indian Mission to Turkey and whose own father was a member of the Mission, for providing support and encouragement since the inception of this project and writing the foreword to this book.

My wife, Şebnem Köşer Akçapar, and our son, Ziya Onat Akçapar, were always there to provide encouragement for the time and energy I spent on this manuscript.

The editorial team of the Oxford University Press, New Delhi, merit special thanks for their meticulous work in producing this book.

I should like to note with great joy that all countries mentioned in this book are considered friends of modern-day Turkey. I have meant this book to stand as my gift to the friendly peoples of the entire subcontinent who rallied to support the Turks at the turn of the twentieth century.

The views expressed in this book do not reflect and cannot be attributed to any government or institution. All views and possible errors and omissions as well as all opinions expressed in this book are solely mine.

1

Introduction

It was an era where sides had to be taken and lines were drawn in people's minds. The Indian Muslims had a salient cause around which to rally. Half a century after the 'first war of independence', they canalized their dissension with their forlorn circumstances onto a common cause. That cause was Islamic solidarity, its object being the Ottoman Empire and the sultan caliph. Its heroes became the members of the Indian Medical Mission. The same cause tied the Turks of today's Turkey and the peoples of the subcontinent in a lasting bond. This bond was catalysed initially by the idea of pan-Islamism and to a degree pan-Asian solidarity. As such, where common ethnic or cultural roots failed for several centuries before, the idea of Islamic solidarity with Turkey succeeded in the time frame of a couple of decades.

At 5.30 pm on 10 July 1913, Delhi was ready for the spectacular welcome of its newly discovered heroes. This was going to be an evening that even the oldest inhabitants of Delhi would describe as a unique experience of their lives. More than six months ago, in mid-December 1912, a group of doctors, male nurses, ambulance bearers, and other staff set sail from Bombay to İstanbul in order to join the effort to treat Ottoman soldiers wounded in the 1912–13 Balkan Wars. Their journey began merely days after the onset of the Balkan Wars, when the charismatic Shaukat

Ali made an appeal to collect funds to send a team of doctors to the Ottoman Empire in order to treat its soldiers. The 1912 surprise attack by Italy on the Libyan territories of the Ottoman Empire had already provoked significant reaction in India, and the most recent news of a coordinated aggression by a group of Balkan countries with avowedly anti-Muslim and nationalistic agendas created a furore in India. Already defeated by European colonialism, the Indian Muslims and non-Muslims coalesced in support of the appeal to send aid. In a matter of days, a team of doctors were joined by a group of volunteers, with no prior medical or paramedical training, to serve in Turkey. Funds were raised from the voluntary contributions of the wealthy and poor alike. The elegant and diplomatic yet unscrupulously professional physician Dr Mukhtar Ahmad Ansari was chosen by the Ali brothers to lead the medical team to Turkey. The Indian Medical Mission led by Dr Ansari reached İstanbul on the last day of 1912 and stayed continuously in Turkey until late June 1913. In the process, the Medical Mission established two field hospitals and conducted other humanitarian and, as this book would argue, political work in support of the Ottomans.

Although members of the Mission were away from India for half a year, their story was brought home through the letters in which Dr Mukhtar Ahmad Ansari detailed their daily activities in the Ottoman Turkey. The letters, published regularly in the *Comrade* weekly news journal in Delhi, demonstrated to the masses that the Mission and the people associated with it were all part of a noble cause and a courageous effort. Maulana Mohammad Ali Jauhar, the fiery Indian Muslim intellectual and the editor of the *Comrade*, would not try to conceal his excitement and pride as he described that exhilarating evening when Dr Mukhtar Ahmad Ansari and several members of the Indian Medical Mission to Turkey returned to Delhi:

Long before the time of arrival large crowds of people had begun to assemble on the platform and along the approaches to the railway station. At about 5 pm the platforms, the cross bridges and every corner of vantage within the station were packed to their utmost capacity, while the vast enclosure of the station and the road beyond were one moving mass of humanity. As the train moved slowly in, the air was rent with glad shouts of welcome. Thousands on the platform pressed forward to catch a glimpse of the man and his lieutenants, who had rendered good services to Islam, to kiss their hands, and offer them flowers and garlands. It was obviously impossible to keep back the eager crowds that thronged all around and the crush that followed was terrible. It was with great difficulty that Dr. Ansari and party could find their way to the main entrance, and enter the carriages that were waiting outside. At last the procession moved, escorted by a body of mounted young Muslims, along the appointed route towards the Jam'i Masjid. The whole route was lined with spectators and thousands accompanied the procession all the way on foot. Dr. Ansari's carriage, in spite of his protests, was dragged by enthusiastic admirers all the way to the mosque. Several Moslem merchants had decorated their shops along the route and had made arrangements for distribution of iced sherbets and milk. The prosperous Moslem community of 'Punjabi' merchants displayed great enthusiasm on the occasion, and spent a good deal in decorations and floral offerings and in dispensing lavish hospitality in sherbet and pan. The procession stopped at the foot of the vast flight of steps leading up to the eastern gate of the Jam'i Masjid. An address on behalf of the Muslims of Delhi was presented to Dr. Ansari in a beautiful casket, to which Dr Ansari made a brief and graceful reply.

As the party entered the vast courtyard of the mosque it was greeted with loud applause by the thousands of Moslems of Delhi, including hundreds from other places, who had gathered there on the occasion. It is difficult to give the exact number of the people in the mosque and of the vast crowds that surged around it. But even according to a most conservative estimate they could not have been much below thirty thousand. They were all inspired by a single sentiment and filled with a single aim—to do honour to the men who had made sacrifices in the cause of Islam.[1]

Dr Mukhtar Ahmad Ansari was likened by Halide Edip Adıvar to a proverbial bridge. She wrote perceptively in *Inside India* that Dr Ansari was the product of Indian soil and became the first Indian to be admitted as the resident medical officer to Charing Cross Hospital in London. This made him a bridge between Eastern philosophy and Western science. Second, his Mission to Turkey made him a bridge between Turkey and India. Last but not least, 'his conception of citizenship was based on equality and cooperation among Indians of conflicting sects and ideas'.[2] This made him a bridge between Hindus and Muslims as well. Mushirul Hasan was to call Ansari Gandhi's infallible guide.[3] Between a bridge and a guide, Dr Ansari lived a memorable life and left lasting legacies. The 1912–13 Indian Medical Mission, which he led in Turkey, was one such legacy. The Medical Mission was, in fact, a turning point in his life. It catapulted the talented physician and humanist to national political spotlight in India. As Mushirul Hasan stated:

> Until 1911, Ansari gave no evidence of his interest in Indian politics. The Balkan Wars, however, brought him to the forefront of public life and carried him to national fame and influence. He, perhaps unexpectedly, found himself as the leader of a Medical Mission to [Constantinople], a position which enabled him to establish close links with leading Muslim figures in north India and to leave his mark as a brilliant organiser.[4]

The Lieutenant Governor of the United Provinces was to report to Viscount Chelmsford, British Viceroy in India, that in Muslim circles Dr Ansari commanded considerable support: 'His work in the Mission during the last Turkish War is a matter of pride to them, as well as the professional position he occupied in India.'[5] His work in Turkey also earned him and Indian Muslims tremendous sympathy and gratitude among the Turks. And not the least, as Mushirul Haq underscored, '[a]lthough the mission was organised by Muslim leaders, it paved the way for the Indian national leaders to put India on the world map by advocating and fostering international understanding.'[6]

In national politics, Dr Ansari built on the stature he acquired as the leader of the Medical Mission to become one of the leaders of the famous Khilafat Movement in March 1919. By then the First World War had ended by effectively wiping the Ottoman Empire off the map, except for a narrow stretch of land. Turkey, including the capital of the Ottoman Empire, İstanbul, was under the invasion of Britain, France, Italy, and Greece. In May 1919 Mustafa Kemal, later to be endowed with the title Atatürk, the father of the Turkish nation and the founder of the modern republic, sailed to Samsun and took the lead of the Turkish War of Independence. Around the same time, the Bombay-based Central Khilafat Committee set out the main objective of the Khilafat Movement as securing a just and honourable peace for Turkey and the caliph. Specifically, they sought to hold the British Prime Minister Lloyd George to his pledge of 5 January 1919 that the British government had no intention of depriving Turkey of the predominantly Turkish lands of Anatolia and Thrace. In March 1922, Dr Ansari and Ajmal Khan published a manifesto setting out the Indian Muslims' demands, which stated that the Turkish portion of the Ottoman Empire should be restored to Turkey with full sovereign rights, and the Arabic-speaking parts, comprising Palestine, Syria, Mesopotamia, and Hijaz, be given full independence without any non-Muslim control, provided that the suzerainty of the sultan is maintained over the Holy Places of Islam.[7] When the British House of Commons met on 26 February 1922, Dr Ansari was to travel to London as a member of the Khilafat deputation together with Seth Chotani, Hasan Imam, and Qazi Abdul Ghaffar to voice these demands.

The Khilafat Movement was more than just voicing solidarity with the Turkish people. For Ansari, it was an opportunity for India as it 'helped the cause of Hindu–Muslim amity [and] provided a unique opportunity to strengthen the alliance between the two communities'.[8] In his capacity as the President of the Delhi Provincial Congress Committee, he championed a united Hindu–Muslim front against the British Raj. However, in the end, the Khilafat Movement, as Halide Edip Adıvar was to observe perceptively, both united and divided the Muslims and the Hindus.[9] No cause save independence from the British rule carried all the Hindus and all the Muslims together. Yet, the Khilafat Movement was to suffer a fatal blow, ironically when Turkey herself first separated the caliphate from the sultanate on 21 November 1922, declared the Republic with the motto 'Sovereignty belongs without any qualifications and conditions to the people' on 29 October 1923, and then abolished the caliphate altogether on 3 March 1924. This was to uproot the Khilafat Movement and cause outrage among Indian Muslims who failed to understand the inescapable logic of the Turkish revolution. Dr Ansari, however, was to bear 'the shock of the abolition of the Khilafat with equanimity'.[10]

Dr Ansari was an Indian nationalist par excellence. He took active part in the Indian independence movement as a leader in both the Muslim League and the Indian National Congress. He served six times as the General Secretary of the Congress and also as its President at the 1927 Madras session. His political career was not an easy ride. He was criticized vilely by the communalists of all sides and bore the brunt of the British rule including imprisonment, which damaged his already fragile health, leading to his early and sudden death.

He managed to squeeze in all this and much more in a mere 56 years of life which began in Yusufpur in the Ghazipur district of the United Provinces on 25 December 1880 and ended with a heart attack on the night of 10 May 1936, aboard a train compartment returning to Delhi from Mussoorie. He is buried at the premises of his beloved Jamia Millia Islamia in Delhi.

After receiving his initial education in India, Dr Mukhtar Ahmad Ansari left India at the age of 25 for London, where he continued his medical training and then settled. He excelled as a doctor at the Charing Cross, Lock, and St. Peter's hospitals in London. It was during this time that Dr Ansari developed a circle of friends, including Jawaharlal Nehru, Motilal Nehru, Hakim Ajmal Khan, and Allama Mohammad Iqbal, who would all become notable independence leaders. He was to return to India nine years later in 1910 and establish a medical practice in Delhi. Living comfortably as personal physician to the princes of Rampur, Alwar, Bhopal, and Joara, he turned his lavish residence in Daryaganj district of Delhi into a happening venue for several meetings and conferences that would be recorded in the annals of Indian history, including the talks between Gandhiji and Lord Irwin, the British Viceroy in India, that led to the Gandhi–Irwin Pact of 5 March 1931.[11]

Dr Ansari remained throughout his life a dedicated philanthropist and an accomplished doctor and surgeon. Revered as a leader of the Muslim community and as a political leader, he staunchly held on to moderation in his beliefs. Dr Ansari persevered as a strong proponent of *ahimsa* and passive resistance, and was blessed with many friendships including one with Gandhiji. In his later years, he devoted his time to establishing and leading the Jamia Millia Islamia in Delhi, which to our day continues the proud tradition of an Indian central university extending light to countless youth. Dr Ansari's house in Delhi was called *Dar-us-Salam* (Abode of Islam and Peace), an apt name given his commitment to the principles of non-violence and Islam throughout his momentous and celebrated life.

Dr Ansari's letters from the field in Turkey appealed to the masses and managed to strike a chord with the popular sentiments, fears, and perceptions among the mobilized Indian Muslim political opinion. Readers of the *Comrade* where the letters were featured regularly must have found significant resonance with their own perceptions of the unfolding events. One could perhaps question the reach of a single journal, or two if one includes *Comrade*'s Urdu counterpart *Hamdard*, yet given the rambunctious welcome that the thirty-thousand-strong crowd had given Dr Ansari upon his return to Delhi, one can surmise that the reach was not negligible indeed. As the Turkish expression goes, the letters became interpreters of the thoughts of the masses. A closer look at Dr Ansari's letters reveals the existence of the early twentieth-century pan-Islamic frame of thinking. Regarding the common sentiments which the letters invoked, one can pinpoint the reverence to the Ottoman Empire and attachment to the sultan caliph. Thus, one month into their arrival in İstanbul, Dr Ansari reported in his letter dated 1 February 1913 that upon their approach from the sea, the members of the team

> could clearly discern the shadowy outlines of the minarets and domes, the old fortresses and the new buildings along the shores of the Bosphorus. There by Istanbul in its proud but sad dignity, and the feelings it aroused in one's mind were difficult to analyse. Those hills and old forts now crumbling down had seen the advent of the mighty Turks, the fall of the Byzantine Empire and the rise and glory of the Osmanli. Now, alas! The time had come when they were watching the gradual dismemberment of their Empire and the Decadence of Moslem rule.

He was to return to the glorified description of the Ottoman rule in his letter published in the *Comrade* on 12 June that in İstanbul

[n]umerous other buildings built by a succession of Sultans carried one back in imagination to those glorious times when the Ottoman power was irresistible and ever on the increase. We were shown Sultan Murad's latest hall where he read out the granting of the Constitution, and the room where the janissaries attacked him. We were shown the golden corridor and the staircase leading to the Harem where, after the murder of Sultan Murad, the janissaries rushed to kill all the royal princes, but they were turned back by the coolness and presence of mind of the Sultan's wife, who threw buckets of glowing charcoal on their faces. The window through which the Sultan made Sultan Mahmud jump out is adjoining this staircase, also the room where he was proclaimed Sultan in the very teeth of the revolt of the janissaries. There were secret ladders, hidden passages leading from one building to another. In fact all those contrivances which were necessary in those days when the palace intrigues and plots were the rule of the day. In passing out of the Harem we were shown the place where the chief of the eunuchs used to punish the offenders. On the gate could be seen the dried scalp of one of the eunuchs hung by Sultan Mahmud. A secret balcony which we entered from the Harem overlooked the hall, where the discussions of Vozara and Vokals [ministers and parliamentarians] used to take place. In this balcony the Sultan used to sit and overhear all the discussions without being seen.

Another related popular sentiment voiced more passionately was the strong esteem accorded to the caliph in İstanbul. This is evident particularly in the letter Dr Ansari wrote on 17 June regarding his audience with Caliph Mehmed V. He stated that this 'is a distinction which we are naturally proud of, for a Muslim it is a great honour to kiss the robes of the Caliph of the Muslims'. Yet another common feeling among the Indian Muslims, of course, pertained to the wrongdoings against the Ottomans. This feeling is manifest in Dr Ansari's response to the characterization of Ottoman hospitals by the European press as 'a tissue of malignant lies'.[12] Accordingly, after inspecting three hospitals in different outskirts of İstanbul, Dr Ansari wrote in his letter dated 11 January that

you would see that not only the general press of Europe was full of a series of calumnies and false reports about the Turkish organization, but even the medical Press was affected by this religious bigotry and fanaticism, and stated facts about the medical organization which on examination one finds altogether incorrect and exaggerated. I do not mean by this that there is no room for assistance in this present unusual situation. It is bound to affect even the best organized country. But what I maintain is that the assistance needed is not true to the extent that it is represented, nor any more than any other European Power would require at the time of war. The story of the Turkish wounded being left in thousands on the battle-field to die is a tissue of malignant lies which is obvious to even a casual observer who visits the hospitals and sees for himself the number of major operations performed on the patients with results which even the best surgeons of Europe would be proud of.

Dr Ansari also skilfully voiced the common concern or fear of extinction that the Muslim public opinion in India and indeed globally held. While deftly avoiding any direct criticism of the British Empire and, in fact, reassuring his loyalty to the British crown at every possible juncture, he still managed to express his alarm regarding the impending collapse of the Ottoman order against the European imperial onslaught. Therefore, in his letter of 10 January, related to his visit to the Persian Ambassador in İstanbul and the discussion there concerning the fate of the Muslims around the globe, Dr Ansari wrote: 'There is no doubt that the events in Turkey and Persia seem to have impressed deeply the mind of all the Moslem world and they are beginning to realise, though, alas! very late, that unless they improve themselves at once they will lose all they possess and be a subject race forever.' In these words, and indeed elsewhere in his letters, Dr Ansari replicates the internal criticism of the Muslims and the cure seen in adopting Europeanness or European modernity. In fact, throughout his letters, Dr Ansari holds Europe, which he obviously knew intimately, as the main reference point for comparison. He upholds his conviction in the superior quality of European modernity. His language is laden with characterizations such as staff consisting 'of teachers and professors of European fame' or military achievement that 'has elicited appreciation from almost every European country'.[13] He nonetheless rejoiced at examples which surpassed the European standard. Comparing the operations by the Turkish surgeons to those by the German, British, and the French Red Cross hospitals, he concluded that the latter's results have been unsatisfactory.[14] Talking about the Haydarpasa hospital, he asserted that 'this hospital would compare favourably with any European hospital and it was certainly much cleaner than the hospitals one has seen in France and Italy'.[15] Overall, he adopted a tone that remained somewhat external to the nation to which he had been deployed or the Indian Muslims that he came to represent. Throughout the letters, Dr Ansari remained viciously critical of things he disliked in the Ottoman Empire, such as the inefficiency with which Ottoman bonds were handled by the Ottoman authorities. He attacked the bureaucracy in one of his early letters dated 20 January, stating, 'I cannot tell you what difficulties are placed in our way here even in arranging a small matter. Our things have all arrived last week, and in any other country but Turkey everything would have been arranged in a day or two.' Even his praise of the adorned capital city which he otherwise admired was never unqualified as was evident in his disenchantment with the cobblestone streets of old Istanbul. Nowhere is Dr Ansari's duality of enduring 'outsiderness' and readiness to sympathize more obvious than in his commentary about the Annual Congress of the Ottoman Red Crescent Society. In his letter dated 6 May, Dr Ansari reported:

> I had never seen Turks looking so interested and keen as I saw on this occasion. It would have convinced anyone who had seen this debate that the quiet and impassive Turk is at times quite capable of getting wound up into an impassioned denunciation or rejoinder. And after all he is not altogether incapable of discussing affairs in a representative assembly as many would have us believe.

These writings invoked some of the shared themes of the Indian Muslim perceptions about what was taking place in the Ottoman Empire during the Balkan Wars. This must have made Dr Ansari's letters influential, especially with the penetrating commentary and discourse of Maulana Mohammad Ali Jauhar, another key personality who had become synonymous with the Indian Medical Mission. In that regard, a quick look at Mohammad Ali Jauhar's political career might be revealing of both his tendencies and objectives as well as his charisma that captured the imagination of the early twentieth-century Indian pan-Islamic movement deriving its strength from the sentiments and concerns reflected in Dr Ansari's letters and amplified by Mohammad Ali's interventions.

In turn, Mohammad Ali was the proverbial intellectual and rhetorical sinew behind the Indian Medical Mission. The Ottoman Empire's ordeal and the well-being of the caliph and the Turks was a popular preoccupation in India since mid-nineteenth century. However, it was the *Comrade*, which Mohammad Ali edited, that generated the focus and organization for the Indian Muslim doctors and medical personnel to initiate and sustain the Mission through the relief funds he helped collect. As such, he captured the sentiments and imagination of the masses that looked to İstanbul 'for political direction and spiritual nourishment'.[16] *Comrade* was launched on 14 January 1911, shortly before the outbreak of the 1911–12 Balkan Wars. During the wars, as the Medical Mission was present in Turkey, when the invading armies came within a threatening distance to İstanbul, Mohammad Ali was tempted to commit suicide, only to be dissuaded by his close friends.[17] Muhammad Ali was to persevere in his support to Turkey during and after the First World War, and he paid a heavy price for this, including the proscription of his journal and his long imprisonment following his criticism of a demeaning 1914 *London Times* article threatening Turkey. Ironically, the last edition of the *Comrade*, before it was banned, published the text of the telegram he and Dr Ansari sent to the Ottoman Minister of Interior Talat Pasha in İstanbul, beseeching 'the strictest neutrality' in the First World War, as the British had wanted.[18] Fearful of being left alone and doubting British intentions, the Ottomans were to side with Germany in that war, which ended with the demise of the Ottoman Empire.

During the Turkish War of Independence that followed the defeat of the German–Ottoman alliance during the First World War and the invasion of much of Turkey by the victors, Mohammad Ali was to lead the Khilafat delegation, which also included Dr Ansari, to Britain to argue in favour of the Turks and the preservation of the Ottoman caliphate. However, he was again to be jailed for his pro-independence discourse and opposition to send Indians to fight against Turks as part of the British imperialist armies. There was already a large number of desertions and much unease with fighting against fellow Muslims, which the British tried in vain to contain by mixing English and Indian forces. Out of this long repeat imprisonment, Mohammad Ali emerged as a gravely ailing man.

His fervour for the Ottomans and the Turks could only be matched by his dedication to Muslim causes and independence from British rule. His initiation to public stage happened in 1904 when he gave a fiery speech in favour of establishing a Muslim university. The same year, he penned articles criticizing the surrender of control of the Aligarh College to the British.[19] The issue was to return in 1911 and this time Muhammad Ali continued his campaign through the *Comrade*. He would later in his life be counted among the leaders who helped establish the Jamia Millia Islamia initially in Aligarh, now a vibrant central university in Delhi.

Mohammad Ali was born on 10 December 1878 in Rampur as the youngest of six children. His grandfather had received large plots of land for having rescued an Englishman during the 1857 uprising, while his mother came from a family that lost many plots of land during the same war because of opposition to the British, both in the Moradabad region. Having lost his 34-year-old father to cholera at the age of two, he was raised by a strong mother who herself was to become active in the Khilafat Movement. Another major and rather permanent influence in his life was his elder brother Shaukat Ali, another talented and charismatic personality. The two were known as the Ali brothers and they were a formidable duo. Mohammad's political charisma showed itself during his time at the Bareilly High School where he showed his promise as a student leader. After a stint in Bareilly, he moved to Aligarh College together with Shaukat Ali. The English education was to leave a strong mark in the intellectual and political development of the Ali brothers as it did on many other talented and devout Muslim youths with strong religious sensibilities at the time. Mohammad Ali joined several other talented youths of his day to move to England for university education and upon return entered irreversibly the political minefields in pre-independence India.

Mohammad Ali was an extraordinary intellectual, and even more remarkable orator and writer. H. G. Wells described him as a man who possessed 'the heart of Napoleon, the pen of Macaulay and the tongue of Burke'.[20] I take it that he intended these words to stand as a praise of sorts. The strength of Mohammad Ali's political passions and oral and written expression proved too much of a threat to the British Raj, which kept him in prison during much of his adult life. Dissemination of his famous article 'The Choice of the Turks' remained banned until 1944.

His vocation in the Indian Independence Movement started with the Indian National Congress, and he was its chairman in 1923. His initial platform was Hindu–Muslim unity in a liberated India. He wrote in *Comrade* of 14 January 1911: 'It is our firm belief that if the Mussalmans or the Hindus attempt to achieve success in opposition to or even without the cooperation of one another, they will not only fail, but fail ignominiously.' When the Ali brothers were jailed, Gandhiji lobbied for their release. There developed a friendship between the two which manifested itself in the Ali brothers lending support to the Congress and Mohammad Ali presiding its 1923 Gaya session. Although this was a rather symbolic position, it nonetheless meant an alliance between Mohammad Ali and Mahatma Gandhi. In fact, Gandhi was to characterize their meeting in 1915 as love at first sight. Together they provided a powerful front of Hindus and Muslims against the colonialists. As Afzal Iqbal wrote, thanks to the association of Mohammad Ali with the Congress, a 'historic phase' began in the history of the nationalist movement, where the climate of Hindu–Muslim unity was pervasive as never before.[21] His contribution to the Congress was immense as he quickly became an engine for spreading revolutionary fervour throughout the country. The love affair between Gandhiji and the Ali brothers was, however, not going to last. Starting with the Kohat riots of 1924, they started falling out. The (Motilal) Nehru Commission Report of 10 August 1928 and Mahatma's support to its rejection of separate electorates for the Muslims and Hindus through reservation of fixed number of seats for the Muslims severed the last links. Mohammad Ali argued that he trusted the majority of neither the Hindus nor the Muslims. And he assumed that Gandhi was caving in to the Hindu extremists and feared Hindu domination of the Muslims in India. Thus, having lost the support of Gandhi, he became sidelined by other Muslims closer to the Mahatma, including Abul Kalam Azad. The biggest irony, however, was perhaps his parting of ways with Dr Ansari, his closest collaborator in defending Turkey and organizing the Indian Medical Mission.

Despite all his reported immoderation, Mohammad Ali was a rare jewel as his 'Jauhar' title suggests. He had the fabric of a hero in the Indian Independence Movement. He also remained a 'Maulana' until his last breath in championing the Muslim community's rights in India and indeed around the world. He was never to understand the Turkish Revolution and how it was to set the Turkish nation on the path of rejuvenation after centuries of decay and pain. He was right, however, that a void would emerge after the Turks yielded the leadership of the Sunni Muslim world to be filled by a cacophony among Muslims. Yet, above all, Maulana Mohammad Ali Jauhar was an uncompromising and incessantly fiery politician. As Syed Tanwir Wasti related:

> In a speech delivered to the Fourth Plenary Session of the Round Table Conference in London on 19 November 1930, as a member of the Indian delegation, Maulana Mohamed Ali Jauhar argued emotionally and eloquently for Indian independence. He was terminally ill, with a dilated heart, high blood pressure and diabetes, but his speech was replete with wit and humour, and he showed no bitterness to anyone. Explaining his allegiances as an Indian Muslim, he said: 'I belong to two circles of equal size, but which are not concentric. One is India, and the other is the Muslim world.'[22]

Mohammad Ali presumed, and not everyone agreed, that the two would not overlap. However, all were to agree when he proclaimed, only a few weeks before his demise, at the Round Table Conference in London in 1930: 'I would even prefer to die in a foreign country so long as it is a free country, and if you do not give us freedom in India you will have to give me a grave here.' When he died on 3 January 1931, instead of India, he was to be buried in Jerusalem. The great poet and thinker Allama Muhammad Iqbal's elegy stated:

The earth of Jerusalem embraced him with desire
To Heaven he went in the path of the Prophet, his Sire.

Together Dr Ansari and Maulana Mohammad Ali steered the Indian Medical Mission towards concrete humanitarian and political internationalist activities that were motivated by a pan-Islamism peculiar to the nineteenth and early twentieth centuries. This book narrates the story of the Indian Medical Mission in the context of the long ethnic, human, religious, social, diplomatic, and geopolitical interactions between the Turks and the Indian Muslims in the run-up to the Balkan Wars of 1912–13. It locates the Mission and the driving ideological force behind it in the context of the geopolitical and ideological wrangling between the colonizers and the colonized as well as within the nascent global Muslim public opinion or the so-called Muslim world.

Instead of providing a conclusive history with exhaustive analyses of each and every angle, the idea has been to acclimatize the reader to the broader circumstances within which the Ansari letters can be read and the Mission understood.

Part One focuses on the historical dynamics at play in the dispatch of the Indian Medical Mission to the Ottoman Empire. It is divided into three chapters which walk the reader through the context of the Balkan Wars, the background of the Ottoman–Mughal diplomatic and strategic interactions, and the roots and manifestations of the idea of Islamic unity or pan-Islamism, both as propagated by the Ottoman leadership and as embraced by the Indian Muslims.

Part One is not meant to be a standalone detailed study of any of the topics touched. There is a vast literature on all the subjects except the Ottoman–Mughal relations. Particularly, the Balkan Wars and pan-Islamism of the nineteenth and early twentieth centuries, including its manifestations in India, have been topics that have been extensively researched and written about. Obviously, a much more elaborate and sustained analysis of these subjects falls beyond the purview of this book. Instead, the intention of Part One is to recall the contours of these topics and thus set the stage for the understanding of the thought processes, perceptions, and the deeds of the Indian Medical Mission.

Part Two focuses on the Indian Medical Mission itself. The chapters in this part introduce the key personalities associated with the Mission, the members of the medical team, their key Turkish counterparts, daily activities in Turkey and the unfolding historic events that the members witnessed, as well as their travels and interactions with Ottoman officials and the Turkish people. In separate chapters, this part also provides an analysis of Dr Ansari's letters as a travelogue and the impact the Mission made on the Ottoman army and society as well as on Indian Muslims.

The book also includes as an appendix the first-ever anthology of the full copies of the letters as they were published in the *Comrade* a century ago. The letters reflect the original voice of Dr Ansari and his colleagues and his unintended yet engaging diary at the time they lived and made history as committed representatives of Indian Muslims aiding the only standing Muslim state.

The Indian Muslims, in fact, dispatched three separate teams simultaneously to Turkey. But thanks, in no small degree, to his regular letters, only the one led by Dr Ansari seemed to have caught the limelight. Supported materially and morally by countless Indian Muslims, those three teams, including the one led by Dr Ansari and fellow members of the Indian Medical Mission, went to aid the Ottomans in the latter's disastrous war against Balkan soldiers who wore a badge on their heads depicting 'a lion rampant [*sic*] prodding over the Crescent and carrying a Cross on its head'.[23] Theirs was an act of mercy sanctioned by the Muslims and Hindus who donated funds for the medical missions.

Yet, against the backdrop of the apex of aggressive imperial expansion that tore deeply into the spiritual, psychological, and indeed geopolitical flesh of the Muslim world, it was also something more. At a time when the whole world was sliding inexorably towards a global war, the Balkans had become not only a prelude to war but also the epicentre of a global confrontation. The Balkan region was also the epicentre of the Christian–Muslim rivalry. The results of the 1912–13 Balkan Wars had been inconclusive and sustained the territorial aspirations of the rival powers in the Balkans and their Great Power allies. As far as the Ottoman Empire was concerned, the Balkan Wars were nothing less than an utter disaster. It came to present the latest episode in the drawn-out assault to the Muslim Turks and their state from European powers, large and small. For the Muslims of India, it was yet another aggression against the Muslim world. During one battle in Turkey, members of the Indian Medical Mission visited the charismatic military commander and political revolutionary Enver Pasha in his field tent. They told him how the whole Islamic world looked to him to retrieve its lost honour and save the sinking ship of Turkey from utter destruction. If you asked the masses that filled up the streets of Delhi on the evening of 10 July 1913, Dr Ansari and his team, through their six-month-long labour in Turkey, had fulfilled an Islamic duty. In the minds of the members of the Indian Medical Mission and the millions behind them in India, the honour of Islamic world and the survival of Ottoman Turkey were one and the same. The work of the Indian Medical Mission in Turkey was nothing short of a political mission to heal the Muslims' pride, not the least back in India. This is their story, reconstructing to the extent possible their thoughts and voices as well as the era that shaped them.

Notes

1. 'Dr. Ansari's Return', *Comrade*, 12 July 1913, p. 27.
2. Halide Edip Adıvar, *Inside India* (London: George Allen & Unwin, 1937), p. 30.
3. Mushirul Hasan, *M. A. Ansari: Gandhi's Infallible Guide* (New Delhi: Manohar, 2010).
4. Mushirul Hasan, *Muslims and the Congress: Select Correspondence of Dr. M. A. Ansari, 1912–1935* (New Delhi: Manohar, 1979), p. xix.
5. 'Meston to Chelmsford, 6 September 1916', *Meston Papers*, cited by Hasan, *Muslims and the Congress*, p. xix.
6. Mushirul Haq, 'Dr. M. A. Ansari', available at http://www.congresssandesh.com/AICC/history/ presidents/dr_m_a_ansari.htm (accessed on 18 October 2012).
7. P. C. Bamford, *Histories of the Non-cooperation and Khilafat Movements* (Reprint, Delhi: Deep Publications, 1974), p. 194, cited by Hasan, *Muslims and the Congress*, p. xxii.
8. Hasan, *Muslims and the Congress*, p. xxiii.
9. Adıvar, *Inside India*, p. 30.
10. Hasan, *Muslims and the Congress*, p. xxiv.

11. It was this pact that Winston Churchill was to irreverently deride as 'the nauseating and humiliating spectacle of this one-time Inner Temple lawyer, now seditious fakir, striding half-naked up the steps of the Viceroy's palace, there to negotiate and parley on equal terms with the representative of the King Emperor'.

12. Dr Ansari's letter dated 11 January 1913.

13. Dr Ansari's letter dated 11 January 1913/Dr Ansari's letter dated 7 April 1913.

14. Dr Ansari's letter dated 11 January 1913.

15. Dr Ansari's letter dated 11 January 1913.

16. Syed Tanvir Wasti, 'The Circles of Maulana Mohamed Ali', *Middle Eastern Studies* 38, no. 4 (October 2002), p. 51.

17. Wasti, 'The Circles of Maulana Mohamed Ali', p. 53.

18. Wasti, 'The Circles of Maulana Mohamed Ali', p. 56.

19. David Lelyveld, 'Three Aligarh Students: Aftab Ahmad Khan, Ziauddin Ahmad and Muhammad Ali', *Modern Asian Studies* 9, no. 2 (1975), p. 237.

20. Afzal Iqbal, *The Life and Times of Maulana Mohamed Ali* (Lahore: Institute of Islamic Culture, 1979), p. 425n5.

21. Afzal Iqbal, ed., *Select Writings and Speeches of Maulana Mohamed Ali* (Lahore: Shaikh Muhammad Ashraf, 1944), p. 186.

22. Wasti, 'The Circles of Maulana Mohammad Ali', p. 51.

23. Dr Ansari's letter published in the *Comrade* covering the period between 11 and 20 February 1913.

Part One

2

The Penultimate War of the Ottoman Empire

On the last day of May 2013, the minister of foreign affairs of the Republic of Macedonia addressed his counterparts from the Balkans and praised joint efforts in the region, particularly emphasizing Turkey's role in promoting regional cooperation. He was speaking at the beautiful lakeside city of Ohrid, famous for its delicious fish, as term chairman for the South-East European Cooperation Process, which brings together Albania, Bosnia Herzegovina, Croatia, Greece, Macedonia, Moldova, Montenegro, Romania, Slovenia, and Turkey. The professed objectives of the Process launched in 1996 upon Bulgaria's initiative comprise a broad spectrum including strengthening the security and economic cooperation in the region, promoting cooperation in human resources, democracy, justice, as well as combating illegal activities. In addition to this and other home-grown initiatives, various international organizations have their own endeavours to promote regional cooperation. Today the region includes countries that are either members of the European Union and the North Atlantic Treaty Organization (NATO) or desiring to become one. The process of acceding to these groupings has played a positive role in addressing contentious issues. All of them strive to strengthen good neighbourly relations and transform the region into an area of peace and stability. Governments are exerting efforts to bury the hatchets for good. They hope to turn the page to a new chapter of history characterized by lasting peace in the region. I have myself played a humble role in the diplomatic efforts to promote lasting peace and cooperation among nations in the Balkans.

Modern Turkey is part of the Balkan family of nations. Every nation in the Balkans has countless of their kin buried in İstanbul and other parts of Turkey decorously and ceremoniously, including as a leading Turkish statesman, general, bureaucrat, artist, architect, or scholar. Most key Turkish personalities mentioned in this book have certain roots or connections with the Balkans. More than the United States of today, the Ottoman Empire of yester centuries did not just attract talent, but also shaped them since their early childhood. For a Christian child born in Belgrade, Sarajevo, or elsewhere in the Balkans, the road could lead all the way up to the post of grand vizier or prime minister of a vast empire once recruited into the Ottoman janissary network.[1]

Contested Historiographies

It was said that the Balkans produces more history than it can consume. Historical knowledge in and about the region differs not only between the Turks and the other Balkan nations but also among perhaps all the various Balkan peoples. In a way, a contest of opposing legitimacies has been at play between the perspective of a nation that was fighting for independent statehood and a polity that was trying to hold its people together. This aspect of disagreement between the old ruler and the ruled can probably be never fully resolved. Hardly ever an easy matter anywhere, conflict and bitterness has to be experienced in the process of secession and independence. However, in the Balkans, the virulence of conflict has long been less between the old rulers and the ruled. Instead, rivalries and overlapping claims have poisoned the region for more than a century since the pacifying grip of the Ottoman Empire started to loosen, replaced by no other viable system of regional politics until the advent of European Union's enlargement in the region.

What made things most complicated was perhaps that in the post-Ottoman Balkans, and indeed the Middle East, the legitimacy of nationhood was sought in all the wrong places. Religious and ethnic as well as militaristic myths were used and abused with alleged historical continuity and longevity as part of nation building for generations since the idea of nationalism reached the Balkans. It was contended that Greeks or Serbs or Bulgarians always resisted an alien rule since the day their king lost in war against the mighty Turk. It was inculcated in the masses that before the arrival of the Muslim invaders, there was once a golden era of Christianity, where the ethnic king was victorious in every battle and he led their nation into prosperity and glory. Not only was there no such golden era, in fact, under the Ottomans the Balkan peasantry, who worked the land, paid most of the taxes, and were liable for military service, were treated much better than before. They were protected by the new landlords and had their feudal services abolished. Apart from the frontier regions, most of the Balkans were spared that cultural and religious destruction usually associated with armies of occupation. Christians, though implicitly encouraged to convert to Islam, were allowed religious toleration and mixed marriages, and the comparative freedom and contentment enjoyed by its people is one of the most important explanations why the Balkans remained under Ottoman rule for over 400 years. The most enduring Ottoman legacy in the Balkans may have been the spread of Islam. Yet even that was owed most of all to voluntary conversions. The Ottomans also brought the advances of a well-functioning administration, attracting talent from all around. The Ottoman administrative edge, not its military yoke, accounted for the longevity of the Ottoman rule. This advantage began to weaken as the Ottomans battled centuries of onslaught against one enemy or the other which, in a protracted attrition, ate away their resources, concentration, prestige, and thus popular support. Against incessant attacks, the Empire had no time to heal its wounds or to see the culmination of the reforms they had begun. Yet it is also true that the historical fallacies that were inculcated among the peoples to mobilize support for nationhood and abandon traditional loyalties have created a lasting distortion and left a deep scar perpetuating conflict and, thus, underdevelopment. Rather than celebrating their centuries together and building a fence around the countless mistakes made in the process of what was inevitable disintegration in the end, intellectuals have continued to drum up mutual hatred. Historiography will need to be addressed in order to build lasting peace in the vast lands that once formed part of the Ottoman Empire. The tired idea of loading every negative aspect onto the Ottoman past has been a favoured approach, but it is gradually making way for more sober scholarship as it should.

Conflicting historical narratives have also poisoned relations among the various Balkan nations. Much blood was spilled based on these fallacies and myths, complicating the issue even further. While the 1912–13 Balkan Wars began with a joint attack of Balkan countries, except Romania, against the Ottomans, it ended with countries changing their alliances and attacking Bulgaria. Thankfully, relations among the countries of the Balkan region are much different now in the early twenty-first century from what it was at the turn of the twentieth century, when not only war but also the modern-day genocide against Bosnian Muslims shocked the world. Yet at least certain tensions have remained simmering under the surface. For instance, Greece has continued to vehemently contest the constitutional name of the Republic of Macedonia, its neighbour, accusing the latter of appropriating symbols such as the Vergina Sun and Alexander the Great as well as of irredentism. The issue would have been resolved long ago perhaps but Greece joined NATO and the European Union before Macedonia did, making it possible for it to leverage its membership against Macedonia and threaten to block accession until Macedonia accepted its demands.

The region of beautiful valleys, forests, historic towns, and remarkably beautiful and sophisticated peoples had been thrown into the abyss of hate, insatiable greed, and senseless violence which exploded in such a cataclysmic fashion when the age of empires was coming to an end that its traces are still to be found 100 years hence. The Balkan region, with its peoples who had lived together in relative peace through much of the last half millennium, has been torn apart by aggressive nationalism and mutually exclusive national myths as well as territorial claims since the nineteenth century. In a way, everyone has been a victim of the ideological trends that were imported and the mutual hatred that were concocted by the very religious institutions that should have promoted reconciliation and peace. Sequestered between İstanbul, Moscow, and various European imperial capitals, the region became not only a theatre of broader geopolitical aspirations and struggles among the empires of the day but also their hapless proxies.

The story of the Balkans in the last 200 years is inextricably related with the final episode of the Ottoman peace that collapsed gradually and painfully. As such, the Balkans was also the theatre where the campaign to annihilate Muslim populations in Europe was played out. This aspect, more than any other, pulled in Indian Muslims into the fold. For, the Indian Muslims were watching intently from afar as the caliph of the Muslims, the sultan of the only remaining bastion, fought to preserve Muslim sanctities. The Indian concern to protect the realm of the caliphate provided the direct reason for the foundation of the Society of the Servants of Kaba, the precursor to the Khilafat Movement of 1919, by Mushir Hosain Kidwai in 1913. The events unfolding in the Balkans, thus, were also a manifestation of a global assault against Islam and the re-emergence of a world view of religious conflict. The Turk was the last bulwark. His or her defeat would mean the loss of all hope for colonized Muslims in India and around the world.

The Assisted Decline of the Multi-ethnic, Multi-religious Polity

By the time the Balkan Wars of 1912–13 were looming large, both Europe writ large and the Balkan states of Bulgaria, Greece, Serbia, and Montenegro were deeply entrenched in a strong desire to avenge their perceived histories vis-à-vis the Ottomans and also expand to their imagined national boundaries. Three key factors help us define the period in question. The first and the obvious is the decline of the Ottoman Empire without which there would not have been the Balkan Wars. The second factor is the vibrant and often conflicting dreams of the newly independent Balkan states and their revanchism, not to mention their overlapping ambitions to expand. Third, in the geopolitical designs and aspirations of the European empires of the day, the Balkans was part and parcel of their broader strategies and competitions. These three factors would combine to form a geopolitical fight that was made more vicious under the intoxicating influences of incoherently articulated nationalisms and imagined revanches.

In fact, as early as 1877, there were learned observers who rebelled at the scheme to libel the Turks as the savage assault was underway to demonize and weaken them only to cannibalize their Empire. Among them, J. W. Redhouse of the Royal Asiatic Society succinctly exposed the game played on the Ottomans which endured all the way to the latter's demise and in the meantime established a strong bias and vilification that still haunts the image of the Turks and distorts human knowledge of the historical experience. Thus, Redhouse wrote with reference to William Ewart Gladstone's racist pamphlet *Bulgarian Horrors and the Question of the East*:[2]

> The 'Atrocities of Bulgaria', referred to in the pamphlet, were entirely the fruit of foreign intrigues … Urged by foreign agents, and foreign gold, distributed by ambassadors and a consular corps, the Bulgarians organized a rebellion, to be commenced by a wholesale massacre of the Turks (even as was the foreign organized plan at the time of the Greek rebellion in 1821, both on the continent and in the islands). They accomplished what they could, most savagely; and they met with such reprisals as their foreign instigator had expected, had calculated on as a means of exciting public indignation in Europe against the Turks. This calculation has partially succeeded—some of the mud has stuck.[3]

The game was clear and was long underway as the Ottoman Empire was sliding painfully down and rather than yielding was still resisting with all that it had to stay alive.

By the end of the nineteenth century, the glory of the Ottoman Empire was long gone. The Ottoman Empire started to experience structural problems as early as in the mid-seventeenth century. As Alan Palmer wrote, the signs of chronic weakness included inflation which was aggravated by the import of cheap silver from Peru and causing a threefold increase in food prices; failings in the tax collection system; growing banditry following a population surge in Anatolia; ruinous fires in overcrowded cities; adherence to old ways of war fighting and governance in captured lands;

and not the least the practice of granting special legal rights and tariff concessions to foreign tradesmen residing in the Ottoman Empire which ultimately ensured that wealth from trade was accumulated in foreign hands.[4] Although all these signs and symptoms went unnoticed at the time, the waning of Ottoman military power became obvious after the botched attempt to capture Vienna in 1683. The siege was an arbitrary attempt of an Ottoman grand vizier who wanted to come to the rescue of Calvinists under Habsburg rule and build prestige by defeating the Habsburg dynasty. Since Sultan Süleyman the Lawgiver decided to return to İstanbul rather than continue his siege, for some 150 years, Hungary was divided between the Ottomans and the Austrians. The forced conversions of Calvinists into Catholicism were creating resistance in Hungary. Repeated calls for the Ottomans to come to the rescue went unanswered. However, in 1683 Kara Mustafa Pasha convinced the Ottoman sultan to let him answer the call of the Hungarian Calvinist leader Imre Thököly. The Turkish army did, in fact, bring down Viennese defences but the grand vizier decided to wait until the city surrendered in order to prevent looting rather than to go forth and complete the invasion. This proved a fateful mistake as in the time gained with the Pope's great efforts a Polish army managed to attack the Ottomans while the reserve forces of the Ottomans did not arrive in time. The routing army of siege abandoned its treasury and supplies on the site and this is how Europe came to know of coffee. The war had nothing to do with Muslim–Christian rivalry. Yet, Austrians and Europeans even to date believe erroneously that the sultan caliph's armies battered on the Christendom in 1683. The defeat was so unexpected in İstanbul that the Grand Vizer Kara Mustafa Pasha who went on an unnecessary war and made mistakes in commanding it was beheaded at Belgrade that same year on orders from the sultan. Now sensing the vulnerability of the legendary 'Grand Turk' against a collective assault, Europeans could not have been able to fathom how resilient the Turkish Empire would nonetheless be. Since 1683, the Ottoman Empire, despite the cancerous developments within its body, continued to be a formidable player in European politics and geopolitics. Two centuries after the failure of the Ottoman siege of Vienna, the European possessions of the empire were finally teetering on the brink of secession by the end of the nineteenth century. The European territories of the Ottomans were by no means a sliver. Up to mid-nineteenth century, the majority of the Ottoman population lived in the Balkans. Due to mass killings and forced expulsions, come 1906, the Ottoman population in the same region shrunk to 20 per cent of the total.[5] Between 1798 and 1922, the empire was in almost a constant state of war, depleting the polity's population, resources, and increasingly also its morale and patience. Its arch rivals Russia and the dual monarchy of the Austrian–Hungarian Empire both had particular designs for the Balkans. As the Ottoman Empire shrank, its domestic squabbles only intensified, which in turn upset any hopes to reform the economy and governance of the state. The state responded by trying to strengthen its surveillance and control over its population through both military and civilian bureaucracy. This, however, only proved to be more counterproductive as it intensified and legitimized the grievances of the people. Domestic rebellions spread, putting the once mighty empire on a downward spiral towards total collapse.

In this context, the conventional Western and Balkan nationalist–dominated literature constructs a narrative of brutal suppression of frustrated nationalist ambitions of the ethnic and religious minorities. In these narratives, the Muslims and the Turks are the oppressors and the 'minorities' are the oppressed. The eternal struggle being between the good and the bad is defined in this narrative in terms of a permanent bad and a permanent good, irrespective of who does what. Moreover, the narrative creates an expectation of a continuous struggle and, thus, tension, until nationalist aspirations are satisfied. Thankfully, this bias is gradually being deconstructed as more and more research is challenging simplistic notions that were an extension of stereotypes (Muslim: bad, Christian: good) rather than hard historical evidence. Indeed, as Blumi argues, 'such narrative tropes have long depended on our uncritical acceptance of a claim that peoples living in such a vast geographic area shared more in common with unknown people living hundreds of miles away because they were categorically of the same "ethnicity" than with neighbours who were often of a different faith and thus a different ethnic group'.[6] Quataert observed:

Seldom, if ever, had the rebels sought to break out of or destroy the Ottoman imperium. There had been revolts but, generally, these had worked within the system, claiming as their goal the rectification of problems within the Ottoman universe, such as the reduction of taxes or better justice. But in the nineteenth century—in the Balkan, Anatolian, and Arab provinces alike—movements emerged that actively sought to separate particular areas from Ottoman rule and establish independent, sovereign states subordinate to no higher political authority.[7]

In this context, Isa Blumi's illuminating study on alternative Balkan modernities demonstrates that 'the western Balkans region covered ... (much of modern-day Montenegro, Serbia, Kosovo, Albania, Macedonia, and northwestern Greece) actually does not warrant being characterized as a "powder keg" of ethnic, sectarian strife'.[8]

To the audience that was bent on perceiving all things Muslim and Turk as inferior, inherently suppressive and violent, and eternally complicit in propagating ancient quarrels and hatreds, this narrative of Ottoman history became conventional wisdom. The fact of the matter was infinitely more complex than a series of ethnic rebellions by long-subdued populations driven by neatly defined nationalisms. Quite to the contrary, the nationalist agitators in their bid to conscript support for their largely peasant armies needed to engage in excruciating ideological indoctrination through the junior but ideologically trained officers. The 'nationalist intellectuals' influenced by the ideas emanating from the French Revolution and emboldened by Napoleon Bonaparte's invasion of Egypt had undertaken a cause to rewrite history with strong underpinnings of a concocted national past. What became agitations for deteriorating living and governance conditions in a failing economy and state have been moulded in such ethnic causes by determined and sustained effort.

That said, the role of nationalism as an ideology cannot be ignored in how the Balkans slided into fire. In the early nineteenth century, the concept of nationalism reached the Balkans from French and German lands initially as a cultural construct. The Serbian and Greek rebellions against the Ottoman suzerains were 'partially in response to the dimly understood western European ethos of nationalism'.[9] As Richard Hall explained,

Intellectuals made great efforts to standardize and celebrate the vernacular languages of the Balkans. In doing so, they frequently referred and connected to the medieval states that had existed in the Balkans before the Ottoman conquest. Soon the emphasis of nationalism became political. A strong desire to achieve national unity motivated the Balkan states to confront their erstwhile Ottoman conquerors. Balkan leaders assumed that only after the attainment of national unity could their states develop and prosper. In this regard the Balkan peoples sought to emulate the political and economic success of Western Europe, especially Germany, by adopting the western European concept of nationalism as the model for their own national development. The Balkan peoples perceived nationalism as a justification for the creation of specific geopolitical entities.[10]

Nationalism, as different from patriotism, differed starkly from the concept of the Ottoman state which was ultimately multi-ethnic and multi-religious, although obviously the Muslim preponderance, but not exclusivity, of the central administration was evident. As Richard Hall indicated: 'This concept of western European nationalism displaced the old Ottoman millet system in the Balkans, which had permitted each major religious group a significant amount of self-administration. The millet system allowed Moslems, Orthodox Christians, Catholics, and Jews to all live in proximity to each other without intruding upon each other.'[11] The millet system of the Ottomans explained why after 500 years of uninterrupted Ottoman rule, the constituent peoples of the empire spoke their languages, exercised their customs, maintained their ethnic names, and practised their religions.

The aggressive Balkan nationalisms did not prosper in isolation. The foreign enemies of the empire manipulated and provoked the domestic discontent to the maximum. Their support was the critical game changer in every rebellion without which all would be doomed to failure. This was arguably not because the Ottoman army or intelligence was all powerful. Rather, it was because the Balkan peoples were initially much divided and hesitant in abandoning their long-held Ottoman loyalties. The main protector of Orthodox Christianity was none other than the Ottoman Empire until Russia stepped into the fold.

People's Mission to the Ottoman Empire

The curtain of Ottoman disintegration was perhaps lifted in 1798 with the French invasion of Egypt which culminated in the coup of Muhammad Ali, an Ottoman Pasha from Kavala, who then set out to consolidate Egypt's autonomy within the Ottoman Empire's possession until the British invasion in 1882 and full annexation in 1914. Serbs followed suit by rebelling in 1804, attracting massive Russian help. They succeeded in establishing a Serbian lord's hereditary rule in 1817. Their independence, however, would have to wait until the end of the Russo-Turkish War in 1878. A pattern was established, as Quataert notes:

> The overall pattern in the Balkans is confusing in its detail but clear in overall direction. Often a local revolt would meet success or the Russians would drive very deep into the southern Balkans. But then a troubled international community, fearful of Ottoman disintegration or Russian success, would convene a gathering, undo the worst results but allow some losses to ensue.[12]

This struggle for domination over the territories recovered from the Ottoman Empire became known as the 'Eastern Question'. The European major powers were, in fact, also conflicted about the fate of the Ottoman Empire. Their subjects included various ethnicities and they were wary of ethnic nationalisms as much as the Ottomans were. At the same time, they were lured by the prospects of expansion that Ottoman disintegration could afford them. However, they could not agree on who would get what from Ottoman demise. There was hardly any other epoch in history when diplomacy was as consequential and as shifting. The Great Power system in Europe was established in 1815 following the defeat of Napoleon Bonaparte's France in order to check primarily French but ultimately all continental European great powers' temptations to expand territory. The system also involved the strengthening of France's neighbours in a bid to halt French incursions into weaker neighbouring states. With Britain throwing its weight behind one or the other European power in a bid to countervail the power of another expansionist power, a system was put in place to maintain the status quo. The unification of Italy and Germany in 1870 and 1871 brought about a new equation which tested the system set up in 1815. Particularly after Austria–Hungary, Russia, and

Prussia formed the Three Emperor's League in 1873, the balance of power system became more precarious. The Three Emperors' League involved the pledge to remain neutral if any of these three states decided to engage any non-member militarily. The Balkans and, thus, the Ottomans were particularly affected by this arrangement given that the region was coveted by two members of the League, namely Austria–Hungary and Russia, and the non-member Ottomans. Being outside the immediate zone of vital interest to Britain and France, the Balkans, thus, became even more a theatre for high politics and geopolitical competition and war. While the preference for Britain was initially to keep the Ottoman Empire intact in order to maintain the balance of power in Europe, the region became a target for Russian subversion which provoked and amplified Balkan nationalisms to set the stage for Russian intrusion. Britain also prevaricated on its policy to maintain the Ottoman Empire. In Quataert's words: '[T]hrough their wars and support of the separatist goals of rebellious Ottoman subjects, European states abetted the very process of fragmentation that they feared and were seeking to avoid.'[13] In fact, to overcome their inherent paradox, they had admitted the Ottoman Empire to the Concert of Europe as of 1856, following the Crimean War in which a coalition of them intervened in favour of the Ottomans against Russia. Had the Ottoman Empire succeeded in reforming its failing economy and stabilized its domestic politics, world history might have fared differently—we will never know. Nonetheless, history took another course and the Ottomans have been left as an outsider, a Muslim other, an enemy of their self-appointed civilized world. And they never failed to subvert, combat, and ultimately devour the ensuing Ottoman decay. The Great Powers of the day were not at all averse to cooperating with the Ottomans when that was in their interest, but equally eager to invoke religious antagonism when cooperation was evitable. We see this pattern enduring through the First World War till date when even the ardent opponents of Turkey's accession to the European Union on the grounds of 'cultural differences' with a Muslim nation would not forsake cooperation with Turkey. In the lead up to the Balkan Wars, the pragmatist yet essentially anti-Turkish and anti-Muslim stance prevailed among the European powers. Yet imperial Russia led the charge.

Lord Kinross observed that 'since 1820 Russia had been assiduous in her policy of encouraging revolt among the Christian Slavs of the Balkan provinces'.[14] Things, however, spiralled out of control by 1876: 'In Bulgaria a rebel leader, visions of himself as a Slav Napoleon, had pledged his followers to terrorist methods. They turned savagely on the Moslem Turks, whom they started to massacre. But within ten days their revolt was suppressed, with a savagery more terrible, by Turkish irregular forces let loose in revenge.'[15] Whether in the Balkans or in other parts of the Ottoman Empire, such violence and counter violence were 'reported' by the European media and American missionaries to the world. In this case, it was the *English Daily News* which also set another pattern of graphic reporting that only helped to inflame European public opinions. Based on the accounts of the *Daily News*, an anti-Turkish fury erupted. A cycle of violence and a culture of Muslim bashing became yet again an order of the era. It proved to be not an exclusively Balkan or Ottoman affair. The two world wars, first unleashed in the Balkans, saw unspeakable savagery and indiscriminate killing which decimated tens of millions of humans around the world. The world had entered into the total war era in which no one was spared from the scourge of war. No distinction was observed between the belligerent and the population. If you ask the Turks, it was the Christians who unleashed this vicious cycle. If you ask the subjects, it was the Ottomans. That debate can perhaps never be resolved. The fact of the matter is that senseless violence was not limited to conflicts between rebellious Christians and the Muslims. A 1913 Carnegie report on the Balkan Wars has given a grave account of the Greek–Bulgarian hatred:

Day after day the Bulgarians were represented as a race of monsters, and public feeling was roused to a pitch of chauvinism which made it inevitable that war, when it should come, should be ruthless. In talk and in print one phrase summed up the general feeling of the Greeks towards the Bulgarians. 'Dhen einai anthropoi!' (They are not human beings). In their excitement and indignation the Greeks came to think of themselves as the appointed avengers of civilization against a race which stood outside the pale of humanity.[16]

In the long list of wars and fighting that ravaged the Ottoman territories during its final century, one of the most consequential was perhaps the 1877–8 Russo-Turkish War. The war pitted an Eastern Orthodox coalition led by Russia, ostensibly to assist a Bulgarian uprising, against the Ottoman Empire. Heavy fighting was waged on two fronts, namely the Balkans and the Caucasus. Russia's main aim was to avenge the 1856 war in which several Great Powers sided with the Ottomans and established themselves in the Black Sea. The Ottomans suffered a decisive defeat, losing Kars and Batum provinces in the Caucasus and conceding Romania, Serbia, Montenegro, and Bulgaria's secession and independence. The two monarchies signed the Treaty of San Stefano which was challenged by the other Great Powers. Chancellor Otto von Bismarck of Germany called for a new meeting in Berlin which ended in diminishing Russia's conquests. The 1878 Congress of Berlin also allowed Britain to take Cyprus and the dual monarchy of Austria–Hungary to occupy Bosnia and Herzegovina. The Congress of Berlin opened new pages in intra-Balkan and intra–Great Power relations. The Bulgarians, the Greeks, the Serbs, and Montenegrins all perceived the 1878 Treaty of Berlin as an impediment to their national ambitions and embarked upon a perilous road towards reclaiming what they regarded as theirs. Hence, the stage was set for the parties to succumb to a long period of competition and fighting which would ultimately culminate in first the Balkan Wars of 1912–13 and then in the First World War, not to mention perhaps the Balkan wars of the 1990s. In the process, 'Balkanization' entered our parlance as a pejorative term that would denote fragmentation of a region or group into mutually hostile units.

Geopolitics under the Shadow of Myths

As Lord Kinross observed, for the Europeans, the prestige of the Ottoman Empire in the military field had already 'suffered an inescapable blow toward the end of the seventeenth century, through the humiliating failure of the Ottoman armies in the second siege of Vienna, and in the campaigns that followed it'.[17] The Ottoman army disintegrated into such a fugitive rabble as to recall those of the West itself in the crusading wars of the past. Europe rejoiced at this palpable turn of the tide, seeing in it the death knell of the Moslem Turks as a threat to the peoples of Christendom. Once and for all the mighty were fallen. Their fall marked the first of a succession of territorial losses which, after further defeats followed by unfavorable treaties, were at regular intervals to continue right into the twentieth century.[18]

The decline of the Ottomans coincided with the rise of the Russian Empire. Peter the Great was an ambitious man who ruled with an iron fist. Turks called this ruler 'Peter the Madman'. Russians under Peter successfully launched a profound military modernization. Russia became Ottomans' main nemesis, which successfully preyed on Ottoman power and lands. From the early eighteenth century onwards, the Russians fought, subverted, and co-opted the Ottomans cannibalizing Ottoman territory.

At the dawn of the twentieth century, the Russian approach towards the Balkans and the Ottomans was moulded by a hybrid ideology that enmeshed religion with geopolitics. 'Russian Orthodoxy is more than a major religion in the country', wrote Dmitrii Sidorov. 'From very early history, it played the utmost political and geopolitical role in the country.'[19] Although Russian popular myth delves deeper into history to find its references, it also attributes particular importance to the conquest of Constantinople by the Ottomans, ending the long reign of Roman and Eastern Roman empires. This was roughly about the time that the Russians were starting to prevail against the Mongol invasions. The Russian princes then came to the curious conclusion that it must have been God that allowed the downfall of Byzantium, or in their perception the Orthodox Second Rome, in order for the Third Rome to arise. Thus, starting with the second half of the fifteenth century and well into the sixteenth century, the idea that Moscow had 'a unique religious and political mission as the successor of Rome and Byzantium',[20] on the one hand, and was the protector of the Orthodox world, on the other, developed among the Russian elite. An apologist for this idea was the Russian clergyman Filofei who in 1511 addressed Tsar Vasily III saying:

The Church of old Rome fell because of the impiety of the Apollinarian heresy; the Church of the Second Rome, Constantinople, was smitten under the battle-axes of the Agarenes; but this present Church of the Third, New Rome, of Thy sovereign empire: the Holy Catholic Apostolic Church ... shines in the whole universe more resplendent than the sun. And let it be known to Thy Lordship, O pious Czar, that all the empires of the Orthodox Christian Faith have converged into Thine one empire. Thou art the sole Emperor of all the Christians in the whole universe ... For two Romes have fallen, and the Third stands, and a fourth shall never be, for Thy Christian Empire shall never devolve upon others.[21]

The Third Rome prophesies did not have much luck in prediction. Obviously, the world did not end either in 1492 or in 1500 as prophesized. Sidorov recounts: When the world failed to end in 1492, the Metropolitan of Moscow marked the event by proclaiming Ivan III to be the 'new Emperor Constantine of the new Constantinople—Moscow'. Russian churchmen also prophesized time and again that the Second Rome would be liberated by the Russians, namely that Russia would capture Constantinople. It is not obvious how popularly or even seriously this prophetic postulation was received at the time. But it seemed to have retained a certain life well into the nineteenth century and early 20th century. In one form or the other such fantasies not only persisted but were also transformed into ideational pretexts for naked geopolitical aspirations. Thus, geopolitically pan-Orthodox 'concept was most often interpreted as the ideal of taking over Constantinople, spiritual leadership in Orthodox Europe and the establishment of a Panslavic union. It was very important in the context of the Russo-Turkish, Balkan wars and the Eastern Question over the straits allowing access to the Mediterranean Sea.'[22]

Pan-Orthodox ideas had resonance in the Balkans, but it must be pointed out that they found a symbiotic existence with ethnic myths in shaping national identities. Ethnic themes or myths became dominant as was the case in Serbia. As Vjekoslav Perica explained, '[T]he cult of ethnic saints, rather than Orthodox theology, helped the creation of the Serbian nation. The Serbian Church commemorated Serbian medieval rulers as saints.'[23] These saints came to stand as hallmarks of not only Serbian Orthodoxy but also Serbian national identity. The church deliberately instilled a cult of Serbian saints by canonizing no less than 76 Serbs including 22 statesmen.[24] As Perica quotes from Milorad Ekmecic, the Serbian Orthodox Church 'turned ethnic nationalism into a religion and fused pravoslavlje (the Orthodox faith) with the ideology of the restored nationhood',[25] giving, in Serbian theologist Nikolaj Velimirovic's words, 'to this nationalism its aura, revolutionary fervor, prophetic vision, and justification'.[26] Yet the same process of legitimating nationalism with religion also separated Balkan nationalisms. Separate nationalisms grew out from within the similar religious identity. Greeks sought the resurrection of the Byzantine Empire; Serbs referred to the times of Stephan Dusan; and Bulgarians yearned for an era of the past two Bulgarian empires. Pan-Slavism might have united Bulgarians, Montenegrins, and the Serbs, but the Greeks and the Latin Romanians were left out. All these nationalisms cohabited not at all peacefully in a narrow stretch of territory sequestered to the point of violent explosion.

The element of space could not be overstated. In the comfort of hindsight, the essentially geopolitical nature of the series of conflicts in the Balkans is as prevalent as the anti-Turkish and anti-Muslim. Several historians agree that far too many pent-up aspirations were created by nationalist ideologies, pushed down on the masses by the intellectuals among the Balkan peoples. However, the boundaries of each of these constructed national geographies overlapped with that of another fellow nascent Balkan state, not to mention the territorial claims of at least Austria–Hungary of the Great Powers.

The actual fighting in the Balkan Wars started on 19 October 1912 when Montenegro attacked the Ottoman Empire. It was immediately after the Turkish–Italian War in contemporary Libya came to an end. The war between the Ottomans and Italy—the latter being left behind in the imperial competition that divided up the globe among a group of empires and which until then had respected Ottoman sovereignty—started abruptly with an Italian ultimatum on 28 September 1911. The Italian government claimed that the state of disorder and neglect threatened its citizens in Tripoli and, thus, Italy would occupy the North African province of the Ottoman Empire. İstanbul responded by trying to placate Rome and seeking negotiations and offering economic concessions. However, the ultimatum given by Italy was intentionally unacceptable. Material interests in an Italy which wanted an empire for itself weighed in and Italy declared war against the Ottomans the next day. The Ottoman navy was not strong enough to defend the seas. Egypt under British occupation also disallowed Ottoman soldiers to cross overland into Tripoli. The Ottoman units in Libya were depleted and could not have offered much resistance. Nonetheless, the Ottomans held up the Italians by an improvised strategic plan which included training the Arab Sanussi tribesmen into military units. As a result, the war stuck in a near stalemate, with the invaders capturing the shore but not being able to penetrate inland. The 1912 Turkish–Italian War saw for the first time the use of aerial bombardment with small hand-held bombs being manually dropped from simple biplanes.[27] Among the individual officers that made their way to Libya despite the effective blockage during this short war were Mustafa Kemal and Enver who would be crucially important in the future course of the Ottoman Empire all the way into the modern Turkish Republic. But, the Ottomans were at the time on the verge of the Balkan Wars and in a dire need for peace. They ceded Tripoli to Italy on 18 October 1912 in Ouchy, one day before the Balkan Wars began. The opportunistic Italian aggression caught Ottomans by surprise and dissipated their focus and capabilities further to put up a strong enough resistance to the invading Balkan League. It also demonstrated the weaknesses of the Ottoman army thus aggravating the Balkan League's lust for war.

The First Balkan War (1912) was the first time in their history when these Balkan states were united. Their discourse line was the liberation of Christians from Muslim rule. Their purpose simultaneously was to fulfil their territorial aspirations. When the Ottomans were preoccupied with the war against Italy and their perennial domestic squabbles, they concluded two founding treaties. Thus Bulgaria allied with Greece and Serbia in two different documents. The demand they conveyed to İstanbul was to appoint a Christian governor general. They also demanded legislatives and constabulary forces to be local. They asked reforms to be instituted under their oversight and wanted the Great Powers to supervise the process. But the Ottoman parliament was dissolved only recently and İstanbul asked for time until it was reconvened. However, the Balkan states were intent on war on the instigation of Russia. Moreover, 'among their own populations the clamour for war was so strong that it could only be ignored at the risk of revolution'.[28] Led by officers that were trained either in Russia or in Europe, and displaying hardly any standardization in their weaponry, the Balkan armies were largely formed by conscripted peasants. As Richard Hall writes, 'All the Balkan armies perceived that the often illiterate peasant infantryman, indoctrinated to some degree with the appropriate nationalist ideology, was the basis for their military posture.'[29] These young men were taking and losing lives in the name of resurrecting ancient glories as inculcated in them by their schoolmasters.What followed was an unspeakable terror that would entail two local and a world war, the first two somewhat linked to the latter.

The War to Which Indian Muslims
Sent Their Doctors

The geopolitical and ideological spaces within which the Balkan Wars were fought were also interlinked. The First Balkan War turned into a complete disaster for the Ottomans. A series of military and political blunders made this feat unavoidable. In retrospect, the confidence of the Balkan armies was well founded, whereas that of the Turkish commanders in their territorial defences proved complacent. Shortly before the war, the Ottoman army demobilized more than 70, 000 soldiers.[30] Large numbers of officers were either already in Tripoli/Trablus or on their way to join the fight—an unexpected war against the Italians. A division was deployed in Yemen and could not join the forces in the Balkan front. The reorganization of the army was still underway. Trained soldiers were lacking, leaving the stage to untrained recruits. Furthermore, vicious domestic political squabbles haunted İstanbul. As Metin Uysal and Edward J. Erickson have explained in their elaborate study of the Ottoman military, the 1878 Berlin Treaty that ended yet another disastrous war against the Russians had already 'shaped the borders of the Ottoman

Balkans in such a way that it was nearly impossible to defend it against multiple enemies'.[31] One faulty presumption was that the Balkan armies lacked the means to launch coordinated assaults. The officers in charge also 'neglected to remember the main lesson of the Russo-Turkish wars, namely, to not spread forces too thinly over the theatres of operation and to avoid the splitting of field armies into composite groups'.[32] The armies in the west and east of the Balkan theatre were largely disconnected. Significant resources were largely pegged down with a view to defending the fortresses in Edirne, Iskodra, and Yanya, as well as Çanakkale (Dardanelles) and the Aegean islands, further depleting means to wage successful battles on other active fronts. The spectre of Italians also joining the war in the Aegean necessitated keeping defensive units in the area. Mobilization continued slower than planned and half of the Anatolian units could not reach the Balkan fronts. That autumn, there was not enough food to stockpile beyond what was the bare necessity for the civilian population. Animals were in scarcity, and hence meat as well. In sum, local supplies to sustain the armies were in much dearth, resulting in the necessity to replenish from Anatolia. The infrastructure also proved to be tragically deficient. Only a single-track railroad was operational. The roads were shabby. And it was a very rainy and cold month creating a sea of mud that made transportation a nightmare. The sea lines, in turn, were blocked by the Greek navy. Even the telephone system broke down initially.

Though the First Balkan War was waged in two main theatres, in practice it was the one in Thrace that was to be the most rancorous, with Macedonia seeing only one major scale military campaign. Thrace is a flat land, conducive to large-scale military movements. It is also the gateway to İstanbul, a determined goal for any Balkan army. The Byzantines too had to defend this city against the Bulgars, Avars, and Serbs in medieval times. Thrace was the most important theatre of the war because of its proximity to İstanbul. 'The war would be won and lost in Thrace', writes Richard Hall.[33]

The Bulgarian command's plan was to capture Kırklareli, aka Kırkkilise, with one army and the fortress city Edirne with the other, and then to unite the two in order to complete their conquest of Thrace. The ethnic Bulgarian and Greek residents in the region were employed to spy against the Ottoman forces. These villagers went beyond spying and actually joined assaults against small units and patrols. The initial engagement with the Ottomans happened in Gerdelli, west of Kırklareli on 22 October. This was a day-long indecisive battle. The same night, however, the Bulgarian surprise raid demoralized the untrained Ottoman reserve forces, which included many Greeks and Bulgarians, who began to flee in panic. The battle of Kırklareli ended with the decision of the army command on 23 October to retreat to a more secure defensive posture. However, the retreat was unplanned and turned into a rout amidst unrelenting rain and swamps of mud. Later on, the same Thracian mud was to hamper the work of the Indian Medical Mission as well, as we will see later. Corps commander Mahmud Muhtar Pasha was to report that during this rout one-third of the Ottoman war materials were abandoned to the enemy. The scale of the loss was not the doing of the enemy but due to the poor organization, command, and control of the Ottoman army.

At this point the Bulgarian army did the inconceivable and stopped to rest rather than to pursue or even effectively screen the routing forces. The Ottoman eastern army command, whose every previous tactic had failed miserably, managed to regroup its forces in Lüleburgaz. But a debate over what strategy to follow next prevented the Ottomans from capitalizing on the time lost by the rival army. And the same natural and man-made factors were still at play. Hunger started to deplete the forces even before the enemy guns reached them. On 28 October 1912, the Bulgarians re-engaged the Ottomans in Lüleburgaz, this time more fatally. Again a rout began. Whatever food stocks remained, those were deserted to the invading armies, with nothing new arriving from the depths of Anatolia. At this stage, sanitary discipline was also lost. A medical disaster set in. An epidemic of cholera, typhoid, and dysentery broke out, spreading in the region by the displaced civilians. There was a dire shortage of doctors and medical personnel. Although sources seem to disagree on the numbers, hundreds or even thousands died as a result. The press reported that a dysfunctional medical system haunted the Ottoman defences against the Balkan League during these battles. It was these reports about medical shortcomings which accounted for the dispatch by the Indians of the Indian Medical Mission led by Dr Mukhtar Ahmad Ansari as well as other medical missions.

A series of other battles was to be fought before the Indian medical team arrived in İstanbul. While the siege of Edirne was already underway soon after the battle of Lüleburgaz, the most important one was perhaps the Çatalca battle on 17–18 November 1912. Between 28 October and mid-November, the Bulgarians again chose to not pursue the routing army, complacent of their strength. The retreating Ottoman eastern army took the opportunity and regrouped, taking defensive fortifications in Çatalca, basically an outskirt of greater İstanbul. Some 40 kilometres away, Çatalca was now the final defence line before the enemy reached İstanbul, the capital city of the Ottomans. As the army prepared for battle along a defensive line that extended some 50 kilometres by 6 from the Black Sea to the Marmara Sea, İstanbul's defences were also being strengthened. The city and its environs stockpiled guns and ammunition and prepared for war. Most importantly, the Ottoman army in the field now received replenishment from the capital, unlike the earlier battles farther in Thrace. Even the telephone lines were reconnected, improving communications lacking in Kırklareli and Lüleburgaz. This was again the Ottoman army coming back to its real self. The Ottoman government led by Kamil Pasha made one more attempt in vain for a ceasefire. Richard Hall reports that the Bulgarian government had, in fact, developed 'serious reservations' over an assault on Çatalca and thence to İstanbul for fear of drawing in the jealousy and reaction of the Russians who clearly wanted the city for themselves.[34] The Balkan command erred on the side of complacency now lusting for İstanbul: 'The Bulgarian military's reluctance to countenance any interference by the civilian government into the pursuit of policy aims once war was declared foreshadowed events in several European capitals in the summer of 1914.'[35] The battle, which also saw the Ottoman navy engaging along the shores, was a disaster for the Bulgarian army. They decimated some twelve thousand of its young men in two days in a vain pursuit of some pent-up ambitions. The advance to İstanbul was stopped, although the Bulgarian command did try again and again later in the spring of 1913, only to face the same defeat.

Faced with unbeatable resistance in Çatalca, the Balkan army focused back on Edirne bordering Bulgaria. Cut off from the main units around Çatalca and the western army deep around Macedonia, the forecast was that the Edirne fortress could not hold for long. The odds were strongly stacked against Edirne, including the lingering cholera epidemic and all the rest of the adverse conditions that plagued the Lüleburgaz battle.

As the drama was unfolding in Thrace, the war on the western front was also not faring well for the Ottomans. The Serbs had captured much of Macedonia including Kumanova, Bitola, and Skopje; the Greeks seized Selanik (now called Thessaloniki) and continued their march towards Yanina, while the Montenegrins penetrated cities in Albania.

However, the Bulgarian Tsar, who had been an ardent promoter of belligerence until then, changed his position after the defeat in Çatalca and ordered Bulgarian diplomats to secure an armistice. Negotiations began on 25 November in Çatalca and an armistice was agreed upon on 3 December. Only Greece decided not to adhere to the armistice and continued its siege of Yanina. Although the Balkans came out advantageous from the armistice, their ambitions were not satisfied, except perhaps in the case of Serbia. The Ottomans particularly proved adamant in not ceding Edirne, Scutari, and Yanina, the latter two mostly in order to not desert the Albanian residents of these cities to Greek rule. Also, around that point, the European major powers decided to intervene upon the call of the Ottomans. A conference began in London on 17 December 1912. During the London conference, trains were allowed by the Turks to go through Edirne to supply the Bulgarian forces. The gesture, however, was not reciprocated in order to supply Edirne.

There were actually two simultaneous London conferences. One was between the Balkan League and the Ottoman Empire. There the Ottomans made an offer to cede all territory west of Edirne. It was a generous offer which the Turkish people were, in fact, not prepared to accept. Nonetheless,

[h]ad the Bulgarians abandoned their dreams of obtaining the city and region, which had only a small Bulgarian population, the Greeks would have been hard pressed to maintain a lone defiant posture

against the Ottomans and ultimately against the Great Powers. The First Balkan War could have ended in January 1913, and the Second Balkan War might never have taken place.[36]

The other London conference was among the Great Power ambassadors. It was there and not at the Balkan ministerial conference that ultimate decisions about the outcome of the war were taken.

As we will see later, the Indian Medical Mission would arrive in İstanbul during this armistice in the wake of the Kırıkkale, Lüleburgaz, and Çatalca battles, as the siege of Edirne was underway, as the London Conference was ongoing, and the Ottoman government was, unbeknownst to them, teetering on the brink of a coup.

The Young Turks staged a coup at that point when the Indian Mission was already in Turkey. The chief of staff of the Strategic Reserve forces in İstanbul, Lieutenant Colonel Ismail Enver Bey, better known as the fiery and charismatic Enver Pasha, led the coup toppling the Kamil Pasha government on 23 January 1913. Nazım Pasha, the minister of war and the alleged culprit of the Ottoman Balkan military blunders, was killed in his office. The Young Turks tabled a new proposal suggesting the partition of Edirne province through the Meriç River, but not yield the city itself, the once capital of the Ottomans. When the Bulgarians snubbed, the second phase of the First Balkan War restarted with a greater Ottoman zeal to protect the motherland against the invaders. Known in Turkish history as the Raid on the Sublime Porte (Bab-ı Ali Baskını), the coup brought a professional military modernizer to the grand vizier's (prime minister) chair, who intensified reforms and mobilization of the army. That said respite was short and there was not enough time to address the deficiencies. When the Balkan League denounced the armistice, fighting restarted on 3 February 1913. Since Macedonia was all but lost, the besieged cities of Edirne, Yanina, and Scutari would become the foci of the military engagements.

The siege of Edirne was recorded in Turkish annals as an epic of bravery and resilience under adverse conditions. The fortress city held up against all odds, having been long cut-off from İstanbul and the rest of the Ottoman forces and unable to replenish its food and war stocks. In order to relieve the city, Ottoman forces launched a daring operation in Çanakkale (Gallipoli), the famous site of another epic Turkish battle to be waged only a year or so later, this time against the imperial British forces composed of a collage of troops from home and colonized territories including India. Dr Ansari would call the Indian soldiers' participation in this war a major inconsistency and the only one at that. But in the February of 1913, the Ottomans were to take the Indian voluntary medical mission along as the Turkish forces raided occupying Bulgarian forces in Çanakkale. In the Bulair part of Çanakkale, in an open field, the two armies came head to head with intense artillery fire. The Bulgarians fielded 78 guns against the 36 of the Ottomans. The plan was to clear the Çanakkale Peninsula and to link up with Ottoman troops making a landing at Şarköy. The Şarköy amphibious landing was, in turn, aimed to encircle the Bulgarian fourth army in front of Çatalca from behind. The Şarköy amphibious landing showed 'a rare combination of leadership, discipline, and courage'[37] write military historians Metin Uysal and Edward Erickson. While the Ottoman forces performed visibly better in February 1913 than in Kırklareli or Lüleburgaz three months before, they failed to alleviate pressure on Edirne. Having upset the Ottoman operations to capture the northern coasts of the Marmara Sea or establish themselves at the rear of the Bulgarian lines at Çatalca, Balkan forces then fired back. But, again, Çatalca defences proved insuperable. Between 24 March and 3 April, 'stubborn and massive Bulgarian frontal assaults were crushed repeatedly by the skilful use of fortifications and centralized fire support'.[38] But these successes were to remain under the shadow of the demoralizing news of the surrender of Yanya on 6 March, Edirne on 26 March, and then Iskodra on 23 April. In effect, by mid-April, the war was lost on the European theatre and the five-century-long Ottoman rule in the Balkan Peninsula came to an end.

The London Peace Treaty of 30 May 1913 ended the First Balkan War but not the full sorry episode of the Balkan Wars. A line was drawn from the west of İstanbul connecting the two seas around İstanbul and every place to its west including Edirne was given to Bulgaria. The treaty maximized Bulgarian gains in Thrace and Serbian gains in Macedonia.

Unsurprisingly, the treaty upset the already unstable Ottoman domestic political scene. The suspicion that the previous government would cede Edirne had been used to legitimize the Young Turk coup only a few months back. Now the new government was signing a treaty formally ceding even more. Although the prospects looked grim for the Committee of Union and Progress–led government, it was going to receive a new lease of life from the collapse of the Balkan alliance.

Politically, the Balkan alliance was a fragile union of convenience. It was only based on lofty, empty ideas about putative ancestral glories and pent-up aspirations of landownership over swathes of multi-ethnic populations. It was a product no less of Russian diplomatic engineering for its own geopolitical ambitions. However, the Russian grand designs abroad reflected a mind-boggling failure of imperial Russian statesmanship. As the Bolshevik Revolution would show only a few years later, the Russian Empire's social and economic order teetered on the brink of collapse as the Russian Tsar was callously seeking adventures abroad. The so-called Great Power balance of power system was itself senescent. And the Balkan League was made possible not least due to the worn-out state of the Ottoman Empire whose rebellions inside became as sinister as the enemies outside, all attacking the body of a once powerful polity. The London Peace Treaty lasted barely a day. On 1 June, Bulgaria saw an alliance of Serbs and Greeks forming against it over the coveted lands of Macedonia. Bulgarian Tsar Ferdinand responded by attacking Serbian and Greek armies on the night of 29/30 June. Left alone, Bulgaria now had to fight its former allies and this time even Romania, which had remained outside the earlier war. Bulgarian army lost on almost every front except Vidin. Ottomans also took the opportunity to join the fight in Thrace and liberated Edirne from the Bulgarians with an ambush operation on 21 July without a field battle. In doing so, the Ottoman leadership chose to ignore the warnings from its friendly and less friendly Great Power peers. This became the wisest decision that the Ottoman leaders made since the advent of the Balkan Wars. The new frontiers of the Ottomans in Europe were thus drawn along the Meriç River.

From the Second Balkan Wars the Bulgarians, thus, emerged with a defeat both on the western and eastern fronts and negotiations for a peace treaty commenced on 30 July in Bucharest. Under the consequent Bucharest Treaty of 10 August 1913, Bulgaria managed to retain its conquests in western Thrace, including an outlet to the Aegean Sea. However, Greece and Serbia effectively cannibalized most of Macedonia while Bulgaria was given a small piece of the region. Yet, Macedonia was the prime object of Bulgaria in the Balkan Wars, even more so than Thrace or İstanbul which were concurrently in the domain of Russian aspirations and British red line. The head of the Bulgarian diplomatic delegation at the Bucharest peace talks voiced its country's fundamental distaste for the deal in non-equivocal terms: 'Either the Powers will change it, or we ourselves will destroy it.'[39]

Bulgarians were going to suffer another blow in Bucharest, this time procedural, from its former allies, when Romania was allowed to refuse Ottoman participation in the peace talks. This meant that Bulgarians would have to negotiate a separate peace agreement with the Turks alone against a still colossal and very much functioning Ottoman state. The Ottomans, now finally gainful in the field and with Bulgaria worn out, concluded the peace treaty in İstanbul on 29 September, more or less consolidating the actual holdings on the ground. The Balkan Wars of 1912–13 ended when Serbia signed the İstanbul Treaty on 13 March, and Greece signed the Athens Treaty on 14 November with the Ottomans.

The wars caused Turkey to lose 150,000 as dead or wounded, Bulgaria 156,000, Serbia 71,000, and Montenegro 11,200. The map of Europe was redrawn. The Ottomans were expelled from Europe. And Macedonia fell to nationalist forces that overturned the Ottoman millet system of autonomy and tried to impose their own cultures on the Macedonians and Kosovars.

The immediate legacy of the Balkan Wars was the forced mass exodus of Turkish civilians in the Balkans. The number of Turkish refugees who fled Greece-occupied Thrace, Macedonia, and Epir reached 240,000 before the outbreak of the First World War on 28 June 1914, barely a year after the Balkan Wars, again with a spark in the Balkans. Large numbers of Greeks also emigrated from the Turkish territories towards Greece. The Balkans had embarked upon a path of forming ethnically homogeneous nation states at great human cost long before ethnic cleansing re-entered our lexicon in the 1990s again via the Balkans. Violence bred counter violence.

Victims sought revenge and became perpetrators. A vicious cycle set in which only fed violent secessionism. Balkan nationalism destroyed the Balkan historical, social, and psychological fabric, uprooting millions, mostly Turks or other Muslims, from their homes in a frenzy of violence and counter-violence in pursuit of expansive yet pure nation states and borders in place of an increasingly decrepit multiethnic Ottoman polity.

The Ottoman Empire's disintegration started taking its toll on the Muslims in the Balkans long before the Balkan Wars. In reality, every rebellion had the tactic of slaughtering Muslim civilians that would create a spiral of violence and end up in the Muslims' displacement. The battles waged by the Christian powers including the larger states almost always involved attacks on the civilian Muslims. These attacks were rationalized by branding the victims as the collaborators of the oppressors. While ethnic purification began in the Serbian provinciality long before and reached unprecedented levels during the Russian war against the Ottomans in 1877–8, the Balkan Wars saw another peak of ethnic cleansing. This was perhaps one of the first examples of all-out warfare, a harbinger of what was to follow in the ensuing wars, where armed civilians participated in the battles. Whether they were called *komitadji*, *četa*, or *fedai*, these armed groups robbed and murdered other civilians. Turks; Muslim Albanians; Slavic, Bulgarian, and Macedonian-speaking Muslims including the Pomaks and the Muslim Roma; as well as Crimean Tatars and Circassians were the target of these armed mobs. Over 400, 000 of them fled to İstanbul only in 1912. Scores died during flight either because they were murdered or because they starved to death or fell victim to epidemic diseases. Alongside Muslims, Jews were also expelled. The tragic history of the deportation and death of millions of Turks and Muslims in the final two centuries of the Ottoman Empire was most adeptly researched and conveyed by Justin McCarthy in his seminal work entitled *Death and Exile: The Ethnic Cleansing of Ottoman Muslims, 1821–1922*.[40] The study lays bare the prejudice that resulted in the Christian world perceiving, articulating, and even concocting narratives always from the standpoint of nations that were carved out of the Ottoman Empire. As British historian

Mark Mazower indicates, one perhaps needed to go as far back as the Crusades to find the enduring roots of this 'martial intolerance in Christian Europe to heretics, pagans and above all, to Muslims'.[41] As Karpat would underscore, the Turks inherited an already negative image existing in Europe for Islam. The Christian clergy felt a threat to their religion from Islam which acknowledged the Bible as the message of God and Jesus as His Prophet and yet went further to reveal the latest message and Prophet through Quran and Mohammad. Islam continues to be the fastest-growing religion in the world perpetuating old fears in the non-Muslim religious establishments. The Turkish lords such as Zengi, Noureddin (the commander and lord of the famed Kurdish general Salahaddin Ayyubi), and Kutuz drove the Crusaders out of Syria and Egypt. Turkish military advances in the centuries following the Crusades only aggravated these perceptions. As Stephen Kinzer notes, since then, 'what made [the Turks] such an awful thing to contemplate was that their forces were battering down across Europe itself'.[42] The Ottoman advances in Europe had, in fact, helped supersede the Catholic–Protestant enmity which ravaged the continent for generations and shifted the axis of conflict back to Christian–Muslim divide. At its peak, the Ottoman Empire, which preceded the modern Turkish Republic, created a duality in the 'Western' mind about the Turk. On the one hand, there has been a persistent and largely religion-based demonization of the Turks and, indeed, all Muslims. On the other hand, there has also been concurrent fascination with the Turks, notably at the heyday of the Ottoman Empire. Mark Mazower noted, 'For all the religious antipathy between Christian and Muslim, sixteenth-century Europeans respected and feared the power, reach and efficiency of the Turks.'[43] English clergyman and historian Thomas Fuller wrote in the seventeenth century that the Ottoman Empire was 'the greatest and best-compacted that the sunne ever saw ... commanding the most fruitful countreys of Europe, Asia and Africa ... its magnificence over-shadowed its squabling neighbors in Christendom'.[44] He was not alone to marvel at the Ottomans. Yet, as the Ottoman power declined and European states rose from backwardness and religious in-fighting to military, economic, technological, and gradually political expansion, the fascination was overshadowed again by scorn for the Turk.

Perhaps the greatest insult to injury was that the European and American public unequivocally took a side as the First Balkan War was glorified in Europe and the United States as a modern crusade against 'Asiatic barbarism'. As Winfried Baumgart observed,

> The inexcusable cruelty of the Bulgarian massacres was preceded by the Bulgarian Christians' equally gruesome massacres of Muslim settlers—these, however, were not reported to the European public at that time, neither by the Russians, who relayed only the information that was useful to them, nor by the English Atrocity Meetings. Moreover, for the estimated 25,000 murdered Bulgarians, the Turks paid with some 1.5 million casualties in the subsequent war against Russia, not counting the hundreds of thousands of refugees who fled the Russians in the winter of 1877/1878 to Constantinople, before dying there of typhus, smallpox and other epidemics.[45]

Such were the conditions and legacy to which the Indian nation responded with indignation. These were the Balkan Wars in which Dr Ansari and his colleagues—supported by donations from Muslims and Hindus from all over India, organized by the *Comrade* journal led by Mohammad Ali in Aligarh and Delhi and supported by several other newspapers—came to serve in Turkey. The Indian Muslims too were bombarded with selective reporting that always showed one victim, the Christian, and one perpetrator, the Muslim Turk. Yet they showed the courage to look beyond the lens put up before their eyes.

At the onset of the twentieth century, the Turks and Indians had more than half a millennium of relations behind them. The next chapter will explain the ethnic and cultural as well as strategic and diplomatic interactions between the rulers and peoples of the Indian subcontinent and the Turkish world. It will show that it was neither cultural affinities nor geopolitical legacies that were the main reasons that culminated in the outpouring of emotional support from India towards Ottoman Turkey. To tell the story we now rewind to the sixteenth century.

Notes

1. The controversial institution of such child recruiting or *devşirme* has been much caricaturized as a tearful and forced separation of the kid from his family. More research is needed on the family reactions to these institutions during the Empire's heyday when being recruited must have been seen, at least by some, as a coveted road for the child to honour and glory. In fact, Noel Malcolm points out in *Bosnia: A Short History* (New York: New York University Press, 1994) that parents in Bosnia were known to bribe their scouts to take their children.

2. William Ewart Gladstone, *Bulgarian Horrors and the Question of the East* (New York and Montreal: Lovell, Adam, Wesson & Company, 1856).

3. J. W. Redhouse, *A Vindication of the Ottoman Sultan's Title of 'Caliph': Shewing Its Antiquity, Validity, and Universal Acceptance* (London: Beffingham Wilson Hoyal Exchange, 1877), p. 4.

4. Alan Palmer, *The Decline and Fall of the Ottoman Empire* (New York: Barnes and Noble, 2005), pp. 6–7.

5. Donald Quataert, *The Ottoman Empire: 1700–1922* (New York: Cambridge University Press, 2005), 2nd ed., p. 54.

6. Isa Blumi, *Reinstating the Ottomans: Alternative Balkan Modernities 1800–1912* (New York: Palgrave Macmillan, 2011), p. 5.

7. Quataert, *The Ottoman Empire*, p. 55.

8. Blumi, *Reinstating the Ottomans*, p. 3.

9. Richard C. Hall, *The Balkan Wars 1912–1913: Prelude to the First World War* (London: Routledge, 2000), p. 2.

10. Hall, *The Balkan Wars*, pp. 1–2.

11. Hall, *The Balkan Wars*, p. 2.

12. Quataert, *The Ottoman Empire*, p. 56.

13. Quataert, *The Ottoman Empire*, p. 56.

14. Lord Kinross, *The Ottoman Centuries: The Rise and Fall of the Turkish Empire* (New York: Perennial, 1979), p. 510.

15. Kinross, *The Ottoman Centuries*, p. 509.

16. *Report of the International Commission to Inquire into the Causes and Conduct of the Balkan Wars* (Washington DC: Carnegie Endowment for International Peace, 1993).

17. Kinross, *The Ottoman Centuries*, p. 618.

18. Kinross, *The Ottoman Centuries*, p. 619.

19. Dmitrii Sidorov, 'Post-Imperial Third Romes: Resurrections of a Russian Orthodox Geopolitical Metaphor, Geopolitics', vol. 11 (2006), pp. 317–47; see p. 320.

20. Sidorov, 'Post-Imperial Third Romes', p. 321.

21. Quote from Sidorov, 'Post-Imperial Third Romes', p. 322, cited from P. Duncan, *Russian Messianism: Third Rome, Revolution, Communism and After* (London and New York: Routledge 2000), pp. 10–12.

22. Sidorov, 'Post-Imperial Third Romes', p. 323.

23. Vjekoslav Perica, *Balkan Idols: Religion and Nationalism in Yugoslav States* (Oxford: Oxford University Press, 2002), p. 8.

24. Perica, *Balkan Idols*, p. 8.

25. Perica, *Balkan Idols*, p. 8.

26. Perica, *Balkan Idols*, p. 8.

27. Palmer, *The Decline and Fall of the Ottoman Empire*, p. 214.

28. Kinross, *The Ottoman Centuries*, p. 585.

29. Hall, *The Balkan Wars*, p. 15.

30. Mesut Uyar and Edward J. Erickson, *A Military History of the Ottomans: From Osman to Atatürk* (Santa Barbara: Praeger Security International, 2009).

31. Uyar and Erickson, *A Military History of the Ottomans*, p. 226.

32. Uyar and Erickson, *A Military History of the Ottomans*, p. 226.

33. Hall, *The Balkan Wars*, p. 22–3.

34. Hall, *The Balkan Wars*, p. 32.

35. Hall, *The Balkan Wars*, p. 32.

36. Hall, *The Balkan Wars*, p. 71–2.

37. Uysal and Erickson, *A Military History of the Ottomans*, p. 231.

38. Uysal and Erickson, *A Military History of the Ottomans*, p. 231.

39. Reported in Hall, *The Balkan Wars*, p. 125.

40. Justin McCarthy, *Death and Exile: The Ethnic Cleansing of Ottoman Muslims, 1821–1922* (Princeton, NJ: Darwin, 1995).

41. Mark Mazower, *The Balkans* (London: Phoenix, 2001), p. 39.

42. Stephen Kinzer, *Crescent and Star* (New York: Farrar, Straus & Giroux, 2001).

43. Mazower, *The Balkans*, p. 7.

44. Quoted in Mazower, *The Balkans*, p. 7.

45. Winfried Baumgart, 'Orientalische Frage', 1999, p. 43. I took the quote from Berna Pekesen, 'Vertreibung und Abwanderung der Muslime vom Balkan', Europaische Geschichte Online, 2 April 2011, available at http://www.ieg-ego.eu/de/threads/europa-unterwegs/ethnische-zwangs-migration/berna-pekesen-vertreibung-der-muslime-vom-balkan (accessed on 4 April 2014).

3

The Ottoman Empire and Hindustan

In 1552 an Ottoman naval fleet under the command of Sidi Ali Reis embarked on a fateful mission in the Indian Ocean, which ended up establishing the Ottoman Empire's diplomatic relations with the Mughal Empire. The mission was abortive not because of the strength of the Portuguese armada it was sent to keep in check but because Mother Nature would prove to be too formidable that year. Thus, the commander of the Egyptian Fleet of the Ottomans wrote in his *Memoir of Countries*:

> God is merciful! With a favourable wind we left the port of Guador and again steered for Yemen. We had been at sea for several days, and had arrived nearly opposite to Zofar and Shar, when suddenly from the west arose a great storm known as Fil Tufani. We were driven back, but were unable to set the sails, not even the storm sail. The tempest raged with increasing fury. As compared to these awful tempests the foul weather in the western seas is mere child's play, and their towering billows are as drops of water compared to those of the Indian sea. Night and day were both alike, and because of the frailty of our craft all ballast had to be thrown overboard. In this frightful predicament our only consolation was our unwavering trust in the power of the Almighty .... We took frequent soundings, and when we struck a depth of five Kuladj [arm-lengths] the mizzen sails were set, the bowsprits ... and ... heeling over to the left side, and flying the commander's flag, we drifted about all night and all day until at

last, in God's mercy, the water rose, the storm somewhat abated, and the ship veered right round. The next morning we slackened speed and drew in the sails.... Meanwhile, the wind had risen again, and as the men had no control over the rudder, large handles had to be affixed with long double ropes fastened to them. Each rope was taken hold of by four men, and so with great exertion they managed to control the rudder. No one could keep on his feet on deck, so of course it was impossible to walk across ... we could not hear our own voices. The only means of communication with the sailors was by inarticulate words, and neither captain nor boatswain could for a single instant leave his post. The ammunition was secured in the storeroom and ... we continued our way. It was truly a terrible day, but at last we reached Gujarat in India.[1]

This event culminated in Sidi Ali Reis travelling to Delhi to meet the Mughal emperor Humayun and which is remembered today as the hypothetical beginning of diplomatic relations between the Ottoman and Mughal empires. However, no permanent embassy was established and the contacts thence remained sporadic until the nineteenth century when the Ottomans founded two consulates on the subcontinent, one in Bombay and the other in Calcutta. That said, the two peoples are also intimately related through kinship ties. The fact was since the third century there was an upswell of Turkic migration out of their ancestral lands in Central Asia.[2] The earliest migrants were entirely assimilated into the ethnic landscape to which they migrated. Later migrations took the form of military incursions and changed the countries they resettled in forever. The subcontinent was among those areas where their impact would prove lasting and deeply transforming.

Ethnic Commonalities and Rivalries

Turkish–Indian historical connections and interactions are grossly understated and are, in fact, largely unknown by many in today's Turkey and India as well as Pakistan. An exception is the common knowledge that the Urdu language owes its name to the Turkish word for army, namely 'Ordu'. Lesser known is that the Mughal Empire, which Turks of Turkey know rather as the Babürlü

(Baburite) Empire, is one of the sixteen stars in the President of Turkey's insignia among other stars which denote the major states in history founded by ethnic Turks. Knowledge about the shared history is astoundingly limited even in otherwise learned circles. It is commonplace to hear, for instance, of an Indo-Persian civilization rather than a more appropriate Indo-Turkish-Persian civilization. The fact of the matter is that the Mughals were not the first Turkish or Turkic rulers in the subcontinent. The ancient ties between the Turks and Indians extend over many centuries and involve interaction and intermingling in the subcontinent. Longworth Dames writes:

> India had long been the coveted object for the men of Turkish race, not Ottoman Turks, it is true, but of the same stock and speaking the same language. Mahmud of Ghazni and Timur were Turks, and Babur, who ... over threw the Delhi kingdom and established the so-called Mughal Empire, was also a Turkish adventurer. Ottoman Turks abounded in India, they were employed to form their body guards by many of the Muhammadan rulers, and were universally found as artillerymen; in fact, all the gunners in India seem to have been Turks.[3]

In fact, Mahmud of Ghazni invaded India 17 times between 999 and 1030. Turks had thus formed part of the elite of India since the eleventh century. As the veteran scholar of the history of religion and South Asia Annemarie Schimmel pointed out, even before the time of the Mughals, Muslims in India were known as the Turks. The word 'Turks' was used alternatively meaning beautiful, fair complexioned, or lively. In clothing, the Mughal period displayed many Turkish features, as can be seen from the miniatures of the early Mughal women wearing Turkish hats.[4] In time, the Chagatai Turkish language, used by Babur and spoken by several of his heirs, was eclipsed in the Mughal court by Persian, although up to both Shah Jahan and Aurangzeb, the learning and use of the Turkish language continued. While Shah Jahan studied Turkish under Tatar Khan, Aurangzeb commissioned several grammatical studies and dictionaries in Turkish. Jahangir read and proudly displayed a copy of the *Khamsa* by Niwai in Turkish. Many Urdu poets also wrote in Turkish.

Turks have always interacted intimately with the cultures of the lands they conquered. They called these geographies home and created a hybrid culture that reflected a mixture of the best from both cultures. The story in India was not outside this paradigm. India absorbed and assimilated Turkish influences. The case of influence in music is rather evident. Musicologist K. C. D. Brahaspati argued that both southern and northern systems had adopted the Persian and Turkish modal (*makam*) system.[5] Te Nijenhuis pinpoints the influence of the fourteenth-century Sufi Amir Kushrao in introducing the sitar and tabla as musical instruments as well as the *qawwali* form into Indian music and even composing new ragas.[6] Amir Kushrao was affectionately called by the venerable Nizamuddin Auliya as 'Turfei Allah' or 'Turc-ullah' or 'God's Turk'. As one goes around India, especially the northern region, one sees the indelible architectural, culinary, and other cultural footprints of the Turks.[7] As such, Turkish peoples have had a permanent impact on the subcontinent through not only the empires they built on Indian soil but also their cultural, social, and even political inputs to their adopted Indian lands throughout centuries. In India, they encountered a uniquely rich, diverse, and proud ancient civilization, or civilizations, and their own contributions to it made it infinitely richer. Turks and other Muslim invaders became Indians. Islam spread in India more effectively through the persuasion of Sufi saints like Kwaja Muinuddin Chisti and Imam Rabbani Shaykh Ahmad al-Faruqi al-Sirhindi than by the sword of the Turkish or Afghan rulers, although their role ought also not to be understated. As M. J. Akbar describes eloquently, 'Islam came to the Indian subcontinent at the beginning of the eighth century, beginning a complex relationship that expressed itself in war, culture, civilization, dialogue, dress, segregation, integration, fantasy, and nightmare. It was a relationship launched by war but not sustained by it.'[8] India is all the more of a gem of humanity because of its multi-cultural influences, a unique tapestry woven through mutual respect and secularism. War and conflict are immutable facts of life but the manifestly unique beauty consequence of the millennial human interactions in the subcontinent is there for the eye, palate, and ear to witness.

Babur invaded India 16 years after the sea-faring Christians established their first colony in India. His heirs came to check the Portuguese advance out of Goa but failed to address the naval incursion in a fatal strategic shortcoming. At their zenith, the Mughals were the greatest political, military, and social power, uniting the largest part of the subcontinent in a millennium. Babur, the founder of the Mughal Empire, was a proud Timurid, coming from the lineage of that formidable Turk. He tended to understate the Mongol strand in his blood from his mother's side. As Annette Susannah Beveridge has shown, Babur reveals his claim to all 'possessions of the Turk' in India in his memoirs, *Baburnama*, originally written in Chagatai (or eastern Turkish). For instance, one would remember his words passed through his emissaries to the people of Behar in today's Pakistan, as Babur's armies were entering Hindustan. As reported in *Baburnama*:

> We rode from Kalda-kahar at dawn next day. When we reached the top of the Hamtatu-pass a few local people waited on me, bringing a humble gift. They were joined with Abdu'r-rahim the chief-scribe (shaghdwat) and sent with him to speak the Bhira people fair and say, 'The possession of this country by a Turk has come down from of old; beware not to bring ruin on its people by giving way to fear and anxiety; our eye is on this land and on this people; raid and rapine shall not be.'[9]

The rulers of the so-called gunpowder empires shared Turkish ancestry. The poetry of the Safavid emperor Shah Ismail stands even today as a fine piece of Turkish literature. However, the shared roots did not engender in any comity or amity between the Ottoman, Safavid, and Mughal shahs. Of the three, historian A. K. Nizami notes, 'The Ottomans were racially closer to the Indian Mughals but diplomatic links could not be forged with them. A feeling of rivalry and jealousy, peculiar to kith and kin, vitiated their relations.'[10] This was, however, true only in terms of the relationship between two polities and their dynastic rulers. Interactions and sympathies continued to exist among the peoples. Traders and, indeed, the Sufi *dargah*s and their sheikhs and followers did interact. Even at the imperial Mughal court, the presence of Turks was considered normal, particularly in the time of Babur and Humayun, both of whom had Turkish as well as Persian and Afghan wives. As historian Naimur Farooqi details,

Babur employed several Ottoman Turks including one of his chief artillery officers and physicians. Babur employed the Ottoman military technique of 'chaining carts together and placing matchlock-men behind these carts'[11] to win his famous Battle of Panipat in 1526. Indeed, after his victory in Panipat: 'In his next important engagement, against the Rajputs, Babur again adopted the same tactics. He arranged the carts "in the Ottoman way" and imitated the "ghazis of Rum" (Ottomans) by posting the tufangchian (Matchlock-men) and radadazan (cannoneers) along the line of carts. Again he came out victorious.'[12] Yet, he was ultimately not as interested in the Ottomans as his closer rivals, the Uzbeks. Babur's territorial ambitions conflicted with the policies of the Ottomans. Well into his last years Babur wanted to invade Samarkand. His plans were thwarted three times by the Uzbeks. The Uzbeks were therefore stood as the arch adversaries of Babur. The Ottomans, in turn, regarded the Uzbeks as the safeguard against the expansionist ambitions of the Safavid Iran. The territorial integrity of the Uzbek state was therefore important for the Ottomans. There is no record of a dialogue between Babur and Süleyman the Magnificent over the issue. Instead the Mughal Emperor appears to have doubted the possibility or usefulness of an accord with the Ottomans and made no effort in that regard. Neither the Mughals nor the other Turks who ruled India before them came to India from modern-day Turkey. The last Nizam of Hyderabad, however, married both his sons to the princesses Durrushehvar and Nilufer, daughthers of the last Ottoman caliph. That said, the common Central Asian Turkish ancestry was unmistakable in the case of numerous Muslim rulers in India including the Mughals. This common ancestry did not culminate in intensive diplomatic interactions, although we now know that the offshoots of the Delhi Sultanate, namely the 1347–1527 Bahmani Kingdom and the 1401–1572 Sultanate of Gujarat, did engage in periodic diplomatic contacts with the Ottomans, to be joined in the latter decades of the Muslim rule in India by others including Mysore.

Ironically, the relationship between the houses of Babur and Osman seemed nonetheless to be haunted, not aided, by kinship ties. In this context, Naimur Rahman Farooqi points to the Timurid–Ottoman mutual distaste of each other. The acrimony between Amir

Timur (the Lame) and Sultan Beyazıd (the Lightning Bolt) was much more intense than what would be considered normal even between two rival rulers. The Mughals, as heirs to Timur, considered themselves superior to the house of the Osman because of Timur's clear defeat of Sultan Beyazıd at the battlefield. The written exchanges between the two rulers stand as examples of non-diplomatic, to say the least, mutual name-calling. Timur, invited to Anatolia by the rival Turkish beys (lords) on the pretext of the empire in Rum (Rome as Turkey was then called by the Muslims) not being devout enough, not only inflicted a humiliating defeat to the Ottoman sultan but also imprisoned him in a cage and toured him around for all to see. Timur then retreated back to Central Asia in a Tzenghis Khan fashion with his true aspiration being conquering China not Anatolia. The success of their ancestor at the Ankara War had left an exaggerated conceit on the part of the Mughals over the Ottomans. This is a pertinent note because, as Lisa Balabanlılar explains, '[w]hile the dynastic founder, Babur, referred to himself as a Turk, ethnic identity clearly was not an important factor in the careful construction of Mughal imperial identity; instead, the Mughals consistently identified themselves dynastically, as descendants of the House of Timur'.[13] One can surmise that this factor could have limited the positive role that cultural commonalities could have played in their relations. At any rate, by the time of Aurangzeb, thanks to the marriages with Persian, Afghan, and Rajput families, the Mughal kings had become more Persian and Rajput in ancestry than Turkish.[14] Overall, Mughal India and Ottoman Turkey looked in different directions most of the time. It may be said that mutual arrogation almost always existed between the two and prevented any serious attempt to build on the countless cultural similarities and possibilities.

Shared Geopolitical Interests and Failures

As noted earlier, the loss of the Ottoman fleet commanded by Sidi Ali Reis, not in a battle against the Portuguese it came to force out of Indian shores but in a massive storm, coincidentally provided a momentous opportunity for the second Mughal emperor to send a letter to Sultan Süleyman the Lawgiver (known as Süleyman the

Magnificent in Europe) to forge an alliance between the two great Muslim empires. Had this occurred, it would have perhaps counteracted the 1455 bull by Pope Nicholas V sanctioning Christians to sail as far as India to form an alliance with the Indians, whom he thought were heretic Christians, as against the Saracens. As Sidi Ali Reis wrote in his memoirs, whether in Gujarat or after he set out on the long travel back to İstanbul via Delhi by road, the admiral was given a magnificent reception involving 100 elephants and 1,000 men by the Indians. He was offered high offices including a governorship which he declined politely. Sidi Ali Reis was given audience with Humayun on the day he arrived in Delhi as was the diplomatic custom at the Mughal Court. Humayun asked which of the two empires was larger, and was impressed upon hearing the extent of the lands controlled by the Ottomans. Sidi Ali Reis also convinced the Mughal emperor of the benefits of alliance with the Ottomans, then at the zenith of their power. Humayun accepted Sultan Süleyman as the caliph of the Muslims and sent a letter to the Ottoman ruler stating: 'It is hoped and expected, that also on your part the gates of mutual communication will be opened by the keys of attachment, and that the channels of mutual correspondence will not be closed; and that in this manner the foundation of the towering fabric of union will be strengthened and kept free from decay.'[15] Although Sidi Ali Reis is not known to have brought a letter from the Ottoman sultan, he wrote about presenting his credentials to Humayun. Therefore, the arrival of Sidi Ali Reis to Delhi in 1555 is credited as the establishment of diplomatic relations between the Mughals and the Ottomans. An alliance, however, never materialized, not the least due to Humayun's demise in a freak accident even as Admiral Sidi Reis was in the country. And the Ottomans apparently did not reply to Humayun's letter possibly because they knew that Humayun was already dead and, one can only speculate, possibly because they were not sure of the fourteen-year-old Akbar's intentions. Whatever the cause, it appears to be a mistake with the benefit of centuries-long hindsight.

At any rate, if there were any doubts about Akbar, they were to be vindicated by Akbar's career. Humayun's heir Akbar, who must have seen the warm letter sent to the Ottoman sultan through Sidi

Ali Reis, would, in fact, remain adverse to the Ottomans during his long reign. The two empires encountered each other during Akbar's reign and while the two did not come to direct armed conflict, competition and even proxy fighting did occur. Akbar was not responsive to the need for strategic cooperation with the Ottomans and the then clear and present threat of European imperial naval power. Nizami notes: 'On the contrary there was tacit acceptance of the Portuguese de facto control of the Indian Ocean. Portuguese visas whether formally sought for or not, were the only safe passport for travel for Hajj. Gujarat tried to form an anti-Portuguese alliance with the Ottomans but Akbar did not realize the magnitude of the problem.'[16] In retrospect, Naimur Farooqi, the author of a rare dedicated study on Mughal–Ottoman relations, appears correct about the flaws of Akbar's strategic choice.

Giancarlo Casale, in fact, argued that Akbar was actually intent on challenging the Ottoman dynasty. His occupation of Surat, then allied with the Ottomans, constituted the opening salvo to that effect. A major motivation for Akbar's conquest of Gujarat was the desire to limit Ottoman influence. The conquest 'had been achieved largely through the connivance of Itimad Khan, the leader of the kingdom's anti-Rumi faction'.[17] Itimad Khan was thereafter to seek Mughal support against the Rumi, or Ottoman, supporters. Even such auspicious sounding acts like distributing massive amounts of alms in Mecca and sending a party of nobility, including his own wife, for an over-extended residence in Mecca were actually part of a strategy to undermine Ottoman hold in the holy cities. After he promulgated the 'Decree of Infallibility' in 1579 to assert his right to be the supreme arbiter in Muslim religious issues and ordered studies on a syncretic interpretation of Islam under the rubric of Din-i Ilahi, Akbar started using titles synonymous with the Ottoman sultan, including the Padshah of Islam, which implied caliphate. He reportedly went to the extent of imparting on Abdullah Khan of the Uzbeks his desire that one day his name be read at the Friday sermons in the holy cities, a privilege accorded only to the caliphs. Naimur Farooqi notes, 'In 1582, Akbar seriously contemplated an anti-Ottoman alliance with the Portuguese. He even expressed willingness to finance a joint Mughal-Portuguese campaign against the Ottomans.'[18]

This nonetheless proved abortive for reasons not entirely clear. However, in the meantime, Akbar was coming under increasing criticism from the Muslims for his 'un-Islamic' behaviour and his totally unrealistic claims to the caliphate. Akbar was not able to maintain his ambition to challenge the Ottomans for long, given the problems he was facing on the home front, including eventually a challenge to his throne from his own son and heir.

It is true that neither the Ottomans nor the Mughals were in the mood for shaping their policies and relationships on the basis of familial, ethnic, or kinship ties. Yet, one can perhaps look at the acrimony during Akbar's reign not from the vantage point of Ottoman–Timurid rivalry alone, but also with reference to the geopolitical circumstances of the time and Akbar's calculations, ultimately faulty, about the opportunities these provided to the Mughals.

When the shipwrecked Ottoman Admiral Sidi Ali Reis landed in Gujarat and was ceremoniously escorted to Delhi, the Ottoman power was at its peak and the Mughals would also peak soon. Yet the peak of a state's power is also the beginning of its downfall, however long the latter may take. The beginning of the end for the Mughals may be found around the period paradoxically marked by the rule of an emperor who assumed the sobriquet 'Great'. For the Mughals, the downwards slide to colonization by a European power, not by Portuguese who had arrived first but by the British, may have had a direct connection to its failure to ally with the Ottoman Empire. The extant historical research is far too limited and appears far too much truncated to put Ottoman–Mughal relations accurately and comprehensively on the canvas which it deserves, namely on the canvas of geopolitical and geostrategic history of multiple basins, one of which arguably extends in one uninterrupted form from the Ottoman to the Mughal capitals. At any rate, it should not be an overstatement to argue that mid-sixteenth century marked a period that was critical for the future fortunes of the Ottoman and Mughal empires and thus of the emerging European imperial powers. The dynamics of the Indian Ocean and perhaps the factor of competition and even hostility between the two Turkish royal houses held Mughal–Ottoman relations hostage.

As Giancarlo Casale brilliantly observed, by the time Sidi Ali Reis arrived in Gujarat and before the Mughal Empire encountered the Indian Ocean for the first time in Surat in 1573, the Ottomans had already built up a vast network of power in the Indian Ocean. Although the Ottomans failed to prevent the Portuguese from building fortification in Goa and were defeated in its naval campaign to oust them at the fateful war in Diu, not the least because they could not receive food and supplies from the shore, they successfully established what Casale calls a 'soft empire' covering the full extent of the Indian Ocean. Rather than territorial conquest, this soft empire successfully built a network of trade and communication, skilfully employing religious connections extending from Zeila in Somalia to Aceh in Indonesia. Casale notes that during the mid-sixteenth century

> [t]rade flourished, with the state itself taking a leading role. Lines of communication had never been stronger, with Ottoman envoys, trade representatives, and secret agents operating throughout maritime Asia. Most important, the Ottoman dynasty's authority as caliph of the universal community of believers was recognized on a scale never equalled before or since, receiving formal expression in the Friday sermons of Muslim houses of worship from the Horn of Africa to Indonesia.[19]

Between 1517, when the Ottomans took control of Egypt and the caliphate from the Mamluk Turks, and 1579, when the legendary Grand Vizier Sokullu Mehmet Pasha was assassinated in Istanbul, the Ottoman statecraft employed soft and hard power not to seize territory but rather to enable free trade in the Indian Ocean. Far-away allies, including the rulers of Aceh and Gujarat, were supported by military resources, and individual merchants were not allowed to disrupt the free flow of goods. So successful was this policy that although by 1517 the region's 'trade-based economy was under the choke hold of Portugal's maritime blockade ... [by the 1570s] the Portuguese embargo had been brought to its knees, allowing the Ottomans to control a far larger share of the Indian Ocean spice trade than the Portuguese Crown ever had'.[20] The Ottoman statecraft failed after Sokullu Mehmed Pasha and perhaps also his successor Koca Sinan Pasha, particularly with regard to appreciating the value of the Indian Ocean connection for the economic fortunes, and thus the very survival, of the Ottoman Empire. Not that efforts, including military, were not made but they were carried out by the remaining few proponents of such emphasis on the Indian Ocean in İstanbul and involved very tentative support from the leadership in the Ottoman capital. After all, İstanbul had to think of its immediate concerns and this required a strong purse. Building strong naval fleets in the Indian Ocean was an expensive affair. Because Arabia and Egypt had no forests, timber had to be brought from the Mediterranean through a punitive logistical ordeal. The repeated plans to build a canal from Suez to the Red Sea port of Tor failed. With political support wavering, no serious enterprise could have been undertaken in the Indian Ocean. Thus, the Ottomans were pushed decisively out of the Indian Ocean. The Ottoman network's strongholds fell one by one. In 1622 Iran's Shah Abbas coalesced with the English East India Company, not yet a formidable force, cut off Basra's contact with the Indian Ocean through the Persian Gulf, and went on to occupy Baghdad. This cut off the Ottomans from the Basra outlet. Then, Portugal annihilated Aceh's navy, which had grown into a regional power by itself, six years later. By 1641, when Portugal lost Malacca to the Dutch, 'the political terrain of the entire Indian Ocean region changed completely. The principal players were now the Dutch, the English, the Safavids, and the Mughals, while the Ottomans and their old network of allies (and enemies) were fading from the picture, never to return.'[21] This might have been a remote affair, with marginal loss, given the increasingly existential threat that the Ottomans were now facing right across their borders in Europe. After all, political and military abstinence in the affairs of the Indian Ocean shielded the Ottomans from some of the local rivalries and prevented them from getting entangled in the intra-European competition and warfare raging in the waters south of the Asian landmass. Trade would continue for some time more and actually grew to a great extent by the 1580s. Yet, what the Ottoman leadership could not see or could not muster strength and concentration to counteract was a basic geopolitical precept. The loss of direct Ottoman state control and facilitation in the Indian Ocean meant losing that very trade route to other powers.

Eventually, as Ottoman merchants lost capacity and connections to those of the emerging imperial naval powers, the empire itself was stripped of essential income. The Indian Ocean connection would have been particularly essential to the Ottomans as the luscious riches of the accidentally discovered New World, America, was never within Ottoman reach. Hence, 'Inexorably, Ottoman commercial fortunes soon followed the same sinking curve, for despite the decoupling of trade and politics of the preceding decades, it was impossible for Ottoman merchants not to suffer the consequences of this comprehensive combination of political disruptions and military defeats.'[22]

However, before this story of decline unfolded, the scene at the time when Akbar took over the empire from Humayun was much different. Whether a Mughal–Ottoman alliance in the Indian Ocean was possible is a subject for further research. Yet, the detrimental effect of its absence was there for all to see. A point to make is that when opportunities present themselves and are squandered, a negative trajectory is established. Such may be the case with regard to Akbar's approach towards the Ottomans and vice versa.

The Ebbs and Tides of Diplomacy

Emperor Jahangir's coming to power created some hopes in İstanbul about a change of policy vis-à-vis the Ottomans. They sent two embassies, in 1608 and 1615, which were embarrassed and refused. The Ottomans did not realize the extent to which Jahangir may have despised them. After all, Jahangir adopted this name in place of his given name Selim because the latter reminded him of the Ottomans. He had a strong affinity for the Safavids and had a particularly cordial relationship with Shah Abbas I of Persia. Jahangir was to err gravely on this account as the Persians, in a move that came as a surprise to Mughals, attacked and captured Kandahar in 1622. Although Jahangir realized his mistake and sought an Uzbek–Ottoman–Mughal alliance, it was too late and did not materialize due to his death.

The next Mughal emperor Shah Jahan sought to remedy the mistakes made by Akbar and Jahangir, and there was an opportunity to do so. Naimur Farooqi indicates that

[h]e had two basic objectives in foreign policy: the restoration of Mughal authority over Qandahar and the conquest of his ancestral domain in Central Asia. The attainment of the former required moral, if not military, support of the Ottomans, while the pursuit of the latter was bound to strain relations with them. Shahjahan had, therefore, to play his cards carefully.[23]

The Ottomans greatly aided the rapprochement with the Mughal king by refusing to support Shah Jahan's rival Prince Baisanghur, who came for Ottoman help to İstanbul in 1632. However, despite the benign beginnings, the relationship dwindled for a decade between 1641 and 1651, due in part to bad diplomacy, but probably more owing to the Mughal capture of Kandahar and the need for Persian neutrality in Central Asian missions. Yet, Shah Jahan too was to follow in the footsteps of his father and grandfather in foreign policy fiascos. Ottoman neutrality allowed Persians to recapture Kandahar and Shah Jahan's Central Asian missions failed miserably. No longer seen as invincible and scorned in the Muslim world, Shah Jahan again fell back to seeking the goodwill of the Ottoman sultan. The Ottomans did seize the opportunity and dispatched an ambassador who was well received in India. Shah Jahan returned the favour by sending his own emissary to İstanbul in 1653. Records show additional exchanges of embassies. A recurrent theme, however, was Shah Jahan's 'acerbity and over-sensitiveness, at minor discourtesies of diction in the Ottoman imperial epistles'.[24] Despite the Ottomans' sincere wish to befriend the Mughals, fixations on the niceties of diplomatic correspondence on the part of Emperor Shah Jahan did not help develop the practical cooperation that was much needed by the Muslim rulers both in India and Ottoman Turkey. The course of history, thus, took a negative turn as India and the Ottomans came under the suffocating pressure of European imperial powers.

The initial Ottoman reaction to Shah Jahan's deposition by his son Aurangzeb was negative. The Ottomans did not send an ambassador to Aurangzeb until 1689. At the time, the Ottoman economy was in decline and a bad crop was causing starvation in parts of the empire. Militarily, they were weakened and were losing against the Austrians in the western Balkans. The Ottoman envoy's letter from the sultan apprised Aurangzeb 'about the conspiracy of the Christian powers to ravage the lands of Islam' and 'recounted the efforts he had made to repel the invaders and to protect the life and property of the Muslims', while pleading to remain united in the effort to annihilate the enemies of the faith.[25] Aurangzeb did not feel the need to engage further with the Ottomans, probably driven by the diminishing threat from Persia and the failure of the Ottomans to extend congratulations or even recognition to his rule for long. Thus, the Ottoman–Mughal relations again did not see any rapprochement. For all his emphasis on religion, Aurangzeb died isolated from the Muslim world. The same atmosphere prevailed also during the reign of Bahadur Shah and Jahandar Shah.

The thawing of the ice had to wait until 1713 when Farrukbsiyar took over the Peacock Throne in a contentious manner and reached out to break Mughal isolation in the Muslim world, including the most powerful among them—the Ottomans. Although devoid of content and frequency, communications were re-established between İstanbul and Shahjahanabad. Muhammad Shah would further develop the relationship and received a positive response from Sultan and Caliph Mahmud I. The Ottoman sultan even admonished the Nizam of Deccan to remain loyal to the Mughal emperor. The Ottoman sultan also ignored a proposal from the Nizam in Hyderabad to jointly invade Persia. The relationship was, however, again to suffer after the death of Muhammad Shah. The study by Naimur Rahman Farooqi notes that '[i]n the 110 years (1748–1857) that the Mughal Empire survived after Muhammad Shah, though in a mutilated and truncated form, there is no record of any exchange of embassies between the courts of Shahjahanabad and Istanbul'.[26]

The Triangular Relationship between Turkey, Britain, and India

It must be noted that the absence of relations and correspondence between the Mughal and Ottoman rulers did not mean that there was no such interaction between the rest of the Muslim dynasties in India. South Indian and Ottoman Muslims were in close communication, to such extent that diplomatic relations were also established. These included the Nizams of Deccan, the Bibi of Cannanore in Malabar, and Tipu Sultan of Mysore. All recognized the caliphate of the Ottomans and sought practical cooperation and cordial ties. By this time, the British had already been occupying the subcontinent and the correspondence included pleas for alliance and assistance against the British. The Ottomans could not entertain these pleas and instead advised the Indians to petition the British representatives to correct their wrongs in India.

A closer look at the case of Tipu Sultan may be warranted. Feth Ali, also known as Tipu Sultan of Mysore, inherited from his father, Haidar Ali, in 1782 an alliance with the French but proceeded to sign a treaty in Mangalore with the British next year. Mysore's invasion of Travancore and its tense relationship with Hyderabad and the Marathas brought Tipu Sultan and the British on a collision course. Upon instigation by the British, the Mughal emperor also declined to endorse Tipu's title as the sultan of Mysore. Even after the signing of the Versailles Peace Treaty between Britain and France, London suspected Tipu's intentions, given his dynasty's amity with the French. Against this background, Tipu Sultan sought the endorsement of the Ottomans for his claim to sultanhood in place of the Mughals. He, thus, dispatched an embassy to İstanbul, which left Seringapatam in November 1785 and reached İstanbul almost two years later in September 1787. The Mysore embassy delivered letters to the Ottoman Padishah Abdulhamid I and his Grand Vizier, which contained an extended eulogy to the caliph of the Muslims. The letters detailed forced conversions and oppression at the hands of the Christians and promoted Tipu's role as the defender of the faith in India. He appealed for assistance from the caliph to help mobilize the Indian Muslims against Britain. His specific proposals included exchanging port facilities in Iraq in return for the same in Malabar, building a water canal in the Shiite holy city of Necef in Iraq, and trade relations between the subjects of the two rulers. He also asked for technical help in manufacturing weaponry, paper, and glass in Mysore.

Sultan Abdulhamid I's response politely prevaricated on these requests, complained about the Russians, and advised Tipu to refrain from acting against the British. The French invasion of Egypt in 1798 honed the alliance between the British and the Ottomans, while Tipu was closing in an alliance with the French against the British. Another round of letters were exchanged between Tipu and the newly enthroned Selim III, which again saw the Ottomans suggesting Tipu to desist from siding with the French against the British. The last Ottoman letter, however, would come too late as by the time it arrived in India, Tipu Sultan was already killed fighting the British, not heeding the advice from İstanbul. However, these correspondences clearly revealed the sentiment of siege on the part of the Muslims in India and Turkey, although perceptions at the time differed as to who was the arch enemy of the Muslims. In the words of Kemal Karpat, 'Tipu was the first Muslim ruler in modern times to reach beyond the borders of his realm, actively seeking broader Muslim political alliances against the "enemies of Islam"—that is, England and France—only to realize that other Muslims regarded these "enemies" as friends, at various times and under certain circumstances and differing views of the interests of Islam.'[27]

The Mughal Empire could not resist the British rule and finally yielded in 1857. The Ottomans continued for another 65 years, albeit in constant decline. As their power over their own territories dimmed gradually and painfully, the Muslims of India and Turkey began to share a comparable feeling of loss. Yet, the Ottomans and the Indian Muslims again had different enemy designations, which obviated any practical alliance. The relationship between the Ottomans and the British were influenced by an altogether different vantage point. Ram Lakhan Shukla in his study entitled *Britain, India and the Turkish Empire*[28] and Raj Kumar Trivedi in *The Critical Triangle: India, Britain and Turkey*[29] set out in great detail the British perceptions and policies in this triangular relationship, which lasted all the way to the proclamation of the Republic of Turkey in 1923 and the abolishment of the caliphate in 1924, albeit in different forms, direction, and content. The Ottomans saw an opportunity in the British hostility against the Russians who were staunchly inclined to bring about the downfall of the Ottoman Empire and descend to the warm waters of the Mediterranean Sea. This cooperation between the British and Ottoman empires benefited the two in numerous instances not the least during the 1856 Crimean War, which the Ottomans successfully fought alongside the British against the Russians. The British, in turn, leveraged their influence in İstanbul to calm the restive Indian Muslims.

As the geopolitical competition between European empires was quickly dressed with religious décor against the Muslims, the Europeans' anti-Turkish and anti-Muslim propaganda only aggravated the Muslims of India. After the Mughals were gone, İstanbul became the sole beacon for Indian Muslims to turn to. Embittered by its own tragic experience with British domination, India set its gaze on the Ottoman struggle for survival against the Christian empires.

The British Empire, in turn, had a particularly unique vantage point into the Indian–Turkish relations. Their policies vis-à-vis the Ottomans were strongly influenced by the awareness of this strong popular connection, especially among the Muslim populations. As Kemal Karpat wrote, 'Apparently, the British were the first to see the caliphate as the potential center that could not only mobilize and unite Muslims—and induce them to fight for England but also soothe some Indian Muslims, who perceived London to be the enemy of Islam.'[30] What appears as a lasting pattern, however, is that Indians and Turks were united at heart but divided in geopolitics throughout the Mughal centuries. There were numerous instances in which the geopolitics also converged, but the lack of frequent and regular contacts constantly undermined formation of practical cooperation against the enemies of the time. The Ottomans and the Indians never sat down to elaborate the potential of an alliance, which could have been infinitely useful to both, though we will never know the full extent of this potential. Notwithstanding all these failures of diplomacy and statesmanship, interest remained. The interactions outside the diplomatic and strategic realm produced unintended consequences—such as the adoption of Ottoman military techniques by Babar, or the Sufi interaction across state boundaries. Religion played a role in drawing Turkish and Indian Muslims closer.

The letter by Tipu Sultan of Mysore to Sultan Abdulhamid I in 1785, which had already proposed an alliance, is only one case in point. Kemal Karpat also notes that the letters by Tipu thus suggested the initial strands of pan-Islamism, the potential of which was unbeknownst to the Ottoman sultan at the time: 'Tipu, his personal political motives notwithstanding, proposed something truly revolutionary: namely, to turn the caliphate into the real political center of Islam and use it to oppose European encroachment.'[31]

The issue of recognition of the caliphate did haunt the relationship between the Mughals and the Ottomans. Some Mughal leaders recognized the Ottoman caliphate, some did not. The Ottoman sultans' claim to the caliphate was not contested in the majority of Muslim lands. The Sharifs of Mecca addressed the Ottoman rulers as the Khalifa or the Messenger of God. The Ottomans were also revered by the leaders of the Uzbeks, the Khans of Crimea, the sultans of Sumatra, and other chieftains in Southeast Asia. Two rulers of Persia recognized the Ottoman caliphate, particularly the Afghan dynasty in Persia. Thus, Shah Ashraf allowed the *khutba* in the mosques to be read in the Ottoman sultans' name in 1727. Nadir Shah also acknowledged the caliphate of the Ottoman sultan. The ruler of the Kashgars issued coins in the name of the Ottoman Sultan in the nineteenth century. The list is extensive. The Mughals, however, until late granted no such recognition and were, in fact, isolated to a large degree in the Muslim lands. The Mughal claim to universal caliphate may have been beyond their reach, yet that nonetheless should have created a dilemma for their Muslim subjects who would be seen as disloyal to their Mughal rulers if they had accepted the Ottoman sultan as the legitimate caliph of the Muslim believers worldwide. That said, coalition among Muslim rulers and peoples was by no means a new idea. It stood at the very core of the Islamic *ummah*, which regarded all Muslims everywhere as belonging to one single nation. While Karpat's thesis on the revolutionary nature of the idea of pan-Islamism may be rather exaggerated, it seems correct in the sense that by the late eighteenth century, there was no Mughal or other power to contest the Ottoman sultan for his title of the universal caliph. The Muslims of India, thus, could accept the Ottoman sultans as their caliph without having to worry about disloyalty to a Mughal ruler.

The Ottomans could not help Tipu Sultan, and, in fact, recommended that he reconcile with the British authorities because of the latter's essential support to the Ottomans against the mounting military pressure of the European powers. However, the Muslim sensitivities in India were irrecoverably in support of the Ottoman Turks and this became a significant factor in how the British Empire came to regard the Ottoman decline. The British feared that decisive Russian advances against the Ottomans brought about the risk of the fulfilment of the Russian dreams of descending on the Turkish shores in the Mediterranean and thereby threatening the connection between Britain proper and their lucrative Indian colony. The French invasion of Algeria in 1830 was another consideration for the British due to the risk this posed to British–Indian communication routes. It was against the background of Russian and French activities in West Asia and North Africa that British preoccupation with sustaining the Ottomans took shape, particularly since the 1830s. The most conspicuous trigger was the Treaty of Hünkar İskelesi of 1833 by which the Russians obtained the permission to dock war ships in İstanbul after the Russians helped the Ottomans to defeat the Egyptian forces, led by Muhammad Ali, which successfully fought against the Ottomans who had developed an ambition to topple the weakening Ottoman dynasty and take over their possessions in Arabia. Before his declaration of secession from the Ottoman Empire in 1838, however, Muhammad Ali's initial starting point in 1832 was to punish the Ottoman refusal to grant his demands, following his decisive support in the war against the Greeks. Facing an assault from Mohammad Ali, the Ottomans first appealed to Britain and France, which were to decline, and subsequently the Russians sent ships and soldiers to İstanbul in support of the Ottoman sultan in 1833. The British, who first failed to appreciate the full import of leaving the stage to the Russians by not aiding the Ottomans themselves, quickly came to question their policy. The analysis by the British Ambassador in İstanbul in 1832 that linked India and Turkey and recommended Britain to consider the two as interrelated had gone unheeded. However, after the Russians landed in İstanbul, thinking in London quickly changed. The British were also apprehensive of the designs of Muhammad Ali in Egypt and saw a potential for Egypt to collaborate with the Russians in Persia after he strengthened his hold in Arabia. If Russia and Egypt divided up Persia, not only the Russians but also an Islamic ruler could physically threaten India. An influential member of the

Board of Control postulated that a 'vigorous state established at the Persian Gulf might form a Mohammedan League comprising all the Muslim rulers of Central Asia for driving out a Christian government from India'.[32] Therefore, in order to safeguard Indian interests, the Ottomans had to be strengthened to check the reach of Mohammad Ali's Egypt. The British Prime Minister Lord Palmerston thus announced the new British policy to the House of Commons on 11 July 1833:

> If Russian conquest should lead to the Christianising and civilising of the inhabitants of that country, these advantages ... would be counterbalanced by the consequences that would result to Europe from the dismemberment of the Turkish empire. I say, then, that undoubtedly government would feel it to be their duty to resist to the utmost any attempt on the part of Russia to partition the Turkish empire; and, if it had been necessary, we should equally have felt it our duty to interfere and prevent the pasha of Egypt from dismembering any portion of the dominions of the sultan. The integrity and independence of the Ottoman empire are necessary to the maintenance of the tranquillity, the liberty and the balance of power in the rest of Europe.[33]

Thus, when the pasha in Cairo and the sultan in İstanbul came to blows again in 1839, Britain would not stand idle in favour of the Russians but rather intervene to support the Ottomans. This British policy was to remain intact until the last quarter of the nineteenth century.

As Lord Palmerston's speech to the Parliament also underscored, the perception of Britain was not divorced of religious zeal, yet, at least, in the early nineteenth century, it was overwhelmed by the geopolitical considerations with regard to the threat it perceived from its rival Russia against its interests in India.

The Crimean War was an important milestone in European imperial history in several aspects. Obviously, the whole affair needs to be cast in the context of the Ottoman decline and the competition among the European powers. However, the immediate reason for the war appeared elsewhere, ironically in another competition that predated the Ottomans. European history is laden with long and bloody religious fights among different denominations. In this respect, the Crimean War was yet another chapter of this history. In this case, it was the competition between the Eastern Orthodox and Roman Catholic churches over the control of the Christian holy sites. The Ottomans had granted the authority over the churches in Jerusalem, Nazareth, and Bethlehem to the Roman Catholic Church. As of 1740, the Roman Catholic monks assumed protection of the holy places. However, the increase in the numbers of the Orthodox as against the Catholics provided for an opportunity for the Russian Tsar Nicholas I to stoke further resentment among the two churches, which resulted in riots between their members. When the Turks entrusted the keys to the Church of Nativity to the Roman Catholics, the Russians sent a mission to Istanbul to threaten the Ottomans. The Ottomans rejected the Russian demands to not only surrender authority over the holy places to the Orthodox but also accept Russia's protectorate over the entire Eastern Orthodox communities in the Ottoman Empire. The British Ambassador in Istanbul, who was to be appointed to St. Petersburg but was refused by the Russians, also appears to have gone out of his way to reassure the Ottomans against the Russian demands. In the war that followed the Russian attack, Britain, France, and Sardinia-Piedmont joined with the Ottomans to defeat the Russians. Austria–Hungary also threatened to join the Ottoman side. The importance of the war for European history was particularly pertinent for the fate of Austria–Hungary, which lost the support of Russia, but also for allowing, as a result of eventual Austrian weakening, the eventual unification of Italy and Germany. The war was beset by rampant epidemics, somewhat heralding those that would claim countless lives during the later Balkan Wars, which the Indian Medical Mission meant initially to help address.

However, apart from its place in European history, the Crimean War was closely followed in India. While the interest was not confined to the Indian Muslims, it was particularly them who circulated heated pamphlets throughout India. The Muslims of India were much content that Britain sided with the Turks and the caliph of the Muslims in Istanbul. Particularly those in the North-West Province were highly excited about the war.

But there appears to be another factor in play in India before and during the Crimean War. About this time, the resentment about the British was mounting in India. The British authorities in India were reportedly concerned before the war about the strength of the British hold in India and were sending warnings to London about the Russian intrigues on the margins of the subcontinent. As the Russian military displayed tenacity during the war, there was widespread anticipation among the Indians about the weakness of Britain and their salvation by the Russians. Some appeared to prefer Russia to Britain, others panicked and in Bombay and Calcutta, some Indians hid their valuables in anticipation of a Russian invasion or at least collapse of British supremacy in India. As Shukla reports, 'During the war most preposterous stories were circulated in the bazaars of India as to the power of Russia and the impending downfall of the British raj. The rumour spread that Russia had conquered even England, and that Queen Victoria had fled and was coming to take refuge with the governor-general of India.'[34] The British officials came to dread the collapse of the sense of Britain's supremacy and invincibility, and saw a need to score an overwhelming victory in the Crimean War. Several British officials suggested the employment of Indian troops in the Crimean War, which the precariousness of the situation in India did not permit. Indian youths would have died in large numbers under the imperial orders of an alien power for a cause that was neither theirs to judge nor to partake in a faraway land. Such a tragedy was averted in the Crimean War, although two regiments, the 10th Hussars and 12th Lancers, did end up in Crimea. Though I am not aware of there being any Indians in these two regiments, Indian losses would become inevitable in the First World War, again under imperial orders.

Ironically, despite the rampant rumours in India of Russian power, after the Russians lost the war in 1856, Tsar Alexander II, who succeeded Nicholas I during the war, was to conclude that Russia needed further modernization to match European armies. And in India, Russian defeat reinforced the perception of the invincibility of the British Empire.

During the Crimean War, British authorities became convinced of the utility of a new instrument that would ensue from the Ottoman gratitude for their support against the Russians. They sought to posit the Ottoman caliph on their side to quell the restive

Indian Muslims, growing inexorably rebellious against their hold in India. The British concern about the mood of the Indians against them was to prove correct in 1857. The mutiny started in Meerut after the rumours that the Enfield rifles used cartridges, of which the *sipahi*s (sepoys or soldiers) had to bite off the ends, were lubricated by a mixture of pig and cow lard. The insult thus perceived brought the Hindu and Muslim anger together against the British. When the sipahis who refused to use the cartridges were shackled and jailed, fellow soldiers rebelled and shot their British officers. Quickly spreading to Delhi, Agra, Kanpur, and Lucknow, the rebellion manifested the explosion of long-contained indignation against the social and religious transformation introduced by the British rule. The religious conversions promoted by the zealous work of the Christian missionaries and ostensibly aided by the British rulers were afflicting both Hindu and Muslim communities. John Kay, in his history of the 1857 rebellion, refers to the 'sensitive state' of the Indian population owing to the threat on their faith, thus recounting:

> Nor was this purely a creation of the Native mind, an unaided conception of the Priests or the People; for the missionaries themselves had pleaded the recent material progress of the English as an argument in favour of the adoption by the inhabitants of India of one universal religion. 'The time appears to have come', they said in an Address which was extensively circulated in Bengal during the closing years of Lord Dalhousie's administration, 'when earnest consideration should be given to the question, whether or not all men should embrace the same system of religion. Railways, Steam-vessels, and the Electric Telegraph are rapidly uniting all the nations of the earth. The more they are brought together, the more certain does the conclusion become that all have the same wants, the same anxieties, and the same sorrows'; and so on, with manifest endeavour to prove that European civilization was the forerunner of an inevitable absorption of all other faiths into the one faith of the White Ruler.[35]

In Delhi, the mutineers reinstated Bahadur Shah II to the Mughal throne. Yet, he was nowhere close to either leading the revolution or quelling it. Northern India fell in the grip of a vicious cycle of violence. The British reaction was even more ferocious than the mutineers could ever achieve, with some British officers protesting the bloodshed inflicted by modern weaponry.

The British forces prevailed, aided by the fact that most of the Indian princes did not join the rebellion. A massive reorganization of the army and governance followed, including the transfer of nominal power from the East India Company to direct rule by the British Empire. Reforms engendered greater Indian participation in the affairs of the state or at least better communication between the rulers and the ruled. Yet the Muslims of India were almost totally uprooted. The 1857–8 rebellion erased all designs to resurrect the past order in India and culminated in the development of a native Indian nationalism. The British win in 1858 proved to be only a mid-point on the road to Indian independence after the Second World War.

The 1857 revolt was a joint Hindu–Muslim rebellion. John Kay summarized the joint grievances which later scholarship widely endorsed:

> The real cause of the mutiny may be expressed in a condensed form in two words—bad faith. It was bad faith to our Sipahis which made their minds prone to suspicion; it was our policy of annexation, of refusing to Hindu chiefs the permission to adopt, with them, a necessary religious rite; of suddenly bringing a whole people under the operation of complex rules to which they were unaccustomed, as in Oudh, in the Sagar and Narbada territory, and in Bundelkhand, and our breaches of customs more sacred to the natives than laws, which roused the large landowners and the rural population against the British rule. This was my opinion then, and it is, if possible, more strongly my opinion now.[36]

However, the British authorities chose to put the blame almost entirely on the Muslims. A reading from the court diary of 16 May 1857 is as follows:

> If we now take a retrospective view of the various circumstances which we have been able to elicit during our extended inquiries, we shall perceive how exclusively Muhammadan are all the prominent

points that attach to it ... Hinduism, I may say, is nowhere either reflected or represented; if it be brought forward at all, it is only in subservience to its ever-aggressive neighbour.[37]

The Court found in 1858 'prisoner Muhammad Bahadur Shah, ex-King of Delhi, is guilty of all and every part of the charges preferred against him'.[38] In the wake of the rebellion, Muslims overall suffered a wave of vengeance by the British authorities. Countless Indian Muslims lost their lives, lands, or status. The Muslim *ulema* were particularly targeted. Several were killed, some had to flee the country.[39] The blow on the Muslims was severe, leaving them distraught in their own country.

One instrument that the British seemingly wielded against the mutineers was the authority of the Ottoman caliph. Indian and British sources refer, including with reference to eye witness accounts, to an 1857 condemnation by the Ottoman sultan for the killings perpetrated by the mutineers and appeal to Muslims to remain loyal to the British.[40] To that effect, an *iradeh* was obtained from the sultan by the British and read in mosques around India. Salah Jang of Hyderabad maintained that this iradeh had proven very effectual and, in fact, played a major role in the ability of the British to defeat the mutiny. Turkish historian Azmi Özcan, however, observed in 1995 that no record of that iradeh from the sultan was discovered at the Ottoman archives. He, nonetheless, concurred that subsequent actions of the sultan corroborated the sultan's disposition towards the British authorities during and immediately after the ill-fated first war of liberation in India. This included granting British troops safe passage from Ottoman ports in Egypt.[41] The Ottomans were, after all, much beholden towards the British for their support against Russia in the Crimean War and the British were naturally eager to capitalize on that debt. Even after the 1857 revolt, the Ottoman sultan continued to intervene to quell the Muslim reaction against the British Raj. The gratitude of the British and the utility they saw in keeping the Ottoman caliph on their side was manifest also in the visit of Sultan Abdülaziz to London in July 1867. The British hosts had made spectacular preparations, but heavy storms resulted in the cancellation of many events. The entire expenses of the visit were met by the India Office to help 'propitiate Indian Muslims'.[42]

However, the Sublime Porte in İstanbul appears to have had little or filtered information about the full nature and scale of the events that unfolded in India during the 1857–8 rebellion. As Azmi Özcan underscores, the Ottoman government had two main arteries of information regarding the rebellion: the British Embassy in İstanbul and the Ottoman Embassy in London. The Ottoman consulates in Bombay and Calcutta were operational since 1849, but the distance, and one can only speculate as to what else, presumably prevented timely dispatch of information from these missions to İstanbul.[43] Sultan Abdulmecid, for instance, is on record stating to the British Ambassador in İstanbul in 1857 that no such assistance would have been rendered should the British have attempted to replace Islam with Christianity in India. This statement may be seen to confirm lack of information in İstanbul about the grievances suffered by the Muslims in India in the run-up to the rebellion.

The reading of the khutbas in Friday prayers in the name of the Ottoman caliph had begun already, following the passing away of Shah Alam II in 1806.[44] However, the Crimean War marked a watershed in Indian Muslims' sympathies towards the Ottoman caliph and their concern for the fate of the Ottoman Empire. The sympathy eventually broadened to the Hindus as well: 'Both the Hindus and Muslims were united in expressing their sympathy for Turkey, much to the surprise of Anglo-Indian observers. It was maintained by the non-sectarian or "Hindu" newspapers that their sympathies for Turkey were because of its being an Asian power.'[45]

Indian Muslims are Pulled in Two Directions

Indian and Turkish destinies were increasingly regarded as intertwined. Indian newspapers began to cover the events in Turkey like never before. Particularly around the 1877–8 Russo-Turkish War, India experienced an ocean of attention, solidarity, and indeed action in support of the Turks. Public rallies demanded British support for the Turks. Funds were collected through various associations (*anjuman* and *mejlis*), and even individuals travelled to Turkey to fight against the Russians. The pro-Turkish zeal and fund-raising was alive throughout the country, whether in Delhi, Calcutta, Bombay, Madras, Hyderabad, Lahore,

Amritsar, Aligarh, or Lucknow. Gladstone and Salisbury's tatty remarks about Turkey only aggravated the Indians, Muslim and Hindu alike. Azmi Özcan notes that religious schools also joined the effort to aid the Ottomans, most notably the Dar'ul Ulum Deoband. Thus, '[t]he Ottoman documents often referred to the efforts of *mouhk* Muhammed Qasim (1833–77), Muhammed Refi ud-Din, Muhammed Yaqub (d. 1886), and Muhammed Abid among the teachers (mudarrisun) of the Daru'l-Ulum Deoband'.[46]

The 1877–8 war began when the Russian and Serbian armies assaulted Turkey crossing the Danube in July on the pretext of assisting Bosnia–Herzegovina and Bulgaria in their rebellions against the Ottoman rule. The background of the war was naturally the continuing Ottoman decline, which vetted the appetite of the Russian and other imperial powers of the day. Having suffered a setback in the 1854–6 war, Russians were intent on cannibalizing the weakening Ottoman Empire. The Russians had used the intervening time well in terms of military preparations and they were initially successful in their campaign in Bulgaria. However, they were soon to confront a determined Osman Nuri Pasha in Plevne, who successfully fended off three attacks, only to surrender in the fourth when he personally suffered a wound. The heroics of Ghazi Osman Pasha and his soldiers did not suffice to halt the Russian advance to Edirne, which also fell by January 1878. Russians were to stop only at the outskirts of İstanbul. The ensuing Treaty of San Stefano in March 1878 guaranteed the independence of Romania, Serbia, and Montenegro while extending autonomy to Bosnia–Herzegovina and an oversized Bulgaria under the protection of the Russian Tsar. Britain and Austria–Hungary had remained neutral during the war. However, the Russian gains prompted them to intervene diplomatically. A diplomatic conference in Berlin in July forced Russians and Bulgarians to yet again yield some of their war bounty.

The neutral stance of Britain created a somewhat heated debate in the British Empire. A severe disagreement emerged between the viceroy in India and his political masters in London. Against the advice of Lord Lytton, the powerful secretary of state for India at the time, Lord Salisbury, who was later to become foreign secretary and prime minister, insisted that the Ottomans were too weak to continue aiding. Although the period saw a detailed and, in

People's Mission to the Ottoman Empire

a way, much intriguing analysis of the British, Russian, Ottoman, and Indian geopolitics, a particular point brought into the debate by Viceroy Lord Lytton pertained to the loyalties of the Indian Muslims. As we read from Trivedi, Lord Lytton wrote to London, stating in unequivocal, even alarming, terms his opposition to British neutrality in the war: 'It is my strong impression that, at the present moment, the lives of all your officers and European subjects in India mainly depend on the course of your Eastern policy and its freedom from all appearance of subserviency to Russia.'[47] However, Lord Salisbury retorted in no less equivocation: 'It is somewhat startling to have our foreign policy in Europe prescribed to us by the people whom we conquered in the East.'[48] Thus, the memorials dispatched to the Queen urging British assistance to the Ottomans had no effect on the British policy. This was the time when Queen Victoria assumed the title of Empress of India concurrent with Empress of the British Empire, thereby turning Britain into a dual monarchy of sorts. In London the British ascendancy was undoubted, the success and virtues of its imperialism unquestioned.

The British thus went in a different direction, partaking in the feast over the Ottoman possessions. The Great Game over the territories and kingdoms that lay between the Balkans and India further intensified in West Asia and Afghanistan. In David Fromkin's words: 'Sometimes as a cold war, sometimes as a hot one, the struggle between Britain and Russia raged from the Dardanelles to the Himalayas for almost a hundred years.'[49]

While London decided to change direction and moved away from supporting the Ottomans, later developments would vindicate Lord Lytton's advice on the need to allay Muslim concerns in India towards Turkey. The loss of the Ottoman ally was perhaps a policy blunder that would create difficulties for the British Empire. Even during the First World War, the Indian office would send stark warnings not to appear hostile to the Turks.[50] After the 1877–8 Russo-Turkish War, the Indian Muslims, and indeed the whole of India, were to embark on a one-way journey away from the British rule, although independence would only come after the British resources were depleted in the two world wars. The origins of the pan-Islamist and pro-independence Khilafat Movement in

India that grew after the First World War in a bush fire had its roots in this divergence.[51] The British change of heart was long in effect before, but 1878 became the representative date when the Ottomans and the British were to increasingly part ways, which brought the Ottomans more and more in tandem with the Germans, now unified and gathering strength but coming in rather late to the imperial 'chessboard' in Eurasia, to quote a famous dictum by Lord Curzon. With the Ottomans no longer obliged to mitigate Indian Muslims' reaction to British rule, they intensified their pan-Islamism under Sultan Abdulhamid II.

Sultan Abdulhamid II remains a highly contentious figure in Ottoman historiography. While the debate is extensive, two points need to be kept in mind when judging the sultan with the benefit of hindsight. Pan-Islamism in Abdulhamid's time was not a matter of course or result of the personal piety of a devout ruler. His views and policies were the product of a particular political context. Firstly, in the intellectual sphere he was under the influence of a rising intellectual current in the Muslim world. As Turkish historian Niyazi Berkes argued with reference to the discourses about unity and regeneration of Islam starting around 1872:

> In these, the nature of the unity was clear only with regard to those Muslims under the rule of the caliph; it meant political unity. Opinions varied on the nature of the unity which was to embrace all Muslims. On the whole, however, the caliph began to appear as the actual or potential ruler of Muslims everywhere. The caliphate was not merely a spiritual power; it was a state. Islam was not merely a religion; it was a nationality, a political community, a civilization. The cause of decline was not only the loss of unity but also the penetration of secular ideas from the outside world. Hamidian pan-Islamism was the child of this trend and not the invention of the monarch.[52]

Secondly, the sultan took action in a particular political and geopolitical context. As such the Hamidian pan-Islamism was a desperate political project to find a lifeline in a senescent state, isolated and cannibalized in its own environment. It is a fact that Sultan Abdulhamid II ascended to the throne at an extremely precarious

time frame when the Ottoman Empire was in an inexorable preci-
pice towards dissolution. Several Ottoman rulers had attempted
to enact reforms to stem the tide but the geopolitics of the time
would not allow the empire either time or room to see these efforts
through. The geographic location of the empire, at the crossroads
of key geostrategic connections, and its close proximity to the rising powers of the age engendered centuries of incessant wars. The
idea of Ottomanism was tried in order to bind the multi-ethnic
and multi-religious polity together in a contractual identity with
no avail. Modernization in terms of Westernization did not reap
any decisive benefits in terms of stemming the tide. The ideas
of the French Revolution reverberated among the subjects of the
empire, distorted irrevocably by religious bigotry and usurpation.
Pan-Slavism, pan-Orthodoxy, and even pan-Germanism had its
toll on the tenets of this particular polity with fatal effects. Having
been stripped of a transcendent contract with all its subjects, the
search of the Ottoman intellectuals for political glue culminated in
the ascendancy of the policy of Islamic unity. As the sultan himself
wrote in his political memoirs: '[U]nity of faith brings us together
as individual members of one large family. Therefore, the stress
must not be on the Ottoman Empire; instead there is benefit in particularly asserting that we are all Muslims. Always and everywhere
the title of Emir-ul-Muslimin [Leader of the Muslims] should come
first and Ottoman Padshah [sultan] be uttered second'.[53]

During Abdulhamid II's reign, with the influential support of
Jamaluddin Afghani and others, Ottomans made an effort to bridge
also the Sunni–Shia divide to engender a pan-Islamic unity. The
famous analogy made by Jamaluddin Afghani, about the ship of
Muslims caught in a storm needing the joint efforts of all on board
despite their differences, resonated well with the Ottoman and
Muslim circumstances.

Abdulhamid's pan-Islamism involved what in today's terminology would have been called robust public diplomacy in Muslim
lands. Ottomans reached out effectively to Muslims outside their
empire and İstanbul quickly became a point of attraction for a
diversity of Muslim thinkers and scholars. The Sufis were particularly welcome, given their direct influence among the people.
Özcan recounts that the sultan personally extended invitations

to influential Muslim figures and treated them well, presenting Islamic textbooks 'as gifts from the Caliph to educational institutions in various Muslim countries'.[54] The Sufi orders including the Shazeli and Rufai sent their disciples to propagate in favour of the Ottoman sultan, the caliph of the Muslims. Abdulhamid II also issued a proclamation to employ Indian Muslims in matters related to Muslim holy places, thereby extending his political reach in practical terms to lands outside his control.

The Indian Muslims overall revered Sultan Abdulhamid II as the leader of the Muslims in the world, including in India. The sultan had been closely following India and had even predicted that 'millions of Indians' when they decided to rid their country of a few thousand Englishmen, could do it rather easily.[55] In his memoirs, Sultan Abdulhamid uses rather exaggerated language on his influence in India, stating that 'everyone knows that one word by the Caliph of the Muslims, Me, would be enough to bring detriment to the English yoke in India'.[56] However, he was not altogether off the mark in his analysis of the strength of the pan-Islamic and anti-British fervour in India at the time. Despite a minority of pro-British Muslims, the reign of Sultan Abdulhamid II between 1876 and 1909 coincided with a frenzy of pan-Islamism that followed the ongoing cannibalization of the Ottoman realm with great disdain.

Where ethnic commonalities and geopolitical interests failed, it was the idea of Islamic solidarity that would bind Indian and Turkish Muslims with a force to reckon with.

Notes

1. Sidi Ali Reis, *Mirat ul Memalik* (*The Mirror of Countries*), available at http://www.fordham.edu/halsall/source/16csidi1.asp (accessed on 5 January 2013).

2. In our day and age, a differentiation is made between the Turks and the Turkic peoples. 'Turk' is used in reference to the dominant ethnicity of the Republic of Turkey. Turkic, on the other hand, is broadly used for the entire family of ethnicities who share not only language roots but also certain historical backgrounds and cultural traits. In addition to the Turks of Turkey, this ethno-linguistic family includes the Azerbaijani,

Kazak, Kyrgiz, Tatar, Turkmen, Uigur, Uzbek, Qashqai, Gagauz, Bashkir, Yakut, Karait, Kyrmchak, Karakalpak, Balkar, Magyar, Bulgar, Nogai, and Chuvash peoples. They have been known as Ottomans, Seldjuks, Mamlukes, Timurids, Khiljis, Avars, Göktürks, Khazars, and so on. The differentiation between Turkish and Turkic is tentative and not entirely grounded given the diversity of the groups that together form the Turkish world. As Carter Vaughn Findley noted in *The Turks in World History*, the emergence of the distinction has a 'guilty history' going back to the desire of the Russian imperialists to differentiate between Turks in the Ottoman Empire and the Turks under their rule. However, the differentiation between Turkish and Turkic comes handy in steering clear of political implications including association with pan-Turkish or Turanian ideology. Nonetheless, since no such ideological context exists here, in this book no care will be given to being politically correct. And in order to avoid ethnic indecision, this manuscript will not try to differentiate between the Turk and Turkic, calling them all Turks or Turkish. Obviously, the reader would understand that Turkish invasions of the subcontinent did not in any period originate from what is now Turkey but rather from Central Asia. Yet, those who settled in India, including the Timurid rulers, shared the ethnic background of the Turks that migrated to the west in modern Turkey. However, all Turkish groups intermarried and were overall influenced by the peoples they came to live with, including in India, changing their traits, while their languages also differentiated over the centuries.

3. M. Longworth Dames, 'The Portuguese and Turks in the Indian Ocean in the Sixteenth Century', *Journal of the Royal Asiatic Society of Great Britain and Ireland*, no. 1 (January 1921), pp. 3–4.

4. Annemarie Schimmel, *The Empire of the Great Mughals: History, Art and Culture* (London: Reaktion Books, 2004), p. 233.

5. K. C. D. Brahaspati, 'Muslim Influences on Venkatamakhi', in G. Kuppuswamy and M. Hariharan, eds, *Readings on Music and Dance* (Trivandarum: B. R. Publishing Corporation, 1979), p. 112.

6. Emmie Te Nijenhuis, *Indian Music: History, Structure* (Leiden, Köln: Brill, 1974), p. 7.

7. For a detailed rendering of this common heritage, see Mansoura Haidar, *Turco-Indian Architecture* (İstanbul: Archaeology and Art Publications, 2010).

8. M. J. Akbar, *The Shade of Swords: Jihad and the Conflict between Islam and Christianity* (New Delhi: Lotus Roli, 2006), p. 137.

9. Zahiru'd-din Muhammad Babur Padshah Ghazi, *The Babur-Nama in English (Memoirs of Babur)*, translation from the original Turki by Annette Susannah Beveridge, vol. 1 (London: Luzac and Co, 1922), p. 381.

10. A. K. Nizami, 'Foreword' in Naimur Rahman Farooqi, *Mughal–Ottoman Relations: A Study of Political and Diplomatic Relations between Mughal India and the Ottoman Empire, 1556–1748* (Delhi: Idarah-I Adabiyat-I Delli, 2009), p. xiii.

11. Farooqi, *Mughal–Ottoman Relations*, p. 20.

12. Farooqi, *Mughal–Ottoman Relations*, p. 20.

13. Lisa Balabanlilar, 'The Begims of the Mystic Feast: Turco-Mongol Tradition in the Mughal Harem', *The Journal of Asian Studies*, vol. 69, no. 1 (February 2010), p. 145.

14. Balabanlilar, 'The Begims of the Mystic Feast', p. 145.

15. Farooqi, *Mughal–Ottoman Relations*, p. 22.

16. Nizami, 'Foreword' in Farooqi, *Mughal–Ottoman Relations*, p. x.

17. Giancarlo Casale, *The Ottoman Age of Exploration* (Oxford: Oxford University Press, 2010), p. 153.

18. Farooqi, *Mughal–Ottoman Relations*, p. 24.

19. Casale, *The Ottoman Age of Exploration*, p. 150.

20. Casale, *The Ottoman Age of Exploration*, p. 202.

21. Casale, *The Ottoman Age of Exploration*, p. 200.

22. Casale, *The Ottoman Age of Exploration*, p. 200.

23. Farooqi, *Mughal–Ottoman Relations*, p. 28.

24. Farooqi, *Mughal–Ottoman Relations*, p. 37.

25. Farooqi, *Mughal–Ottoman Relations*, p. 55.

26. Farooqi, *Mughal–Ottoman Relations*, p. 68.

27. Kemal Karpat, *The Politicization of Islam: Reconstructing Identity, State, Faith, and Community in the Late Ottoman State* (Oxford: Oxford University Press, 2001), p. 52.

28. Ram Lakhan Shukla, *Britain, India and the Turkish Empire: 1853–1882* (New Delhi: People's Publishing House, 1973).

29. Raj Kumar Trivedi, *The Critical Triangle: India Britain and Turkey: 1908–1924* (Jaipur: Publication Scheme, 1994).

30. Trivedi, *The Critical Triangle*, p. 51.

31. Trivedi, *The Critical Triangle*, p. 51.

32. Ram Lakhan Shukla, *Britain, India and the Turkish Empire: 1853–1882* (New Delhi: People's Publishing House, 1973), p. 3.

33. Shukla, *Britain, India and the Turkish Empire*, p. 5, referencing Donald Southgate, *The Most English Minister: The Policies and Politics of Palmerston*, p. 65.

34. Shukla, *Britain, India and the Turkish Empire*, p. 44.

35. Colonel Malleson, ed., *John Kay, Kaye's and Malleson's History of the Indian Mutiny 1857–58*, vol. V (London: Longmans, Green and Co, 1914), p. 346.

36. Malleson, ed., *John Kay, Kaye's and Malleson's History of the Indian Mutiny 1857–58*, pp. 282–3.

37. Malleson, ed., *John Kay, Kaye's and Malleson's History of the Indian Mutiny 1857–58*, Appendix C, p. 349.

38. Malleson, ed., *John Kay, Kaye's and Malleson's History of the Indian Mutiny 1857–58*, Appendix C, p. 350.

39. Azmi Özcan, '1857 Büyük Hint Ayaklanması ve Osmanlı Devleti', *İslam Tetkikleri Dergisi*, vol. IX, p. 271.

40. Raj Kumar Trivedi, *The Critical Triangle: India Britain and Turkey: 1908–1924* (Jaipur: Publication Scheme, 1994), p. 11. See also Sayyed Suleman Nadvi, 'Khilafat Awr Hindustan', in Sayyed Sabah al Din, M.A., ed., *Maqalat-i-Nadvi*, vol. I (Karachi: National Book Foundation, 1989), p. 177; Syed Mahmud, *The Khilafat and England* (Patna: Sidaqat Ashram, 1921), pp. 50, 80.

41. Özcan, 'Büyük Hind Ayaklanması', p. 272.

42. Trivedi, *The Critical Triangle*, p. 12, citing *The Friend of India*, 1 August 1867, p. 913.

43. Özcan, 'Büyük Hind Ayaklanması', p. 272.

44. Farooqi, *Mughal–Ottoman Relations*, p. 139.

45. Trivedi, *The Critical Triangle*, p. 12.

46. Azmi Özcan, *Pan-Islamism: Indian Muslims, the Ottomans and Britain, 1877–1924* (Leiden: E.J. Brill, 1997), p. 68.

47. Trivedi, *The Critical Triangle*, p. 4.

48. Trivedi, *The Critical Triangle*, p. 4.

49. David Fromkin, *A Peace to End All Peace: The Fall of the Ottoman Empire and the Creation of the Modern Middle East* (New York: H. Holt, 2001), p. 28.

50. Fromkin, *The Critical Triangle*, p. 66.

51. Trivedi, *The Critical Triangle*, p. 5.

52. Niyazi Berkes, *The Development of Secularism in Turkey* (Montreal: McGill University Press, 1964), pp. 267–8.

53. Abdulhamid, *Siyasi Hatıratım* (İstanbul: Dergah Yayınları, 1975), p. 180.

54. Özcan, *Pan-Islamism*, p. 29.

55. Abdulhamid, *Siyasi Hatıratım*, p. 155.

56. Abdulhamid, *Siyasi Hatıratım*, p. 155.

4

A Portrait of Pan-Islamism

Although numerous sources refer to the Indian Medical Mission almost entirely in passing, various authors have successfully linked the origins of the Mission with the growing tide of pan-Islamic ideological fervour among the Indian Muslims. However, designating the endeavour as pan-Islamic runs the risk of embroiling the Indian Medical Mission of 1913 in the profound confusion that has been reigning unabatedly until today about what pan-Islamism as a political ideology does or does not entail. Hence, a specific narrative of pan-Islamism needs to be set out in order to help contextualize the Indian Medical Mission to Ottoman Turkey during the first Balkan War. For this, I draw a figurative portrait of the idea of Islamic unity, which would be applicable to the Mission in general and the key personalities leading the enterprise. In so doing, I rewind the cognitive clock to history as it was perceived at this time, marking thoughts, personalities, events, and indeed the international system as it was experienced at the turn of the twentieth century. I thus reconstruct a narrative that I believe would not be entirely alien to the protagonists in India who set sail towards İstanbul in December 1912.

Flirting with European Modernity

After a long and painful nineteenth century, the twentieth century lifted its curtain with a desolate act for the Muslim world. It was as early as the eighteenth century that the European ascendancy became too obvious to deny. Yet, by the 1900s, which were to become the bloodiest in the history of human civilization, 'a small white minority radiating out from Europe'[1] already controlled most of the world's land territories and maritime routes. They developed an unparalleled aptitude to travel, slay, and exploit around the world, and used their capabilities unreservedly. Their industrialized cruelty was hardly matched in history by another civilization since the Mongol invasions. The Europeans simultaneously helped advance and shape human civilization profoundly, excelling in arts, letters, engineering, and sciences. A sophisticated body of knowledge was produced in political systems, philosophy, and jurisprudence. Ideas and ideologies were propagated around the world, sometimes at gunpoint, with consequences for the bodies they entered. This rise involved both a military and geopolitical advance as well as a civilizational challenge. The Europeans offered a new modernity not only in warfare but also in sociopolitical organization and cultural systems. They embarked on a civilizing mission, which created a certain epistemology which denigrated the historical self of the colonized peoples and professed construction of a new identity and history.[2] For instance, in India, 'English writers, bureaucrats and missionaries conveniently presented a negative image of the Muslim rule to legitimize the British seizure of India from the remnants of the Mughal Empire'.[3]

One reaction of the Muslim and other non-Western peoples was to confront the challenge of European modernity by striving to adopt European means to modernize their own societies. The success of European modernity bred appreciation and created legions of aspiring Asians and Africans. Their intellectuals presumed that their societies could be reformed through Western education and by embracing European ways and means. They promoted adoption of European science and way of life. Scores emerged who thought like the Europeans, spoke like them, wrote like them, acted like them, and most of the time, even dressed like them. Europeanness came to define modernity, the civilizational currency that needed to be attained. Those who had the opportunity to imitate formed the new elites in their countries. Historian Cemil Aydın wrote that 'many intellectuals of the existing non-Western empires (Ottoman, Chinese, Japanese and Persian) accepted the idea of a universal European civilization and even the benevolence of European imperialism in offering to uplift the level of civilization in the rest of the world'.[4] The Ottomans, the Japanese, and the others tried to imitate European empires and societies, acquire their sciences, education, training methods, and curricula, and even their culture. They ultimately sought acceptance by the Europeans and Americans into their 'civilized' ranks. Muslim intellectuals recalled the shared Hellenistic and monotheistic roots with the Europeans. They attended international gatherings to convince their European counterparts of the compatibility of Islam with the European form of modernity. They countered European scholars who argued that the Muslim societies were inferior.[5] At home, they pushed forward reforms to catch up with modernity. In Aydın's words, 'Appropriation of the notion of a Eurocentric but universal civilization by the Ottoman, Chinese, Egyptian, Persian and Japanese elites also empowered these same elites in domestic politics, as they could justify centralizing radical reforms over their own populations as a civilizing mission.'[6] Thus, the Tanzimat Movement in the Ottoman Empire between 1839 and 1876 introduced reforms to modernize the state along European lines, with significant support from the Ottoman elite. The 1839 Royal Edict of the Rose Chamber (Gülhane Hattı Hümayunu) guaranteed life, property, and dignity for all citizens of the empire irrespective of their religion or ethnicity. It also instituted reforms of the taxation system and conscription for the army. A new secular school system was established alongside European-inspired commercial and criminal codes. Judiciary control of these codes was given to state courts independently from the Islamic religious councils. The Ottomans became a full-fledged member of the Concert of Europe in 1856. They implemented the Gülhane Royal Edict until 1876. They continued refashioning their state and army along European lines. They hoped that this would stem the disintegration of their polity, and prevent bloody uprisings, foreign instigations, and indeed military interventions under the guise of a civilizing mission. After all, the civilizing mission of European powers implied that being backward legitimized their intervention as a corrective. To the targeted non-European peoples, modernization was a product of hope for a peaceful and prosperous future.

Colonialism in Crisis of Legitimacy

As reforms and the surrounding debate were underway in a vast geography ranging from the Ottoman Empire to Persia, Egypt, and India, colonial expansion took an intense and aggressive form around the world. In the wake of the division of Africa among several European empires around 1882, colonization took an even uglier turn. Concomitantly, reassured of their superiority, soon the pride of the imperial mind turned into outright contempt for other races and societies. Many groped backwards to reconstruct their own justification for the ascendancy of their empires and welfare of their societies, presenting it as a historical inevitability arising out of their innate racial and civilizational superiority. Thus, 'European empires were embracing the ethos of white race's superiority over the colored races or the superiority of Christianity over Islam in its legitimacy claims', notes Cemil Aydın.[7] It is, of course, easy to write exaltations to the successful. The 'Euro-Americans', to use Indian sociologist Benoy Kumar Sarkar's terminology, had been doing what every dominant group before them also did by taking success as pre-ordained. Yet, Euro-Americans showcased their superiority with an intensity of conviction and flair that was hardly matched by any other dominant civilization in the thousands of years before their time. Rudyard Kipling, a Mumbai-born Anglo-Indian literary figure, was one name most associated with the eloquence of the naked imperial contempt towards the subject races. His controversial and well-known poem 'White Man's Burden', dated 1899, was initially authored for the diamond jubilee of the British monarch and rewritten to address the American colonization of the Philippines: 'Take up the White Man's burden/Send forth the best ye breed/Go send your sons to exile/To serve your captives' need/To wait in heavy harness/ On fluttered folk and wild/Your new-caught, sullen peoples/Half devil and half child'. In addition to poets and politicians, scholars also rushed in to legitimize European Christian empires. In 1883, Ernest Renan would argue that whatever great scientific and cultural achievements might have existed in medieval Islam, these were to be credited to Christian Arabs or to the Iranians whose Aryan race eclipsed the shortcomings of their Semitic religion. If Arab Muslims wanted to be civilized, he argued, they needed to convert to Christianity.

As Euro-America slid down the path of a self-indulgent sense of racial and religious superiority, a dichotomy emerged between what the West exacted at home and as against what they applied in the world, deepening the legitimacy crisis of European imperialism. At home, they moved towards greater public participation, accountability, individual rights, and the rule of law. Progressively since the eighteenth century, religious authority in Europe retreated as the church lost political and indeed economic ground. The European and American populations marched towards greater secularization at home. This was to reach a level beyond institutional separation of the church and state, moving away from the 'ultimate' towards 'proximate' and from 'metaphysical' to 'positive'. Theoretically, secularization and liberalization could have culminated in forming a bond among various faith groups. A new communization around institutional values could have united Christians and Muslims, overshadowing differences of the faiths of the individuals. Yet, as this secularist liberal trend was being established within Europe, outside the colonial armies and administrations continued to forcefully subjugate increasingly restive subject nations. At the same time, European and American missionaries vehemently promoted their own allegedly 'superior' forms of religion through vast networks, despite the fact that at least in India the colonial government did make reluctant and ultimately frail attempts to curtail the influence of missionaries. Colonial governments, in turn, took for granted a civilizational mission to legitimize the hegemony of superior Western Christian societies over backward non-Western ones. Thus, to the Muslim, Hindu, and Buddhist peoples, the pervasive and fervent Euro-American hegemony meant an all-out offensive, including a religious, assault. The European effort unavoidably demarcated 'civilized' Christians from the 'philistine' Muslims,

Hindus, Buddhists, Sikhs, Jains, Parsis, and others. All vessels of mass communication joined in the parade, bending and distorting history and even current facts to suit their own perceptions and world views. Hence, Benoy Kumar Sarkar wrote in *The Futurism of Young Asia* in 1918: 'Christian missionaries and even scientists of research societies take a morbid delight in picking up the worst features of Oriental life and thought. Ultimately through the movies, theatres, and journals, Asia has become to their nationals a synonym for immorality, sensuousness, ignorance, and superstition.'[8] The inherent contempt was not lost on the non-Western peoples including Muslims. Thus, Sarkar concluded: 'If it is possible to generalize the diverse intellectual currents among the Turks, Egyptians, Persians, Hindus, Chinese, and Japanese of the twentieth century into any suitable formula, probably it should be called the "critique of Occidental Reason".'[9] That 'Reason' established an insuperable separation between the separate identities of the East and the West. 'East is East, and West is West, and never the twain shall meet', argued Kipling. The world view of permanent bifurcation obviated the hopes of transcending a vision of permanent conflict between the white Christians and the Muslims, Jews, and the so-called coloured races. In the process, the world was demarcated between putative categories of the civilized and the non-civilized. The clash of civilizations thesis finds its roots in this demarcation.

Eclipse of the Civilizing Mission

The immediate victim of the intensification of the imperial onslaught and its cultural, racial, and religious supremacist pretensions was the optimism in the non-Euro-American world about the potency of the European-inspired institutional reforms to help transcend the racial and civilizational divide between Euro-America and their own societies. They would not be shedding their faith, as Ernest Renan had proposed, in order to civilize their societies. Conversions remained largely involuntary and very rare. After abortive attempts on Ottoman Jews as well as Muslims, protestant missionaries in Ottoman Turkey, in fact, had to focus on non-Protestant Christian subjects of the Ottoman Empire, including the Greeks, Armenians, and Bulgarians, as well as Catholic Arabs. Their influence went beyond proselytizing their own version of the Christian faith and included, in a manner yet to be objectively explained, sedition and provocation against the İstanbul government. Their own ideology was pan-Christian or pan-Protestant in nature, which implied a reorganization of the international order in their image, a feat that confirmed every doubt in Muslim minds about the ill-will of the whole enterprise. The countless good deeds that many missionaries did in fact make, including in the fields of education and medical care, were eclipsed by that obviously abortive wild attempt to refashion a Christian world order out of a chaos which they helped instigate among the already restive sections of the Ottoman polity under geopolitical siege. Preaching on the basis of the strength of their message rather than on instigating rebellion, including through communicating biased reports about unfolding events to galvanize world public opinion, would have been more respectable. However, Protestant missionaries were most definitely not the only group conjuring up the blind date of geopolitical ambition with religious zeal and reinvigorating a clash of religionists at the turn of the catastrophic twentieth century. Similarly, the Ottoman Empire was not the only stage where this drama played out, nor were the Muslims its only target. The stage was indeed global. Jews, Hindus, and Muslims suffered comparable ordeals, although the Holocaust of the mid-twentieth century would take suffering to a unique category of evil.

Segregation on the basis of culture and religion was bad enough. And by the second half of the nineteenth century, pseudo-scientific racial theories became popular particularly in Europe but also in America to justify the superiority of the white race. Race is the most inescapable exclusionist when it is exploited as such. Unlike culture, biological characteristics could not be changed. Thus, racism implied a permanent demarcation of the white from the non-white which condemned the latter to stigmatization. Racism had added another complication into the mix. The Turks considered themselves to be of the white Caucasian stock and the ruling Ottoman dynasty and elites had over the centuries numerous mothers of white European Christian descent. Insofar as racism was concerned, they would not suffer as much as the black Africans or the coloured Indians. At some point, the Ottoman intelligentsia even sought to escape stigmatization by accentuating the shared white race. Many Africans and Asians discovered that excelling, as they did, in European languages, arts, and sciences may win some of them some respect, but they still would not be admitted to the first-class couch at Pietermaritzburg or could get beaten up by the conductor for not giving their seat to a white European passenger, as a bright London-educated lawyer Gandhi was to find out decades into the twentieth century.

Several European or American educated Muslim, African, and Asian intellectuals, well versed in the Euro-American scholarly literature and media, came to build on the clash of civilization theories they had learned in the West. European-inspired education helped articulate another intellectual and indeed political discontent and dissent to imperialism and colonialism. For the Muslims, pan-Islamism grew alongside other Asian and African pan-isms as one form of such dissent.

While the nineteenth century began with an order based on empires in the European theatre, ideas of the 1789 French Revolution, including a reconstructed ethnic nationhood, began to contest the identities formed on the basis of allegiance to the empires. A dynamic was unleashed that forced a redefinition of the identities based on ethnicities and ultimately 'civilizations'. The supremacist ethos of the European societies helped reinforce this dynamic. Thus, the Russian Empire reached across its borders towards Orthodox Christians and Slavs at the cost of ignoring its own vast and largely loyal Muslim populace. The Asian empires of China and Japan came to be associated with the 'yellow' race. The Ottoman Empire bent on preserving itself by underscoring Ottoman imperial identity moved into association with the Muslims around the world as it lost ground to nascent separatist identities among its non-Muslim populations. Successful nationalist integrationist movements added strength to other integrationist ideas. While Slavs followed up with pan-Slavism, other variants spurted in various formulations around much of the world, emboldened by the German example. The anti-colonial 'primary resistance', to borrow Ranger's terminology,[10] spread around Asia and Africa. Accordingly, shortly before the onset of the twentieth century, feeling pushed away by Euro-America through insurmountable racial and so-called civilizational barriers, transnational movements began to gather momentum in which 'Pan-Islamic, Pan-African and Pan-Asian ideas were produced as a rethinking of the relationship between civilizing processes, the international order and predominant forms of racial and religious identities'.[11] This rethinking no longer regarded Western expansion as a potentially benevolent modernizing feat. Instead, a near consensus developed outside Europe and America that there was instead an aggressive assault that established an international order based on a pattern of unfair and lopsided relationships. A geopolitical vision was cast in opposition to another that was promoted by the expanded Euro-American politicians, generals, administrators, scholars, journalists, missionaries, and indeed laymen. As such, the restive world entered a dangerous epoch of 'popularization of geopolitics'.

Assertion of national and transnational identities was the sign of the times and not limited to the disaffected 'East'. Pan-Europeanism as well as many other global identities were also emergent. Yet as Nikkie Keddie observed, unmistakably 'Pan-Islam, like Asian and African nationalism, was primarily a reaction to Western imperialism'.[12] It is no coincidence that pan-Islamists often formed close collaborations with leaders and organizations of other religions and causes around the common theme of anti-imperialism. Being a committed member of both the Indian National Congress and the Muslim League was possible. Pan-Islamists could be at the same time pan-Asian, sympathizing strongly with China and Japan. The loyalties were painlessly plural in the non-Euro-American world.

Pan-Islamism as a Form of Dissent

Pan-Islamism, like many other 'pan' variants, cannot be used even today without raising confusion and alarm. The fact is that almost all pan-isms are controversial, some more so than the others. Being mostly utopian and erected upon mythical and imagined foundations, they are also not conducive to infallible definitions. The fact of the matter is that pan-Islamism is a concept that has meant different things to different people and has been used and abused to the fullest extent, both by its proponents and its opponents.

An encyclopaedic definition is furnished by the *Oxford Dictionary of Islam*, in which John Esposito has defined pan-Islamism as

an ideology calling for sociopolitical solidarity among all Muslims. Has existed as a religious concept since the early days of Islam. Emerged as a modern political ideology in the 1860s and 1870s at the height of European colonialism, when Turkish intellectuals began discussing and writing about it as a way to save the Ottoman Empire from fragmentation. Became the favoured state policy during the reign of Sultan Abdulhamid II (r. 1876–1909) and was adopted and promoted by members of the ruling bureaucratic and intellectual elites of the empire. With the rise of colonialism, became a defensive ideology, directed against European political, military, economic, and missionary penetration.[13]

This definition locates pan-Islamism as a politically active dissent, solidarity, and cooperation among Muslims across the world against foreign intrusion.

At the roots of the concept, one sees that the unity of all believers as well as their common action against the threat posed by the rival non-Islamic world is more or less an established doctrine. Similarly, the idea of loyalty to a caliph is almost as old as the classical era of the Islamic nation. In the Sunni tradition, the institution of the caliphate began with the election of Abu Bakr as the first caliph after the death of the Prophet of Allah in 634. Abu Bakr's most imminent challenge was to keep the Muslims of Mecca and Medina together in one community of faith. An institution thus came into being out of practice. The other pious and rightly guided caliphs included Omar, Osman, and Ali, who were also elected to the leadership position of the fledgling Islamic nation. Being compared to the Rashidun caliphs of Islam's earliest years, as Sheikh Ahmad al-Damanhuri of al-Azhar assessed the Ottomans in the 1770s, is regarded as the highest praise any Muslim ruler could receive. Since the caliphs between 632 and 661, all close companions of the Prophet, governed a single political entity, the doctrine reflected that the caliphs represent political, theological, and economic unity among different tribes that adopted Islam. The theory would hold during the Ummayyad dynasty's caliphal lead. The dynasty would, in fact, run a polity of Muslims, now members of an established religious community. The Umayyad dynasty was followed by the Abbassid family from 750 CE until the Mongol invasions in 1258. The largely Turkish slave warriors (Mameluks) in Egypt allowed the fugitive members of the Abbasid dynasty fleeing Baghdad to use the title of caliph, thereby keeping the institution alive. However, these Abbasid royalty had retained no power to exercise. The fact is that since the very beginning, the issue of the caliphal succession became a point of competition and a bone of contention. The emergence of the Sunni–Shia split too traces back to the issue of who was the rightful successor of the Holy Prophet.

The universal acceptance of the caliphal authority was not extant since the classical period. Various doctrines and ideas grew, all with tentative bases. The Britishers in a bid to counter Istanbul's influence would strive to popularize the thesis that the caliph had to come from among the members of the Qureish tribe. That theory did not win much support. Others at different times would argue that Muslim monarchs righteously implementing sharia law would become caliphs in their own territories. These included prominent jurists and sociologists like Gazzali in the twelfth and Ibn Khaldun in the fifteenth century. Ottomans would use the title since the rule of Murad I in the early fourteenth century in accordance with the theory that righteous Muslim rulers can be caliphs in their own domains. In 1517, Selim would bring Arabia within his empire and become the protector of the two holy mosques in Mecca and Medina. Thus, the Ottomans would claim universal caliphal status between 1517 and 1924. The futile contestations and argumentations mattered little as no one within that period would ever aspire to greater legitimacy and acceptance to the caliphate of the Muslims than the Ottoman sultans. This was a point that Akbar learned through experience in India when he forwarded unsuccessfully a claim to the caliphate. The fact is that the idea of a single leader would become increasingly improbable and impracticable as the number of believers exploded around the world, including onto geographically incontiguous territories, and comprising men and women of mutually unintelligible languages. However, the hope for unity remained and transformed into political aspiration as the Muslims started feeling the encroachment of the resurgent Christian empires.

Pan-Islamism of the late nineteenth and early twentieth centuries was both similar to and also distinct from the yearning for a period where the righteous companions of the Holy Prophet were almost unanimously believed to have led the Muslim nation after his passing. It was similar in that it invoked the established Koranic principle that Muslims belonged to a single nation. It also built on the practice of a monarch claiming leadership of the universal Muslim nation, although the actual authority over all the believers did not exist uniformly throughout centuries. Mutual support and common action including jihad against the aggressors were also part and parcel of the Islamic nation's religious and political doctrine. A revival of coalescence around these principles, however, did not suffice to define and explain the late nineteenth to early twentieth century ideology of pan-Islamism. The task is made harder by the fact that there never existed a single authoritative text or person to streamline the panoply of views under a single ideological pan-Islamic movement. There never was a *Das Kapital* of pan-Islamism. One should recognize that the spectrum of pan-Islamist thought is so vast and diverse that the term remains fluid even after countless valuable studies. Explaining the phenomenon also suffers from vastly different vantage points or levels of analysis adopted in countless studies by eminent scholars.

In one of the most authoritative studies of the pan-Islamic idea, Gail Minault argued, in her 1982 book *The Khilafat Movement: Religious Symbolism and Political Mobilization in India*, that the leaders of pan-Islamism in the Indian subcontinent used symbols, such as the caliph, that were meaningful to all strata of the Muslim community, in order to generate political unity among the heterogeneous community of Indian Muslims on the issue of nationalism. She showcased how pan-Islamism brought religious revivalist *ulema* of different opinions together with nationalists. Her study provided an elaborate account of the internal divisions and machinations of Indian Muslim politics. However, Minault seemed to understate external impulses of Indian pan-Islamism, including the legacy of Indian Muslim interaction with the Ottoman and Central Asian Turks—and I would argue Iranians—over many centuries.

In a uniquely elaborate and well-documented study, Naeem Qureshi, among others, offered a corrective to Minault's focus on the internal divisions. While the strength of this legacy varied significantly within India, Qureshi and several other authors including Naimur Rahman Farooqi and Ram Lakhan Shukla have documented its strong imprint. I would argue that another such external impulse was the profound suffering of the Turkish and Muslim populations documented by the Muslim Indian press and indeed various delegations that travelled to Ottoman Turkey during the Balkan Wars. Valuable treatises on the subject, such as those by Jacob Landau, Nikkie Keddie, Peter Hardy, Azmi Özcan, and indeed several other accounts in the Indian and other contexts, shed considerable light on a pheonomenon whose past and future impact was questionable.

Perhaps one could best understand the nineteenth- and early twentieth-century pan-Islamism by acknowledging that in the late 1800s pan-Islamism as a political agenda was a product of its times, aiming to respond to the extant challenges. Parting from the traditional conceptions of Islamic *ummah*, the new wave was based on an analysis of the contemporary challenges of the very historical epoch in which it was formulated. Pan-Islamism's objective was to generate a political reaction to save a perceived global community of faith. It was a tool to forge an alliance among the like-minded against the existentialist colonialist threat. It was as much about protecting the other Muslims as it was about protecting oneself. However, the question was how to generate a political agenda and action when Muslims within any community displayed myriad traditional and teleological as well as theological differences. As Edmund Burke argued, 'A major drawback of Islam as a focus of political loyalty was the gradual accretion of a host of local beliefs and practices, including saint worship and maraboutism. In order for resistance to be successful, some means had to be found to transcend these particularistic interests.'[14] In turn, Terence Ranger has shown in the East African context that the problem of attaining scale and momentum could not be resolved by appealing to anti-colonial resentment or indeed Islam alone. It needed a transient ideology that bridged the perceived past with the aspired future. It also needed the appeal of commonly accepted, albeit vaguely defined, symbols that would unite the community behind political action.

Thus, pan-Islamism sought to attain scale by invoking a universalistic notion of the Muslim nation and the more or less, although not entirely, the universally accepted Ottoman caliphate. The expansion of Christian supremacist empires at the cost of the caliph and the last remaining independent Muslim polities, as well as the suffering of the Muslims, were all symbols that helped build scale by forging unity. This worked both within Muslim communities, whether in the Ottoman Empire or India, and across the political boundaries. In concurring with this analysis, I do not call into doubt the sincerity of the pan-Islamist ideologues or masses in responding to the political tribulations of the Ottoman Empire or its sultan caliph or the human sufferings of the Turks and other Muslims. I nonetheless argue that the depth of these sensitivities helped propel individualized anti-imperialist primary opposition to national and indeed transnational scale, thanks in no small degree to the ability of the religious symbolism to garner politics of scale.

Emergence of a Global Muslim Public Opinion

The concept of a 'Muslim world' is an ancient construct, which re-emerged alongside other identities in the context of the legitimacy of imperial legacy in the second half of the nineteenth century. As we have seen, in this period, 'there developed an increasing awareness of how the expansion of European power was increasingly subjecting Muslims to Christian rule'.[15] The onslaught of European imperialism was documented and interpreted through the print media, including newspapers and travelogues. The state of affairs of other Muslim lands was brought home through these writings. Modern technology obviously helped bring about the ease and speed with which the Muslim peoples had come to interact. The travel time was signficantly cut, thanks to the steamship. As a result, Muslim intellectuals ventured to travel more easily to other Muslim lands, most notably to the Ottoman Empire, and wrote in eloquent terms their observations about the culture, society, economics, politics, as well as the responses to imperial challenge, including modernizing reforms. Hajj travels always helped people-to-people contacts and the dissemination of contemporary Muslim thought among believers from around the world. However, Hajj's role in this regard was supplemented by direct journeys to various lands, which had become more extensive and faster than ever before, thanks to modern transportation technology. While almost all print media was censured in any empire they were published, significant information and commentary was nonetheless passed through newspapers and travelogues. The advances in technology was augmented by the advent of modern postal systems, which further aided the dissemination of the written word. The modern construct of the Muslim world, or a transnational public opinion of Muslims, became uniquely possible as a result.

However, it would be wrong to believe that this public opinion was a self-contained and exclusive unit detached from other concurrent identities. At any given moment in the late nineteenth and early twentieth centuries, Muslim public opinion co-existed with anti-colonial and non-Western identity developing simultaneously. This marked a diversion from the previous era when 'Ottoman, Iranian and Egyptian elites saw monotheistic Christian Europe, with whom they shared the Hellenistic legacy, closer to them than East Asians'.[16] European imperialism towards the 1890s culminated in the linking of Muslim with Asian or African destinies. The 'Eastern' as opposed to its Hegelian counterpoint, namely Western, identity engendered cooperation between various political constituencies. For instance, the Japanese and the Muslims were drawn closer against the background of a transnational anti-colonial nationalism.[17] Japanese advances in development and technology and Chinese nationalism became objects of Muslim sympathy. The 1905 victory of Japan over Russia was celebrated widely, including in the Muslim world. This was hardly due to the acknowledgement, let alone support, of imperial Japan's geopolitical ambitions over Manchuria or Korea, yet the struggles against the white man, as depicted in Tokutomi Soho's 'Yellow Man's Burden', which inversed the idea of Kipling's 'White Man's Burden', touched a common chord with the Muslims. Similarly, pan-Islamist discourses of the Ottoman intellectuals received support from geographically detached lands such as China and India. Again, also in this larger context, the modern press and travel facilitated dissemination of ideas and information as well as contacts among different constituencies.

If the transnational Muslim public opinion was not self-contained, it was also not monolithic. The Muslim world may have agreed on the nature of the European challenge to their culture and sovereignty, even faith, yet they continued to espouse different explanations and responses. The acceptance of the need to reform and modernize too could be more or less acknowledged across the Muslim public opinion. Several modernizers espoused a return to the classical golden age when Muslim societies and polities were ahead of the European ones, curiously sounding similar to their Salafist co-religionists. The modernists and Salafists, while coming from different ideational backgrounds, seemed to converge on the need to revive the pristine Islamic values. Thus, in 1916 Şemseddin Günaltay wrote:

> The Muslim peoples were once the most powerful and most advanced nations of the world while today they live in misery. The Islamic lands were once centres of civilization, while today they are in ruin ... In olden days their religion bestowed upon them the light of endeavour and knowledge, while today their beliefs drag them toward the abyss of cruelty and disappointment.[18]

One inherent aspect of this convergence was, of course, the blaming of fellow Muslims for the woes of the contemporary Muslim societies. The decline of Muslim societies was the consequence of the practices of fellow Muslims who had walked away from the precepts of Islam. They had abandoned the teachings of the rightly guided caliphs and jurists and adopted novel practices including Sufism. Even those that did not necessarily espouse a return to the fundamentals of early Islam did nonetheless levy criticism on fellow Muslims for falling behind. Part of the blame was directed on Muslim women, as if this was and still is not a male-dominated world. A representative account of this widely shared point of view is presented, in fact, in one of the letters by Dr Mukhtar Ahmad Ansari from İstanbul. In his letter dated 10 January 1913, Dr Ansari relates his visit to the Persian Ambassador in İstanbul where the state of the Muslim world became a subject of discussion. Thus reports Ansari:

> Whilst our friends were having tea at Shaikh Chawish's house, I went to see the Persian Ambassador with a few members ... The First Attaché to the Embassy spoke English very fluently, and

discussed in a very animated fashion the causes of the gradual decay of Islam. He took the view of Mr. Garvin that the great cause of decay was to be found in the backward conditions of Moslem women both mentally and physically, and the only way to salvation lay in the emancipation of women. His Excellency intelligently followed the discussion and gave his approval to what his Attaché expressed to us. There is no doubt that the events in Turkey and Persia seem to have impressed deeply the mind of all the Moslems in the world and they are beginning to realise, though, alas! very late, that unless they improve themselves at once they will lose all they possess and be a subject race for ever.

It may be interesting to note that while this debate was ongoing at the Persian Ambassador's residence, several other members of the Indian Medical Mission were entertained by Shaikh Abdul Aziz Chawish, discussing similarly the fate of the Muslim world. Although Ansari does not provide details on that meeting where he was not present, he does nonetheless report in his letter dated 9 January that 'Dr. Esad Pasha, a very famous Turkish Ophthalmic Surgeon of European reputation, was present at the tea and made some pregnant remarks regarding the condition of Turkey and the Moslem world in general. Our Manager replied and made a great impression on those present by his weighty words'. The intra-Muslim discussion on the state of the Muslim world and how to catch up with Euro-America continues to date with the successor of the Ottoman Empire—the modern democratic, secular, free market Republic of Turkey, widely presented as a successful model.

In the development of the transnational Muslim public opinion the role of the newspapers merits further emphasis. The press was indeed the singularly most important contributor to the evolution of vastly different political agendas in Muslim nations into a more or less coherent public opinion around the turn of the twentieth century with the Ottoman Empire at the core of shared concerns. If Muslim publications played the central role in disseminating ideas and information, thus promoting a more or less shared opinion and an alternative epistemology, the newspapers were at the forefront of this phenomenon, thanks to their reach and speed of delivery. As Khaleed Adeeb points out, the Muslim 'public sphere was the product of print, of course, and its most important form was the newspaper'.[19] In the nineteenth century, newspapers and journals entered wide circulation in all Muslim geographies, thanks to Euro-American shipping, railway, and telegram technologies. As a primary form of dissemination, they were read widely and exerted significant influence. The press thus became a milieu for competition among various thoughts. Pan-Islamists excelled in their use of this medium. The imperial governments were fully aware of the potential of newspapers to reach across borders and exert influence on various constituencies. As they guarded against negative publications, they simultaneously promoted favourable ones. They also sought to impose censure on the newspapers and journals published in other countries. Thus, when an Indian Muslim Nusrat Ali Khan started publishing *Peyk-i Islam* (Follower of Islam) in İstanbul in 1880, the British Empire's Embassy in İstanbul lobbied vigorously for its closure.[20] The main theme of the journal was the propagation of the Ottoman sultan as the caliph of all Muslims around the world including in India. This went against the emerging British propaganda in the direction of challenging the Ottoman sultan's legitimacy as caliph, forwarding through a minority the opinion that the Muslim caliph had to be an Arab from the Quresh tribe. This viewpoint much to the consternation of the British was not gathering much force and the majority of Indian Muslims continued to endorse the Ottoman caliph as the leader of the believers. The publisher Nusrat Ali Khan from India himself was known to the British authorities as a fiercely anti-British journalist whose previous newspaper in India was closed down by the British government and who had collected funds for the Ottomans during the 1878 Russo-Turkish War. However, whatever its message, the *Peyk-i Islam*, published in Turkish and Urdu versions, had very limited circulation. So much so that only 18 copies were received in India. Nevertheless, its publication did cause a furor in London, possibly upon Ambassador Layard's instigation and Prime Minister Gladstone's avowedly anti-Turkish and anti-Muslim prejudice. Kemal Karpat notes that the financial support given to the journal was not due to a calculated ploy by the Ottoman Sultan Abdulhamid II to undermine the British rule in India. Instead, 'Ottoman documents indicate that the Peyk-i Islam matter resulted from Ottoman bureaucratic carelessness and disregard for the possible implications of the decision to help Nusrat Ali publish his newspaper'.[21] The Ottoman government appears not to have studied the petition of the publisher carefully while donating a small sum out of benevolence towards an Indian Muslim journalist.

The *Peyk-i Islam* affair resulted in a counter salvo from a variety of British newspapers including the *Statesman*. It also culminated in a closer scrutiny of the press on both sides. However, perhaps the most important impact was the exaggeration of sensitivities against pan-Islamic allegiance to the Ottoman caliph, an idea which they initially upheld and promoted. Karpat underscores that the newspapers were taken by the British authorities at face value whenever they claimed activities allegedly instigated by the Ottoman sultan against the British rule in India. As Karpat writes, 'The "activities" range from secret anti-British committees supposedly established in India at the sultan's orders, through Osman pasha's pan-Islamic conspiracies, to the activities of the Turkish consul in Bombay, and other similar exaggerations based more often on rumor than fact.'[22] The Ottoman newspapers were indeed full of writings in favour of pan-Islamic thought since the concept of 'unity of Islam' was first used by Namık Kemal in the 10 May 1869 edition of the *Hürriyet* newspaper in İstanbul. The British Empire after the *Peyk-i Islami* row joined the other European imperial powers in their exaggerated fear of the pan-Islamic press as well as their efforts to suppress it. However, these efforts would not succeed as the pan-Islamist newspapers would continue to sprawl both in Ottoman Turkey and definitely in India. In India, in fact, the pan-Islamist ideas would become the mainstay of the Muslim press and their focus would lie squarely in the developments taking place vis-à-vis the Ottoman Empire and its sultan caliph. They would report on the human trials and tribulations about the wars against the Ottomans, counter the distortions about the Muslims and the Ottomans by the Euro-American press both through a network of reporters they dispatched and through very capable and eloquent commentators back home. Whether in India, Iran, Egypt, or Turkey, political theorists and ideologues, including the much-studied Jamaluddin Afghani, would also make use of the newspapers as an outlet to disseminate their views. The newspapers would not only lead the formation of a national and transnational Muslim public space and public opinion, but also spearhead mass mobilization to support concrete activities in support of the Ottomans. The role of the newspapers, including the *Zamindar* and *Comrade* among countless others, in collecting funds to help the Ottoman war effort against the coalition of European powers cannot be overstated. Such vanguard role by the Muslim press would continue all the way to the abolition of the caliphate by the modern Turkish Republic and leave in its wake such concrete manifestations as the 1913 Indian Medical Mission and the Khilafat Movement of 1919.

The Internationalism of Pan-Islamism

Recent scholarship forwards the concept of religious internationalism which may prove useful in locating the emergence of the Muslim public opinion within the development of a broader international society and its mobilization towards concrete objectives through specific endeavours. More importantly, the introduction of the term liberates those activities and deliverables from the contemporary wear and tear of all pan-isms including pan-Islamism, which is heavily polluted, including by the Muslims themselves. Accordingly, religious internationalism is defined as a new configuration of the modern era involving 'a cluster of voluntary transnational organizations and representations crystallizing around international issues, in which both "ordinary" believers and religious specialists could serve as protagonists'.[23]

The panoply of international/transnational religious activity considered in this regard include international organizations, communities of action, sects and religious brotherhoods, global and transnational religious publics, interrelated kinship groups, and diaspora organizations, not to mention ideologies. Despite their deep roots in the nineteenth and twentieth centuries, these internationals 'drew upon traditional communal institutions and practices, while remaining distinct from them'.[24] The utility of this concept arises in particular with reference to the emergence of the global civil society, by charting its religious origins and nature. Accordingly, the ascent of religious internationals are aided by modern communications and transportation, mass migration, challenge of colonial expansion, as well as the spread of the European nation-state model and secular ideologies. These international religious activities projected religious energy into both modern society and the global arena simultaneously. Thus, it is argued, 'the interaction of traditional religious structures and identities with wider processes of political, social, cultural, technological and economic change promoted the transformation of communities of believers into communities of opinion'.[25] In other words, although religious association takes place in a non-voluntary manner, in the sense that people are born into religious communities, the distinctive feature of religious internationalism involves mobilization based on voluntarism.

Students of religious internationalism have identified that single issues, such as abolitionism for Protestants, defence of the Papacy for Catholics, and international relief for Jews, have 'catalysed a process of politicization and transformed these creeds into globally visible forces in civil society'.[26] In the case of the Muslims, the assault against the Ottoman Empire and the caliph was the focal reference for the emergence of Muslim internationalism. The Islamic Internationalism took shape in the form of 1919 Khilafat Movement, although the archetype could be seen as the Organization of Islamic Cooperation that boasts a permanent structure with 57 member states across the Muslim world.

How pan-Islamism and Muslim internationalism relate and interact is a worthy question that needs further analysis. On one level, pan-Islamism as an ideology is a broader concept. Pan-Islamism encompasses Muslim internationals, which are not the only manifestations of it. It can also be argued that Muslim internationals are produced by a pan-Islamic ideology. In the case of the Indian Medical Mission, the pan-Islamic ideology of its sponsors was instrumental in their participation in the funding and manning of the enterprise. However, one can also argue against this position, especially given that the vast literature on the mobilization of the Indian Muslims does not appear to suggest unanimously that the masses have been moved by ideology. Instead, feelings of sympathy and solidarity with a fellow Muslim community and their suffering was the overarching motivation at least in 1912. In fact, the participation or support of the Hindus to the Medical Mission was shaped obviously not by pan-Islamism but sympathy for the afflicted. However, by 1919 it could be argued that the Khilafat Movement had arisen on more solidly defined and propagated ideological bearings in support of the caliphate.

At another level, one can argue that pan-Islamism and Muslim internationalism not only coexist but also mutually reinforce each other. Their coexistence, not obvious under the classical notions of the unity of the Islamic ummah, is natural under a particular definition of pan-Islamism as an ideology current in its period. The emergence of a global Islamic state under one political direction was as incredible at the turn of the twentieth century as it is today. The modern political ideology of pan-Islam, therefore, inherently acknowledged separate national or multinational boundaries traversing the Muslim world. Notwithstanding other suggested formulations, pan-Islamism of the late nineteenth century meant supporting the caliph and thus the Ottoman Empire against Christian assaults, not necessarily re-establishing a single political entity under Ottoman rule. As such, pan-Islamism created a communicative space between the national and international domains. Being part of a broader Muslim world facing common challenges did not foreclose national identity and agendas. The former instead reinforced the latter. The plight of the Muslims elsewhere strengthened the awareness of the challenge at home and provided dissent with mass appeal.

The Muslim internationals have thus translated the Muslim political ideational space into action through international activities to aid the Ottomans and the Muslim world writ large. Although mobilization included all strata of the societies, the educated middle class was the vanguard which negotiated the communicative space between the national and the international, between pan-Islamism as an ideology and the Muslim internationals as its actionable outcomes. The press was basically led by the educated middle and upper-middle classes, several of them having English education. The middle classes were empowered by the skills, such as language training and the press, as well as the cross-fertilization of ideas from other secular and religious internationalist processes, thanks to their 'cosmopolitan' education. These educated middle classes had realized that individually they were as competent as the best of their peers in the West. The fault for the weakness of their religious community should then be sought, in their eyes, elsewhere. At that point, however, views diverged; while some blamed the education of the masses, others resorted to other theories including alleged conspiracies. This confusion, in turn, was not peculiar to the Muslims, but was experienced by others feeling the brunt of colonialism.

Ottoman Uses and Ruses of Pan-Islamism

The Ottoman sultan and Caliph Abdulhamid II is not the person who invented pan-Islamism. Nor is he the first Ottoman sultan to have seen its potential use. However, he remains one name that is singularly associated with its effective utilization as a state policy. Ironically, he would be criticized in some quarters for not possessing all the religious, political, and moral requisites that should be present in a sultan and caliph. Abdulhamid II to this day remains a much-debated ruler who oftentimes received much criticism for his domestic policies. Tunali Hilmi, as one such critic contemporary to Abdulhamid, thus scolded the ulema including the madrasa staff, students, teachers, and judges, as well as the sheikhs and members of Sufi brotherhoods for being passive and indifferent to the wrongs of Abdulhamid's rule. He argued that their commitment to forbearance meant avoidance of social leadership against a tyrannical regime.[27] His primary motive in drafting these harsh words was to topple Abdulhamid II and bring back constitutional rule by recruiting the legitimizing support of the ulema. Tunali Hilmi, like many before and after him, realized the potential of religion to mobilize masses and thus attain scale, in his case, for the political agenda of the Committee of Union and Progress. Feeling besieged by both the modernist bureaucracy and the ulema now moving into opposition, Abdulhamid responded by appealing to the traditional loyalties and indeed the faith of the masses. Karpat observes that 'monarchy's search for alliance with the masses was something unprecedented in the past'.[28] Abdulhamid II, aware of the potential strength of the ulema, responded by increasing pressure on the religious leaders, including through vigorous surveillance and banishment as well as rewards and government positions—carrots and sticks. The pan-Islamic thought of the learned religious leaders including the Sufi orders were thus brought under his control by Abdulhamid. Abdulhamid II, and others after him, remained intent on taming and supervising the religious establishment and their public pan-Islamism. A dichotomy which existed between the state policy of pan-Islamism and its public version was made as consistent as was possible.

Although Abdulhamid II is almost unanimously credited for the employment of Islamic themes as an instrument in service of political goals, one must recall that the Ottomans had appealed to Muslim populations both within and outside their imperial domains and sought to extend their political influence over them in varying degrees throughout Ottoman history. Many of the Ottoman rulers used 'Ghazi' and 'Khan' as part of their official titles. They considered themselves as spreading the message of Islam and protecting the faith. The first international treaty that codified the Ottoman sultan's responsibilities over the Muslims was in fact the Treaty of Küçük Kaynarca with Russia in 1774, which dissected Crimea from the Ottomans but acknowledged the Ottoman caliph as the recognized religious leader of the Muslim Tatars in the independent Khanate of Crimea. In turn, of course, the Russians also codified their privilege to represent in religious matters the Orthodox Christians in Wallachia and Russian Tsars would later interpret this priviledge as a mandate to intervene on behalf of all Orthodox Christians anywhere in the Ottoman realm as they saw fit.

In the run-up to, and indeed during, the reign of Abdulhamid II, four main factors arguably brought the propagation of an Islamic or pan-Islamic identity to particular limelight. One was the fact that following the successive losses of Christian-populated territories in the preceding decades and the migration of Muslim populations into the new boundaries of the empire, the Muslim share in the Ottoman population grew to 73 per cent by the 1880s. Therefore, Muslims became the primary audience in a multinational empire which was quickly losing its non-Muslim populations.

Second, a debate raged within the Ottoman Empire, and indeed among the Muslims around the world, about how to salvage their own polities from the subjugation of the European empires. The debate included a diversity of views regarding how to treat the woes of the Muslims. The modernists who espoused Europeanization, religious revivalists from various Islamic schools of thought, the emerging middle class, as well as the nationalists were among the panoply of contenders for public opinion if not actual political power. One can add to the mix those who clung on to traditional loyalties as opposed to those which aimed to uproot them. Furthermore, another cleavage existed among the supporters of the British, French, or German empires, although not so much the Russian tsar. The Sublime Porte, in fact, contained representatives of all the various viewpoints and Weltanschauungen taking root among the Ottoman population and intelligentsia.

Third, a new international environment or international system emerged that was marked by expanding and more aggressive European imperialism, which not only threatened further territorial constriction but also greater contacts and indeed sympathies among various Muslim peoples, thanks to modern transportation and communication means.

As such, the new Ottoman state 'pan-Islamism' credited to Abdulhamid II took account of these factors and sought to employ them purposefully in the service of İstanbul's efforts to preserve the imperial realm and the Sublime Porte's efforts to hang on to power in a polity that became accustomed to rebellions and coups, one of which ultimately brought Abdulhamid II himself to power. Thus, as Şükrü Hanioğlu has argued, Hamidian pan-Islamism involved a two-pronged policy. One was to knit together the Ottoman Muslims into a more or less cohesive and governable populace. The other involved state-sponsored international propaganda directed against colonial powers ruling over Muslim populations and, I would add, threatening the Ottoman state. Abdulhamid's foundational premise was that the Ottoman Empire needed a breathing space in its attempts to reform and redeem itself, without the constant subversive and corrosive interventions of outsiders with the connivance of their agitated domestic collaborators and, I would add, threatening the Ottoman state. Without that breathing space neither economic, political, and social nor indeed military reforms underway since the early nineteenth century had held any chance of success. The first prong of Hamidian pan-Islamism thus aimed to forge a new national identity of the Ottoman Muslims. In turn, the second was a deterrent posture to create a space to rebuild the Ottoman polity without the destructive influences of external meddling. Together they were to make a coherent and mutually supportive whole in defence of the empire. It must be this conviction and sense of purpose, as much as any other alleged sociocultural or psychological factors, which led to the repressive reign that Abdulhamid II's period turned out to be.

Ideas and stratagems do matter, of course, but they need actionable instruments in order to produce effect as a state policy. Both tracks, therefore, employed a toolbox of activities and instruments which need to be highlighted in order to explain and trace the nature and impact of the Hamidian and post-Hamidian pan-Islamic state policy and Indian as well as British reactions to it.

Therefore, domestically Abdulhamid set out to build a centralized modern nation state of a sort, in this case the nation being not undergirded by an ethnicity but rather the construct of an Ottoman nation with its constituent elements moulded into a unitary polity with the caliph at its centre. He sought to institute the Hanefi strand of Islamic jurisprudence as the official school.[29] The Islamic intellegentsia was put in a straightjacket in order to streamline the debate and reinforce the particular official school of thought. Religious debate was stiffled. Instead a uniform interpretation as well as strong devoutness was encouraged through educational institutions and curricula. The official Ottoman Printing Office was mobilized to publish and disseminate approved texts chosen by a group of state-recognized religious authorities.

Abdulhamid went ahead to build up a particular personae of the caliph as a central figure by extensive utilization of Islamic symbols as well as architecture. The buildings of religious institutions, tombs of saints, and holy sites were renovated. Loyal devout Muslims were appointed to ranking judiciary positions. The salaries and pensions of the loyal ulema were increased. Abdulhamid returned the palace to the position of central executive office, subordinating the Sublime Port and the government offices and bureaucracy. The palace built a network of technocrats appointed on the basis of loyalty to the sultan caliph.

Reforms were introduced that furthered this centralization, deviating from the constitution, which was eventually to be discarded by the sultan. The palace treasury was reinforced to fund the activities directed by the sultan.

The palace promoted a number of Arab Ottomans to key positions in numbers unprecedented in Ottoman history. Similarly, Arab provinces received officials with higher pay and qualifications. A circle of Arab advisers provided advice as well as interface with the Arab local populace, which reached some 30 per cent of the entire population of the remaining territories of the empire. Various Sufi orders of particular appeal in Arab lands, including the Rifai and Kadiri, were coopted by providing government jobs, rewards, and honors to their members as well as granting of endowments. The idea of Islamic unity or pan-Islam as well as the caliph's centrality was propagated veherociously by hosting religious dignitaries from North Africa, Bosnia, Central Asia, as well as India in İstanbul.[30] The visibility of the caliph in Mecca and Medina was strenghtened. Massive propaganda for Islamic unity through newspapers, pamphlets, and free Korans supported the cause and indeed the imagery of universal caliphal authority. The Central Government strove to arrest separatist tendencies in the peripheral domains of the empire through the propagation of the idea of unity of the Muslims and the image of the authority of the sultan caliph.

The state policy cut deeply into the social life of the Ottomans. Alcohol ban was enforced, women's dress was regulated, judiciary defence against insults to religion was strengthened, and rules of moral behaviour were imposed through the state machinery. In a bid to indoctrinate the state interpretation of Islamic jurisprudence and instill a devotion to the caliph, not only religious educational establishments but also public education schools and textbooks were engineered and directed from the capital. Ethnic nationalism was strongly discouraged, albeit with little success.

As this social engineering, which Selim Deringil aptly calls the invention of tradition, was underway, the Hamidian rule also modernized the local administrations, the judiciary system, taxation, communications and transportation infrastructures, as well as the security establishment including a vast network of spies and informers. Yet modernity was going to have its toll on the big thorn in the flesh of the Ottoman polity, namely the resistance of the Muslim tribes and feudal autarchies, which proved too daunting a challenge for the Ottomans to address effectively all the way to the British subversion of the Arab desert bedouins against the Hicaz railway.

The international dimension of Hamidian and indeed Ottoman pan-Islamism could not be seen as the primary purpose and axis of their state policy. Instead various international manifestations of Ottoman pan-Islamism were a necessary corollary of the essential objective of preserving the Ottoman Empire against European imperial assault. In a bid to strengthen the sultan's legitimacy, the idea of the unity of Islam, with the caliph as the central authority, was propagated intently vis-à-vis the remaining Muslim populations of the Ottoman polity. International Muslim acceptance and indeed support of the caliphal authority strengthened the hand of the sultan both at home and also against the imperial powers which all contained significant Muslim populations within their colonial domains and, thus, were wary of any other source of legitimacy beyond their control. The pan-Islamic discourse was primarily directed towards both the Muslim populations residing in territories lost to European invasions and to the other Muslim communities which were never part of the Ottoman Empire. The real objective was never a single geopolitical Muslim entity governed by the Ottoman sultan caliph. As such pan-Islamism had to address a dual agenda. First, it needed to build up the acceptance of reverence to the caliph and thus win concrete support to the Ottoman cause across the Muslim communities in the world. Second, pan-Islamism had to sustain an aura of fear among the imperial powers against the caliph's potential political influence among their colonized populations.

The instruments of pan-Islamism in the international arena overlapped to some degree with the instruments used within the Ottoman state. As such, contacts, propaganda, religious propagation, employment of rewards and honours, and avoiding administrative and advisory positions—all found their place in the Ottoman pan-Islamic toolbox, both domestically and internationally. Thus, the Ottoman sultan caliph hosted prominent figures and ulema from other Muslim nationalities in Turkey. Making use of the caliphal authority, the sultan appointed *mufti*s, *qadi*s, and *mudarris*es to former Ottoman domains including in Egypt, Crimea, Bulgaria, Bosnia, and Cyprus. Missions were dispatched, such as the one led by Baghdad-based Seyyid Süleyman Efendi, during the 1877–8 Russo-Turkish War, to seek support from Indian Muslims. Similar missions were also sent to Algeria, Tunisia, and Morocco. The Islamic treatises and textbooks printed in İstanbul were dispatched to religious institutions around the world. Letters were exchanged between Ottoman statesmen and prominent Muslim thought leaders. The caliph stood up for the rights of the Muslims even in Liverpool.[31]

The transnational networks of the Sufi brotherhoods carrying favour with the caliph's court played a major role in advocating worldwide the ideal of Islamic unity and propagating in favour of the Ottoman sultan as well as the inspirational and rightful Ottoman fight against the European imperialists. As Özcan highlights, the Sufis helped in fostering communication with Muslims elsewhere, including in India, and cultivated loyalty to the caliph and sympathy to the Ottomans.[32] Landau underscores that the Ottomans sent preachers, messengers, and emissaries to advocate Islamic unity, including in a clandestine fashion.[33] Deringil notes that students from other Muslim lands received scholarships in Ottoman schools.[34] Consular officials were activated from North Africa to China and assumed active part in spreading sympathy towards the Ottomans and the caliph as well as raising funds. The particular effort that was made to increase the visibility of the caliph at the cities hosting the two holy mosques and during the annual Hajj pilgrimage served the domestic and international audience simultaneously. Ottomans made good use of the Hajj and distributed pamphlets and placards, which the pilgrims carried back to their home countries.[35] A massive effort was underway to refute the industrial scale disinformation pouring from various European imperial quarters, missionaries, and orientalists through the press. Another effort also involved the newspapers and aimed to counteract the propaganda that sought to undermine the caliph's acceptance by Muslims. Thus, when the *Al-Khalifa* newspaper published in London launched a campaign that confronted the Ottoman hold on Islamic caliphate and called for a rebellion of the oppressed Arabs, Ottoman Ambassador Musurus Pasha responded by sponsoring the *al-Ghayrat* newspaper which emphasized the Ottoman caliphate.[36] In order to showcase the global sympathies for Abdulhamid II and the Ottomans, the Ertuğrul frigate toured the Indian Ocean in 1889–90 to much popular acclaim in all the harbours it visited, yet sank on the way back from Japan at a storm. Even this cursory listing of various instruments employed by Abdulhamid II and his successors demonstrate the vast spectrum and busy practical content of pan-Islamist Ottoman state policy.

Whether in the domestic or in the international track, the specific set of activities that sustained Ottoman state pan-Islamism involved close interaction, communication, alliances with specific eminent minds, dispatch of overt and covert missions, and, above all, playing to the fears of the domestic or international enemies. The latter point needs an example and an emphasis. The test of pan-Islamism's success was not whether it engendered a global Muslim state led by the Ottoman caliph, which was not its real or realistic purpose in the first place. The test was instead the impact these activities had made in the perceptions of the European imperial powers regarding İstanbul's remaining political influence in the last decades of the Ottoman Empire's long existence. From that vantage point, the Ottoman use of pan-Islamism did provide significant value to their efforts to galvanize international support for their fight against extinction in the face of a determined and relentless physical and psychological attack by European imperialism. Given the considerable attention that the use of Ottoman pan-Islamic instruments of statecraft received in rival countries, their actions must have yielded credibility to their defensive claims of influence. Perhaps nowhere was the influence of specifically Ottoman based pan-Islamic proclivities more credible and strong than in the late nineteenth- and early twentieth-century British-ruled India. One would see in the context particularly of the British Empire that the Ottomans quickly became aware of the European fear of the idea of Muslim unity, which acquired a phobic dimension.

One can argue that the European fear of Islamic unity was not the making of the Ottomans or other Muslims. In fact, whatever the discourse, in reality the idea that Muslims everywhere would simultaneously rebel and topple the British rule could not have convinced even the sultan caliph himself. The Ottomans could not have called for jihad until the First World War and that too at misguided German advice. The call fell on silent ears in India where Muslims did not see this as an opportunity to reclaim what they lost in 1857. While Abdulhamid II did not invent fear-mongering among the Europeans, neither he nor his successors shied away from capitalizing on it in order to strengthen their hand in their dealings with European empires. I would argue that the Europeans fell victim to suspecting of the Ottomans the subversion that they practised against the Ottomans and indeed each other.

An example in that regard could be the dispatch of a high-level delegation in 1877 to Afghanistan in order to seek the support of the Afghan Amir Shir Ali Khan against Russia. The Ambassadorial Mission of Şirvanizade Ahmed Hulusi Efendi to Afghanistan, as the mission was chronicled,[37] was sent by Abdulhamid II soon after the Russians started the 1877 war in April. For the Afghans and the Ottomans, Russia was a common enemy as the Russians were pressing hard against Afghanistan and eastern Turkestan after Bukhara, Kokand, and Khiva came under their control. The British had responded only a year earlier by occupying Quetta. Afghanistan was suffering as a buffer zone as the Great Game of competition and rivalry between the British and Russian empires unfolded in Central Asia. The Afghans, however, had adopted a policy of balance between the two formidable empires. They had refused the British demand to open a resident embassy, whose aim would be to influence, if not direct, the external policies of Afghanistan. Thus, the Ottoman diplomatic mission in 1877 to Afghanistan was encouraged and supported by the British authorities and was, in fact, received in Bombay by the British mayor and escorted to Afghanistan by British authorities. The mission failed to obtain its objective of convincing the Afghan ruler to maintain cordial relations with England as the Afghan ruler rightly and rather expectedly insisted on British withdrawal from Quetta. Wasti relates, 'The Amir stated that his desire was to see an independent and neutral Afghanistan, although his country had to contend simultaneously with the enmity of Russia, Iran and Great Britain, of which the most pressing and aggressive was that of Britain.'[38] However, the Afghan amir seemed to have promised support to the Ottomans should they be attacked by the Iranians. The Afghan ruler was to pay dearly for his refusal to comply with British demands put nicely through the Ottoman delegation. He would be deposed by the British next year and die soon after in Mezar-i Sherif. His appeal for help from the Russians would not be heeded.

The point one needs to make here, however, is that the warm reception accorded to the Ottoman diplomatic mission by the Indian and Afghan Muslims made the British authorities apprehensive even though the mission itself was conceived due to the pressure of the British authorities in the first place. Thus, Syed Tanvir Wasti quotes a contemporary account of the Ottoman mission by one of its members, Ahmed Behai Efendi:

> [T]he Ottoman mission reached Bombay where the party was received with a salute of 15 guns by [Ottoman Consul General] Hüseyin Hasib Efendi and the Mayor of Bombay, a Mr Grant. Hüseyin Hasib was an active Consul-General and, as a representative of the most important Islamic state of the time, was the focus of much popular attention. The Bombay Muslims therefore gave a rousing and vociferous welcome to the envoys of the Sultan-Caliph.[39]

The Ottoman envoys would be spirited away from Bombay by the worried local British authorities in order to wait for the appointment with the Afghan amir in Rawalpindi in today's Pakistan. Azmi Özcan writes that the British authorities had planned a chance encounter in Bombay with viceroy Lytton who would suggest the inclusion in the delegation of Syed Ahmad Khan as the only thoroughly loyal and trustworthy Mahomedan. That, however, apparently that did not materialize.[40] The delegation did, however, travel to Aligarh on their return from Afghanistan and met Syed Ahmad Khan. Ironically, the Afghans perceived the diplomatic mission as a British ploy to advance its interests, as the British themselves came to believe that the outpouring of sympathy shown to the Turkish diplomats acquired an anti-British tinge. In fact, the project to use and bolster the Ottoman Sultan Caliph Abdulhamid II's influence was suspect from the beginning. First, it went against the British policy of neutrality in the 1877–8

Russo-Turkish War. And second, the British viceroy in India had reservations about its longer-term impact in India from the outset. The weapon that the British sought to develop, they feared, could also turn against them. I would reminisce the seminal question in Mary Shelley's 1818 classic *Frankenstein*, the story of a creature which turns on its creator: 'Why did you create me if you were not ready to love me?'

Pan-Islamism and the Ottoman sultan's prestige and influence in India was used and abused by the British Empire even before the Ottoman Sultan Abdulhamid II gave it a certain shape and vigor. One would recall the British use of that instrument since the revolt of Tipu Sultan and his call for support from the Ottoman caliph. However, pan-Islamism or the politics of Islamic unity and the associated global Muslim public opinion against colonialism became a true headache for the British authorities in India.

Nonetheless, it would be a mistake to confine the Hamidian statecraft and its use of pan-Islamism to the diplomatic overtures here and there. The real manifestation of Abdulhamid's politics was internal reform that was accompanied by heavy-handed implementation and the internationalist coalition his government managed to deploy behind the strategic project of the Hicaz Railway. His pan-Islamism cannot be construed as a reactionary conservatism. Abdulhamid II was a reformer of first degree and his most prominent achievements were not only political, such as the first Ottoman constitution promulgated on 23 December 1876 soon after he came to power by replacing his deranged brother and suspended in February 1878 following the disastrous war with Russia. The modernist reformism of this much-assailed ruler was manifest most prominently in the 11 vocational and professional schools, the Dar-ul Fünun later to be known the İstanbul University, and the vast network of primary, secondary, as well as modern military schools he spawned over the 32 years, 7 months, and 27 days of his rule in a tumultuous world of conflict and war. His modernism was also manifest in the railways and telegraphic lines that his government built around the empire.

The internationalist *piece de resistance* of his geopolitical but also pan-Islamist policy was, in fact, the Hicaz railroad from Damascus to Medina, which was financed without any European debt, thanks to some degree the subscriptions from Muslims from outside the Ottoman Empire including the Indian subcontinent, although most of funds were raised within the empire. The funds collected by the Indians covered 15,000 out of the total of 3 million Ottoman currency needed to complete the railway.[41] The 800-mile-long railroad was built in eight years between 1900 and 1908. As James Nicholson wrote:

> [T]he reputation that it truly deserves is for the epic story of its construction, a monumental feat of engineering, requiring enormous imagination, skill and resolve. Here was something breathtaking, combining the romance of steam locomotion with the grandiose vision of the last years of the mighty Ottoman Empire ... It was to lay its tracks across pitiless, wadi-fissured deserts and the unforgiving mountains of the Hejaz, from which the line would earn its name.[42]

The railway which was announced at the twenty-fifth anniversary of Abdulhamid II's accession to the throne on 1 May 1900 was completed under the supervision of German engineers. The main artery between Damascus and Medina was supplemented by an offshoot to Haifa, thereby turning this small town into an important exit for Damascus to the Mediterranean sea.[43]

Although due to the attacks by the Bedouin tribes and the sabotages instigated by the British agent provocateur T. E. Lawrence, much of the railway suffered damages, limited remaining sections of the railway continued after the end of the First World War to provide a lifeline to the regional economy. Lawrence's fixation on destroying the railway was not without a reason. First, the railway became an object of pride for Muslims both in the Ottoman Empire and outside. After Abdulhamid II made the first donation and appealed to all Muslims to raise funds, contributions poured in from all quarters. Whether in Tajikistan or Egypt, people contributed what they could. In India, Mohammad Inshaullah established the Central Committee of the Hejaz Railway 'which appealed to both Muslims and Hindus all over India to donate for the project by highlighting both the difficulty of the pilgrim route from Damascus, and the commercial benefits which might come about as a result of the railway'.[44] The Indians did respond passionately.

Özcan states that some Indians reduced the cost of their weddings and funerals in order to contribute to the funds for the railway.[45] The Ottomans rewarded the major donors in India by awarding gold medals.

Another reason for the British government's targeting of the Hicaz railway was because it was believed to be part of the Ottoman and indeed German efforts to find alternative routes to the Indian Ocean, given that the British had taken control of the Suez Canal, another Ottoman project, but one which they could not carry out. It also could help extend Ottoman reach deep into Arabia including militarily. The geo-economic considerations did indeed play strongly in İstanbul's determination to build the Hicaz railway. As the private secretary to Sultan Abdulhamid II wrote later, the intention of the Ottoman ruler was to reinstitute the 'ancient road' which connected India and Europe through which the bi-directional trade flourished.[46] Shifting the axis of trade from the British-dominated Indian Ocean back to the land of the Silk Road would bring significant Ottoman control over a voluminous trade and thus accrue economic benefits to the empire. The Silk Road was a network of routes for caravans for a thousand years, controlled by the Turks and Mongols and generally running in the east–west axis, with branches in all directions: 'Between China and Samarkand in Central Asia, the traveller had a choice between a route that went north of the Tienshan mountains through Jungaria, or south of them through the Tarim basin and its city-states.'[47] Hardly any tradesman would venture the entire length of the network of roads, more than 6,000 kilometres long. The one who did was Marco Polo from Venice and his travel would fascinate the world all the way to our day and age. In addition to being a trade route carrying silk, porcelain, amber, furs, pharmaceuticals and slaves, the Silk Road was a system of communication and exchange, the most important such network in the world until the sixteenth century. Reviving that route today in the twenty-first century would change the fortunes of inner Asia linking the zone between Europe, Turkey, China, and India to a world of opportunities by removing the region's relative insularity. But that is another story.

The story of the Hicaz Railway simultaneously demonstrates the appeal and the limits of pan-Islamism. The limits became obvious with the violent reaction of the Muslim Bedouin tribes of Arabia who took up arms to thwart the extension of the railway to Mecca, which would destroy their traditional source of income, namely renting camels to the pilgrims en route to the holy city of Mecca. Facilitation of the Hajj for the pilgrims, the strong pan-Islamic support behind the project, and other religious considerations did not matter for the Bedouin Muslims who only wanted to carry on renting camels. This clash of mundane interests which the Ottoman government could not resolve finally turned into an explosive bomb in the hands of the rival British Empire that provoked and supported the rebellion of 1916. Abdulhamid II had fulfilled his dream by building the Hicaz Railway, which served his policy to centralize government, facilitate İstanbul's reach into Ottoman territories in the Muslim Middle East, and prove the utility of appealing to Muslim solidarity across the Muslim world. Yet, the same dream culminated in the final blow to the Ottoman Empire, the loss of its Arab possessions by giving the British Empire a useful instrument, the tribal opposition to the Hicaz Railway and the modernity it would bring to their ancient way of life and subsistence.

Indian Muslim's Embrace of Pan-Islamism

As part of the global Muslim public opinion, Indian Muslims embraced pan-Islamism almost instinctively. The long nineteenth century was unkind to the Indian Muslims. The Great Rebellion of 1857 culminated in the final deposition of a Muslim empire which had ruled over that glittering microcosm of human civilization called the Indian subcontinent, home as it was to a colourful melange of nations, castes, and almost every religion known to mankind. What was once the mighty Mughal Empire was first diminished to nothingness by the East India Company, which came first to trade and then to subjugate. The process of subordination was slow in the making and incremental. Over a period of centuries, multiple actors, including the Portuguese, the Dutch, and the French, diluted the empire's power, downgraded its revenues, co-opted its domestic rivals, and ripped up the empire step by step. The arch domestic enemy of the Mughal Empire, the Maratha Empire, could not hold on to power for long. Having been defeated first by the Afghans and then by the British, the Marathas too were subjugated.

By 1857, the last remnants of the indigenous Indian empires, whether Muslim, Hindu, or Sikh, disappeared from the face of the subcontinent. India was again shattered into pieces, only held together by a system of alliances overseen by the British Empire, without a uniting, shared political contract between the rulers and the ruled. This was not unique to the Muslims in India. In his detailed study of the Khilafat Movement in India, M. Naeem Qureshi noted: 'What made pan-Islam more intelligible to Indian Muslims was the growing consciousness among them that they were the members of a world-wide ecumenical community, stretching from the shores of the Atlantic to the Straits of Malacca in one unbroken chain.'[48] This community shared a perception of attack against its core values and indeed against its own very existence.

The genesis of the pan-Islamist idea and its appeal in India owes directly to the fears associated with the long and painful cannibalization of the Ottoman Empire, which intensified, albeit unrelatedly, around the time of the end of the Mughal Empire. Ishtiaq Ahmad noted that the idea of pan-Islamism in India, beyond the traditional concept of the single Islamic nation (ummah), culminated in the 1919 Khilafat Movement, which 'was an expression of the Subcontinent Muslims' sentimental attachment to the Ottoman Turks, who were perceived as not only the last stronghold of Islam but also their Sultan was viewed as the Caliph of all Muslims'.[49] Naeem Qureshi also underscored that 'in the political turmoil of the early twentieth century India, renewed challenges to the daru'l-Islam from strident imperialism fuelled still further Indo-Muslim enthusiasm for the Ottomans'.[50]

Education's Role in Empowering Dissent

At one level the British Raj, as the British rule in India had come to be known, at its apogee directly governed only half of India, the other near half being administered by allied Indian nobility.

As M. J. Akbar reminded, 'School maps did show the whole of India painted red, but the princely states were not technically a part of British India. A separate accession treaty had to be obtained from each one of the 565 princely states on this subcontinent at the time of independence.'[51] However, this did not mean that Indians ruled the subcontinent. The Raj had the prerogative to grant or withhold recognition of individual rulers, who either had few rights or their rights were handed to them by agreements with the British authorities. The power-sharing arrangements, particularly in regional legislative affairs, announced by the Secretary of State for India Edwin Montagu in August 1917 was in the words of London-born President of the Indian National Congress and the Theosophical Society Annie Beasant, 'unworthy of Britain to offer and of India to accept'. Although the British Indian Civil Service included Indians, separated by race, their ranks were low and their contribution to policymaking negligible.[52] Matters of high politics such as diplomacy or national defence were outright beyond the Indian reach. Jawaharlal Nehru was to famously ridicule the British Indian Civil Service 'as neither Indian, nor civil, nor a service'. The so-called Government of India was not in any way the government of the people, by the people, for the people of India. Until it won its independence in the mid-twnentieth century through determined civil resistance, India was part of a non-Asian but European empire whose peoples never saw the sun the same way.

The British power was, nonetheless, pervasive and transformative in intent, deeply penetrating into the social, economic, and political fabric of the country, under the rubric of the civilizing process. The introduction of European education owed as much to the mundane needs of the colonial administration for appropriately trained manpower as the strivings of an elite to demonstrate their civility and equality. The East India Company assumed responsibility in the area of education as early as in 1813. The purpose was the 'encouragement of the learned natives' and the 'revival and improvement' of literature as well as 'introduction and promotion' of sciences. Two years later, the Company started to focus its funds on 'the best means of improving the education of more respectable members of Indian society' rather than education of the masses starting with primary levels.[53] Shanti Tangri explains that '[f]or the next two decades the Government encouraged classical learning in Sanskrit, Arabic and Persian, the missionaries promoted the vernaculars and primary education, while the native urban gentry (mostly Hindu tax farmers, landlords, nouveau-riche businessmen, civilian and military government officials in Calcutta and Bombay) sponsored Western education through the medium of English.'[54] In 1835, English and Western education became the new official policy of British authorities in India.[55] Owing in no small degree to the need to find suitable recruits to the Indian cadres of the British government in India, in 1854 a policy was set out to 'spread European knowledge among all classes of people' by establishing universities and teacher training colleges, supporting private educational institutions, government schools and colleges, developing primary education, and encouraging education of females, Muslims, lower castes, the poor, and the backward.[56] This policy also secularized English language education. By 1857, three universities were established along the model of the University of London. Economic and social transformation gathered pace around the time. Railroads began to crisscross the subcontinent. The cotton textile industry was introduced to Bombay and jute to Bengal. By the 1890s, India had already embarked upon a rapid course of industrialization and urbanization. University education picked up so much so that 'between 1885 and 1900 college students increased from 11,000 to 23,000 and secondary students from 429,000 to 633,000'.[57] Emigration also occurred in large numbers although many were to return due to harsh conditions faced abroad. The number of Indian youth who had travelled outside India or completed their higher education in England reached thousands in the final four decades of the nineteenth century.[58] As Tangri noted, '[M]odern education resulting from contacts with the West, created a whole class of people who found new avenues for advancement, new mobilities, new techniques, new perspectives and new goals. They were not only opinion makers in their societies, they were the makers of new societies.'[59] However, at the same time, Western education also helped create and empower dissenters. Whether it was the conditions of indentured labour on indigo plantations, depicted forcefully in Dinabandhu Mitra's novel *Nil Darpan*, or the nascent ideas and resentments that returning migrant workers brought back home, or numerous other tribulations that colonialism engendered—these were more skilfully voiced, thanks to European education.

Tangri notes that 'Westernized Hindus, Parsis, and Christians, had learned the value of public meetings and political organization and were demanding representative government' in India.[60] Yet until 1886 not a single Muslim went for education to England.[61] Observing that the rejection of Western education had been causing the Muslim youth to stay behind in commerce, industry, as well as government jobs, Sir Syed Ahmed Khan established the Madrasatul Uloom Musalmanan-e-Hind or Mohammedan Ango-Oriental College at Aligarh in 1875 to modernize the education system of the Indian Muslims. During his travel to England he was impressed by the orderliness of Europe. He noted that the Ottoman Egypt was more developed technologically than India. As Wasti underscored, 'Sir Syed did not prescribe a blind imitation of European institutions and paraphernalia, but opted for what might be called "the Turkish model". He recognized that the Turks had already gone down the route of his first, diffident steps. He did not wish to undermine the Islamic curriculum but to update it.'[62] The Mohammedan Anglo-Oriental College, which later transformed into the Aligarh Muslim University, has rendered great service to the education of countless Muslim youth. These included several members and organizers of the 1912–13 Indian Medical Mission to Ottoman Turkey. The college also turned into an incubator for pan-Islamism and nationalism in India.

The drawn-out campaign to establish a Muslim university between 1898 and 1920 is instructive of how education was seen as a means for the enfranchisement of the Muslims of India or, as the Aligarh College's English principal Theodore Beck put it, the passport to government service.[63] However, Syed Ahmad Khan's own interpretations of reformist Islam as well as his unflinching loyalty to the British Empire put him at odds with the Ottomans when London started to drift from friendship with the Turks to outright hostility. In the meantime, some Indian Muslim religious scholars were exploring the option of an alliance with the Ottomans against the British Raj. This gathered pace with the advent of the twentieth century when the religious seminaries at

Deoband and Firangi Mahal were fervently pursuing anti-British political thought. The Muslim public opinion was inexorably coming under the grip of the pan-Islamic, pro-Ottoman movement aided by the establishment of the Anjuman-i Islam in 1876 and the Anjuman-i Khuddam-i Ka'ba in 1913.

Ottoman Travails and the Indian Muslim Public Opinion

At the turn of the twentieth century, the geopolitical competition was among various European-based empires including the Americans and Russians. No Asian or African geopolitical power entertained any hope of challenging this total domination by the Christian white men. Among the rare remaining pockets of resistance, the Ottoman Empire was the only Muslim state. The Ottomans may be called the 'Romans of the Muslim World', as historian Albert Hourani was to write.[64] They were part and parcel of the Eurocentric balance of power system. As of 1856 they acceded to the Concert of Europe alongside other European empires. The Ottomans' encounter with nineteenth-century European imperialism, however, positioned them as a leading anti-imperialist empire.[65] Their fight against European imperialism became an inspiration to the colonized peoples around the world, not the least in India.

Ultimately, the Ottoman Empire was demolished in a long and sustained collective assault by its enemies from the outside and inside. Yet, it died hardly as a 'sick man' as the popular European derisive moniker suggests. Instead, as Elie Kedourie indicated, the Ottoman Empire 'for all his alleged sickness,... did not die of disease, but was violently destroyed in a long and bitter war in which he proved a formidable opponent and gave quite a good account of himself'.[66] Even after its demise the empire left behind enough vision, will, and manpower not to allow colonization of its Turkish heartland. However, its breath did not suffice to help establish a stable order in its former West Asian territories in place of the shattered Ottoman one. We are still to witness the painful ramifications of this in our day and age. The fight of the Ottomans and then the Turks inspired anti-imperialists everywhere, including the

Muslims as far as in India and Indonesia. The ideas the Ottomans produced and debated in the process was spread around, discussed, and indeed followed by Muslims in different geographies. Outside the Ottoman realm, all discussions on the future of Islamic peoples seemed to revolve around the struggle of the Ottomans.

Pan-Islamism in India at the turn of the twentieth century fulfilled and derived strength from the function of uniting the Indian Muslim community around a political and humanitarian cause. They came closest to uniting around a single cause when the news of atrocities against the Balkan Turks started dominating their newspapers since the late nineteenth century. The news of coordinated 'Christian attack' against the Turks reached India with the twentieth century's telegraphic speed; it was disseminated through eloquent newspapers and wrought havoc among the masses. At the beginning of the century, Indian Muslims were as divided as ever. There was, however, 'an increasing awareness of how the expansion of European power was increasingly subjecting Muslims to Christian rule'.[67] The idea of pan-Islam filled a certain ideational vacuum across the Muslim world, including in India. 'Because Turkey alone of all Moslem countries is free, because, the Turks alone have power to defeat enemies not overwhelmingly strong and the manliness to prefer death to slavery', wrote Dr Ansari retrospectively in 1935, 'the imagination of the Indian Moslems converted them into as convinced Pan-Islamists as they themselves, and placed on their shoulders the burden not only of defending their hearth and home, but the honour of Islam and all Moslem peoples as well'.[68] This sentiment produced public mobilization towards concrete outcomes. As Slyvia Haim Kedourie noted, pan-Islamism made 'Islam into the mainspring of solidarity, and thus ... placed it on the same footing as other solidarity-producing beliefs'.[69]

Thus, writes Özcan, 'The Deobandis, the Barelvis, the Farang-i Mahalis, and the *Nadvatu'l-Ulema*, as well as the Shiis, came together. The Deobandis issued a fatwa declaring that support for the Turks was incumbent on Muslims and that *zakat* (alms) should be given to relief funds.'[70] K. H. Ansari explains that pan-Islamist opposition to the British rule in India was represented by four major strands.[71] All of them had a connection or at least sympathy to Turkey. The first was led by Muhammad and Shaukat Ali (the Ali brothers), as well as Maulana Hasrat Mohani and Zafar Ali Khan from Aligarh. These young and Western-educated Muslims edited the *Comrade*, *Hamdard*, *Urdu-i Mu'alla*, and *Zamindar* newspapers, harping on Muslim issues, such as protesting against the bulldozing of Muslim shrines as the British built New Delhi with imperial grandeur. All of these newspapers passionately supported the Ottomans as European powers took turns to dismember the only remaining independent Muslim state and the seat of the caliph. The second strand was led by Abul Kalam Azad, who was to become independent India's first minister of culture. He signed the first-ever cultural cooperation agreement of the nascent Republic of India, which was with Turkey. Following Jamaluddin Afghani, Azad was a strong proponent of Muslim–Hindu alliance and promoted political organization in revolt againt the British. Azad visited Iraq, Egypt, Syria, and Turkey towards the end of Abdulhamid's reign in 1908, and started publishing the *Al Hilal* newspaper, which expressed strong sympathy with Turkey and 'exhorted Muslims to do their duty to struggle against British power which did not respect Islam'.[72] The third strand was led by some members of the Deoband religious seminary including Mahmud al-Hasan who underscored the need to return to the original precepts of Islam and the possibility of the purification and renewal of Islam after independence was achieved. The fourth strand was composed of those who left India, including Qidwai, Yaqub Husain, and Nazir Ahmad, for Europe, West Asia, and Afghanistan, some settling in İstanbul. These strands and indeed the masses were united around the core issue of the protection of the Ottoman Empire against colonialist assault.

Pan-Islamism and Indian Nationalism

Pan-Islamism defined an agenda to counter or aid the targeted Muslim nations. It was, however, not about defining a religious identity or a religious space at home. This was instead negotiated by a budding nationalism which was increasingly avid on its criticism of the British rule. As historian Nikkie Keddie pointed out, 'on closer examination, pan-Islam seems to have more resemblance to modern nationalist movements than to older Islamic feelings' and as such it 'was an important step in the transition from Islamic to national loyalties'.[73] The feeling of solidarity with fellow Muslims was a manifestation of the strong pan-Islamist sentiment of a mobilized Indian Muslim civil society entering a political space. Such comity risked the very existence of European colonialism, which depended on insatiable exploitation of far-away, including Muslim, wealth and resources. This concerned foremost the British Empire that counted by far the greatest number of Muslims within its dominion. Ironically, the initial reaction of the British rulers of India was rather supportive of pan-Islamist movement. After all, the British Empire was able to deploy the coveted help of the Ottoman caliph to calm the restive Indian Muslim population. This could work as long as Britain supported the Ottoman Empire. Yet, when Britain changed course in late nineteenth century and then, in fact, joined in the feast in the twentieth, pan-Islamism became a problem for its own survival as an empire. As such, the movement would grow from pro-Turkish to include anti-British, from pro-caliph to pro-independence like bush fire within mere decades. Keddie appears correct in suggesting that pan-Islamism functioned as proto-nationalism. The national agenda was not yet unequivocally defined. This would have to wait for a few more decades of debate and action comprising all segments of the Indian population of the British Raj.

The British Empire's apprehension of the fervour for pan-Islamic solidarity was, therefore, not without reason. Humayun Ansari notes, 'Between 1908 and the outbreak of the first world war, Pan-Islamism in India, which had been simmering steadily beneath the surface, erupted into active opposition to the British.'[74] On 17 October 1912, the New York Times was reporting from Simla: 'The fear that the British Government has of a Moslem outbreak in India as a reaction against the defeat of the Turks by the Christian nations in the Balkans has been betrayed in the speech made by the British Viceroy in adjourning the Legislative Council this week.' In that speech, Lord Hardinge would praise the Turkish soldiers and state: 'I would add a word of friendly warning to the Moslem community in India not to forget that they form

a part of a great empire, and not to give an unreasonable interpretation to the idea of Islamic solidarity. Nor must the Hindu
community here make a similar mistake.'[75] The latter statement
demonstrates in small degree the existence of strong feelings
towards the fate of the Ottoman Turkey also among the Hindu
community of the British Raj. Yet the events of the Balkan Wars
and the subsequent First World War, which led to the final demise
of the Ottoman Empire, unleashed the figurative Indian Muslim
genie out of the lantern. Thus, writes Mushirul Hasan, 'Money
and ornaments poured into the Khilafat fund, thousands flocked
to the Khilafat meetings, and some even left the fields and factories to migrate to the Dar al-Islam in response to a call for hijrat.
Students quit their studies and joined the swelling ranks of non-
cooperators, while many of their elders gave up their lucrative
jobs and high-sounding titles.'[76] Sufi orders, including the Shazeli
and Rufai, sent their disciples around to propagate in favour of
the Ottoman caliph. However, as far as the Indian Muslim community was concerned, the crystallization of a nationalist agenda would need to wait until the abolishment of the caliphate in
Turkey, which destroyed a unifying theme and shifted the focus of
the Indian Muslim community inwards to India. Increasing divergence about the religious space and the feasibility of co-habitation
with the majority Hindus would gradually strengthen the movement for separation of the two communities, culminating in the
1947 partition of independent India. This debate became as much
within the Indian Muslims as it was *between* Muslims and the
Hindus.

Commenting on the tumultuous last decades of the Ottoman
Empire and the Indian Muslims' passionate sympathy and sup-
port for the caliphate in İstanbul, Dr Mukhtar Ahmad Ansari
would bemoan in hindsight that '[i]t is difficult for anyone not an
Indian Muslim to realise what Pan-Islamism means to the Indian
Muslims ... It is a sentiment of which the prayers for Turkish success in the Tripolitan and Balkan wars, the Relief Fund, the Medical
Mission and even the Khilafat movement were but weak and fal-
tering expressions.'[77] On the long road to Indian independence, the
Indian Medical Mission during the 1912–13 Balkan Wars would be
an unacknowledged station.

Among the several medical teams deployed in Ottoman Turkey, Dr Ansari's Mission was one that became particularly revered and trusted and seems to have overshadowed the others. The letters of Dr Ansari were instrumental in Mohammad Ali's efforts to rally continued support and provide essential feedback to the masses back in India who contributed morally and financially to the Mission. One could argue that the success of the Indian Medical Mission owes in large part to the efficiency of Dr Ansari and his colleagues in running the Mission and liaising with the Turkish authorities, and Maulana Mohammad Ali Jauhar's influence in publicizing the work of the Mission with admirable power of the written word. In other words, the personalities involved in this particular medical team had made all the difference in distinguishing their effort from the other and perhaps equally useful medical interventions.

This chapter has outlined the pan-Islamism of 1913 involving both a shared public opinion and a defensive strategy that was internationalist as well as proto-nationalist in nature. It has underscored the common themes that generated profound sincerity about the sympathy towards the Turks, the Ottoman anti-imperialist and anti-Christian supremacist struggle, the concern for the future of the caliphate and the state of the Muslim world, as well as awareness and distaste towards the deliberate and latent reconstruction of the Muslim past and the denigration of Muslim culture. It has also highlighted the appeal to action to resurrect the dignity of the Muslim nation both at home and in the rest of the Muslim world. In terms of strategy, the foregoing sections have drawn attention to the quest for attaining scale to empower the primary opposition to colonial rule and emerging nationalist focus as well as the successful use of modernity and modern technology and media. The chapter has also introduced the Muslim internationalist framework of action in a bid to rid the legacy of the Indian Medical Mission of the corruptive formulations of Islamic unity or the Western pejorative counterpart term of pan-Islam that had held sway to our day and age.

The following Part will tell the story of the Indian Medical Mission from the eyes of the leader of the team and provide a rudimentary analysis of their labour of love in Turkey.

Notes

1. Pankaj Mishra, *From the Ruins of Empire: The Revolt against the West and the Remaking of Asia* (London: Allen Lane, 2012), p. 42.

2. Dipesh Chakrabarty, *Provincializing Europe: Postcolonial Thought and Historical Difference* (Princeton: Princeton University Press, 2000), pp. 3–9. Also, Gyan Prakash, 'Postcolonial Criticism and Indian Historiography', in *Social Text*, vols 31–2 (1992), p. 17.

3. Jose Abraham, 'A Discussion on the Possibility of a Subaltern Reading of Indian Muslim History', Association of *Muslim* Social Scientists of North America (AMSS) 35th Annual Conference 'Muslim Identities: Shifting Boundaries and Dialogues', co-sponsored by Hartford Seminary, Hartford, Connecticut (27 October–29 October 2006), p. 4.

4. Cemil Aydın, 'Islamic Traditions of the Muslim World: The Legions of the Late 19th Century Intellectual History', AMSS 38th Annual Conference 'Islamic Traditions and Comparative Modernities', 25–26 September 2009, p. 4.

5. Carter Vaughn Findley, 'An Ottoman Occidentalist in Europe: Ahmed Midhat Meets Madame Gulnar, 1889', *American Historical Review* 103, no. 1 (1998), pp. 15–49.

6. Aydın, 'Islamic Traditions of the Muslim World', p. 5.

7. Aydın, 'Islamic Traditions of the Muslim World', p. 5.

8. Benoy Kumar Sarkar, *The Futurism of Young Asia, and Other Essays on the Relations between the East and the West* (Berlin: Julius Springer, 1922), p. 12.

9. Sarkar, *The Futurism of Young Asia*, p. 1.

10. Terence Ranger, 'Connexions between "Primary Resistance" Movements and Modern Mass Nationalisms in East and Central Africa', *Journal of African History* 9, no. 3 (1968), 437–53.

11. Aydın, 'Islamic Traditions of the Muslim World', p. 6.

12. Nikki R. Keddie, 'Pan-Islam as Proto-Nationalism', *Journal of Modern History* 41, no. 1 (March 1969), p. 18.

13. 'Pan-Islamism', in John L. Esposito, ed., *The Oxford Dictionary of Islam*, available at Oxford Islamic Studies Online, http://www.oxfordislamicstudies.com/article/opr/t125/e1819 (accessed on 17 January 2013).

14. Edmund Burke, 'Pan-Islam and Moroccan Resistance to French Colonial Penetration, 1900–1912', *Journal of African History* 13, no. 1 (1972), p. 99.

15. K. H. Ansari, 'Pan-Islam and the Making of the Early Indian Muslim Socialists', *Modern Asian Studies* 20, no. 3 (1986), p. 510.

16. Aydın, 'Islamic Traditions of the Muslim World', p. 13.

17. See Selçuk Esenbel, 'Japan's Global Claim to Asia and the World of Islam: Transnational Nationalism and World Power, 1900–1945', *American Historical Review* 109, no. 4 (October 2004), pp. 1140–70.

18. M. Şemseddin (Günaltay), *Hurafattan Hakikate* (From Superstitions to Truth) (İstanbul: Tevsi-i Tıbaat Matbaası 1916), pp. 3–5.

19. Khaled Adeeb, 'Pan-Islamism in Practice: The Rhetoric of Islamic Unity and Its Uses', in Elisabeth Özdalga, ed., *Late Ottoman Society: The Intellectual Legacy* (New York: Routledge Curzon, 2005), p. 205.

20. Azmi Özcan, 'Peyk-i İslam: 1880'de İstanbul'da Çikarilan Bir Gazete ve İngiltere'nin Kopardiği Firtina', *Tarih ve Toplum*, no. 99 (March 1992), pp. 169–73.

21. Kemal Karpat, *The Politization of Islam: Reconstructing Identity, State, Faith, and Community in the Late Ottoman State* (Oxford: Oxford University Press, 2001), p. 212.

22. Karpat, *The Politization of Islam*, p. 213.

23. Abigail Green and Vincent Viaene, eds, *Religious Internationals in the Modern World: Globalization and Faith Communities since 1750* (Houndmills: Palgrave, 2012), p. 1.

24. Abigail Green and Vincent Viaene, eds, *Religious Internationals in the Modern World: Globalization and Faith Communities since 1750* (Houndmills, 2012), p. 1.

25. Green and Viaene, *Religious Internationals in the Modern World*, p. 1.

26. Green and Viaene, *Religious Internationals in the Modern World*, p. 8.

27. İsmail Kara, 'Ulema–siyaset ilişkilerine dair metinler-II, Ey Ulema! Bizim gibi konuş!', *Divan*, no. 7 (1991/92), p. 14.

28. Karpat, *The Politicization of Islam*, p. 165.

29. Selim Deringil, *The Well-Protected Domain: Ideology and the Legitimation of Power in the Ottoman Empire, 1876–1909* (New York: IB Tauris, 2009), p. 48.

30. Jacob M. Landau, *The Politics of Pan-Islam: Ideology and Organization* (Oxford: Clarendon Press, 1990), p. 35.

31. Cezmi Eraslan, *Abdülhamid II ve İslam Birliği* (İstanbul: Ötüken Neşriyat, 1992), pp. 206–8.

32. Azmi Özcan, *Pan-Islamism: Indian Muslims, the Ottomans and Britain, 1877–1924* (Leiden: E.J. Brill, 1997), pp. 52–3.

33. Landau, *The Politics of Pan-Islam*, pp. 64–5.

34. Selim Deringil, 'Osmanlı İmparatorluğu'nda "Geleneğin İcadı", "Muhayyel Cemaat" ("Tasarımlanmış Topluluk") ve Panislamizm'

(Invention of Tradition in the Ottoman Empire, Imagined Group and Panislamism), Toplum ve Bilim, Sayı 54–5, Yaz-Güz 1991, 47–64, pp. 53–4.

35. Eraslan, *Abdülhamid II ve İslam Birliği*, pp. 147–8.

36. See Azmi Özcan, 'The Press and Anglo-Ottoman Relations, 1876–1909', *Middle Eastern Studies* 29, no. 1 (January 1993), pp. 111–12.

37. M. Cavid Baysun, 'Şirvanizade Ahmed Hulusi Efendi'nin Efganistan Elçiliğine Aid Vesikalar', *İstanbul Üniversitesi Tarih Dergisi*, vol. IV (1952), pp. 146–58.

38. Syed Tanvir Wasti, 'The 1877 Ottoman Mission to Afghanistan', *Middle Eastern Studies* 30, no. 4 (October 1994), pp. 959–60.

39. Wasti, 'The 1877 Ottoman Mission to Afghanistan', pp. 958–9.

40. Özcan, *Pan-Islamism*, pp. 81–2.

41. William Ochsenwald, 'The Financing of the Hijaz Railroad', *Die Welt des Islams* 14, no. 1/4 (1973), p. 142. See also Ufuk Gülsoy, 'Bağışlarla Gerçekleşen Eser: Hicaz Demiryolu', *Tarih ve Medeniyet* Sayi 16, Haziran (1995), pp. 35–7.

42. James Nicholson, *The Hejaz Railway* (London: Stacey International, 2005).

43. Walter Pinhas Pick, 'Meissner Pahsa and the Construction of Railways in Palestine and Neighboring Countries', *Ottoman Palestine 1800–1914*, edited by Gad G. Gilbar (Leiden: E.J. Brill, 1990), p. 193.

44. Rashed Chowdhury, 'Pan-Islamism and Modernisation during the Reign of Sultan Abdülhamid II, 1876–1909', unpublished PhD Dissertation, McGill University, 2011, p. 333.

45. Özcan, *Pan-Islamism*, pp. 109–10.

46. Ali Vehbi, *Avant la debacle de la Turquie: Pensées et souvenirs de l'ex- Sultan Abdul Hamid* (Paris: Attinger, 1913), pp. 46–7.

47. Carter Vaughn Findley, *The Turks in World History* (Oxford: Oxford University Press, 2005), p. 14.

48. M. Naeem Qureshi, *Pan-Islam in British-Indian Politics: A Study on the Khilafat Movement, 1918–1924* (Leiden: Brill, 1999), p. 5.

49. Ishtiaq Ahmad, 'From Pan-Islamism to Muslim Nationalism: The Indian Muslim Response to the Turkish War of Liberation', International Conference Turkish War of Liberation, 12–13 May 2005, National Institute of Cultural and Historical Research-Pakistan, available at http://www.ishtiaqahmad.com/downloads/Paper_Khilafat_05.pdf (accessed on 17 January 2013).

50. Naeem Qureshi, *Pan-Islam in British India: The Politics of the Khilafat Movement 1918–1924* (Oxford: Oxford University Press, 2008), p. xxiii.

51. M. J. Akbar, *India—The Siege Within: Challenges to a Nation's Unity* (Suffolk: Penguin Books, 1985), p. 18.

52. Michael J. Nojeim, *Gandhi and the King: The Power of Non-Violent Resistance* (Westport: Greenwood, 2004), p. 50.

53. Shanti S. Tangri, 'Intellectuals and Society in Nineteenth-Century India', *Comparative Studies in Society and History* 3, no. 4 (July 1961), p. 386.

54. Tangri, 'Intellectuals and Society in Nineteenth-Century India', p. 369.

55. Tangri, 'Intellectuals and Society in Nineteenth-Century India', p. 369.

56. Tangri, 'Intellectuals and Society in Nineteenth-Century India', p. 386.

57. Tangri, 'Intellectuals and Society in Nineteenth-Century India', p. 387.

58. Romesh C. Dutt, *England and India: A Record of Progress during a Hundred Years, 1785–1885* (London: Chatto and Windus, 1897), p. 155.

59. Tangri, 'Intellectuals and Society in Nineteenth-Century India', p. 394.

60. Tangri, 'Intellectuals and Society in Nineteenth-Century India', p. 391.

61. Referenced in Tangri, 'Intellectuals and Society in Nineteenth-Century India', pp. 390–1, quoting Mir Shujaat Ali, p. 180.

62. Syed Tanvir Wasti, 'Sir Syed Ahmad Khan and the Turks', *Middle Eastern Studies* 46, no. 4 (July 2010), pp. 529–42, see p. 530.

63. Gail Minault and David Lelyveld, 'The Campaign for a Muslim University, 1898–1920', *Modern Asian Studies* 8, no. 2 (1974), pp. 145–89.

64. Albert Hourani, 'How Should We Write the History of the Middle East?' *International Journal of Middle East Studies* 23, no. 2 (1991), p. 130.

65. Cemil Aydın, 'Emperyalizm Karşiti Bir İmparatorluk: Osmanli Tecrübesi Işiğinda 19. Yüzyil Dünya Düzeni' (An Anti-imperialist Empire? Ottoman Lessons on the Nature of 19th Century World Order), *Divan* 12, no. 22:1 (2007), pp. 39–85.

66. Elie Kedourie, 'The End of the Ottoman Empire', *Journal of Contemporary Society* 3, no. 4, '1918–19: From War to Peace' (October 1968), p. 19.

67. Ansari, 'Pan-Islam and the Making of the Early Indian Muslim Socialists', p. 510.

68. M. A. Ansari, 'Introduction', in Halide Edib, *Conflict of East and West in Turkey* (Delhi: Maktaba Jamia Islamiya, 1935), pp. v–vi.

69. Sylvia G. Haim, ed., *Arab Nationalism: An Anthology* (Berkeley: University of California Press, 1962), p. 15. She made the reference regarding Afghani, but I believe it is an equally valid point for pan-Islamism writ large.

70. Özcan, *Pan-Islamism*, p. 106.

71. Ansari, 'Pan-Islam and the Making of the Early Indian Muslim Socialists', p. 511.

72. Ansari, 'Pan-Islam and the Making of the Early Indian Muslim Socialists', p. 512.

73. Keddie, 'Pan-Islam as Proto-Nationalism', p. 18.

74. Ansari, 'Pan-Islam and the Making of the Early Indian Muslim Socialists', p. 510.

75. *New York Times*, 'Balkan War's Effect on India: British Viceroy Hastens to Reassure Both Moslems and Hindus', 19 October 1913.

76. Mushirul Hasan, 'Pan-Islamism versus Indian Nationalism? A Reappraisal', *Economic and Political Weekly* XXI, no. 24 (14 June 1986), p. 1074.

77. Ansari, 'Introduction', in Halide Edib, *Conflict of East and West in Turkey*, pp. v–vi.

Part Two

5

The Unintended Travelogue

In one encounter early in the 1990s, a senior German official said to me: 'We have learned about Turkey through Karl May.' Karl Friedrich May, born in Saxony, was the prolific bestselling nineteenth-century German writer who published numerous much enjoyable and equally simplistic adventure novels and travelogues taking place in northern America and Muslim lands. His books were detailed verbal feasts about other cultures, whether they were the American Red Indians or the Muslims from Egypt to Sumatra. He told his readers that he travelled extensively and that he spoke 40 languages including Kurdish, Malay, and Swahili. His house was full of exotic pieces, which he said he brought from his travels in the Orient and the New World. He captured and indeed shaped the imagination of tens of millions of people, mostly young readers. However, while writing those travel books, which sold more than 200 million copies, he had not stepped his foot once outside his native lands. His travelogues were a complete sham. As Jan Fleischauer wrote:

> May had a studio photographer in Linz make portrait photos of him, dressed in an Old Shatterhand costume against exotic backdrops. A rifle maker in Dresden made the Silberbüchse (Silver Gun), the Bärentöter (Bear Killer) and the Henrystutzen (Henry Rifle), the most famous weapons from his books, according to his specifications.

They were proudly displayed in his house, the 'Villa Shatterhand', which the author bought in 1896 with his now handsome royalties. But the guns could not be used because they probably would have exploded.[1]

In his only travel outside Germany, much after he became rich and famous, Karl May and his valet sailed to Egypt and thence to Sumatra via Sri Lanka. Then an aging man, he was shattered by the gap between reality and the fiction he created and vowed never to travel again. He died as an exposed con artist, fighting legal battles only a few months before Dr Ansari and the Indian Medical Mission set sail towards Turkey.

May catered to a public that was already predisposed to believing any image that would confirm their preconceived ideas. A mental image of the Orient existed much before Karl May and countless others in various forms of their Orientalism reinforced and nurtured public prejudices and fascination in the exotic land of the 'uncivilized' others. The impact of these blurred lenses has been beyond the realm of the rational and comprehensible. A 2003 English language reprint of Karl May's 'travel tales' in the Kurdistan region claim that although written more than a century ago, 'his thoughts and ideas deal with issues that are as relevant today as they were more than a century ago'.[2] Obviously not all travelogues are fictitious. In fact, the field is full of intimate accounts of direct observations of every corner of the Orient visited and studied by the European traveller. Since the conquest of İstanbul and the later conquests of Syria and Egypt, the Ottoman Empire was the favoured subject of countless travelogues by European and particularly Venetian diplomats, clergy as well as artists working for embassies, nobility, merchants, and seamen. The rising importance of the trade route to India in the mid-sixteenth century was among the key factors that increased the demand for information about the Ottoman Empire, which was growing as a major power. Turks have been a permanent factor for Europe as the object of fascination, fear, or disdain for many centuries. European travellers in the empire since the sixteenth century wrote extensively about their observations about this mesmerizing society, culture, and polity, not to mention its military prowess. Nineteenth century saw an explosion of both travels and spread of the written word.

It also saw the emergence of Orientalism as an established academic discipline alongside archaeology, philology, and ethnography, enabling systematic treatment of data collected by travel accounts. However, the data about the Ottomans and the Muslim world was utilized as an element of power projection in support of colonialism. That point has now become an established fact since Edward Said's *Orientalism* and the whole corpus of postcolonial scholarship have exposed it, particularly in the last three decades. Lesser known is that a misconception about the Muslim travels has fed a pedigree of intellectuals in Europe and America that ascribed an insular world view to the Muslims. In this regard, long before Richard Rorty and Gianni Vattimo[3] suggested that Muslims only travel to destroy and not to learn, Bernard Lewis suggested that the insularity of Muslims owes to their lack of curiosity to find out about others beyond their own borders. This lack of curiosity, in turn, was the outcome of their sense of superiority over the infidels.[4] Learning from the Christendom and indeed studying and adopting at least the material, if not the moral, aspects of their civilization was, however, a formula advanced since nineteenth century by reformists in the Ottoman and Muslim world. Many of those intellectuals travelled to Europe and benefited from their observations. Furthermore, there is now significant scholarship that has brought to limelight Arab travels before the nineteenth century to Europe in order to study in great depths the European culture, society, and polity.[5] When the Muslims did not travel, it was in no small part due to the threat of violence perpetrated against the Muslims or the refusal of the English seamen to carry Muslim passengers.[6] The resistance against Muslims was so strong that the Ottomans had to employ Christian diplomats in Italy.[7]

Whereas Muslim travels into Europe were less frequent, travels between the Muslim countries have existed for centuries. The most established form of travel was for pilgrimage to Mecca both for the annual Hajj and for the Umrah which can be made throughout the year. The nineteenth century facilitated travel from Europe to Muslim lands and vice versa as well as within the Muslim lands. The travels within the world of Islam were not restricted to visits to holy places and included 'a "grand tour" in which sightseeing, observations of the social, cultural and political scenes in the countries visited, and the simple, enriching joy of moving about in a friendly but unfamiliar environment began to gain importance'.[8] If travel is a medium for sharing experiences and communication of ideas across boundaries, travelogues and newspapers formed the communicative space within which this interaction was facilitated. As essential complements to newspapers, these travelogues made the other more distant Muslim peoples more familiar and accessible. Although historians have sought to chart a new genre of writing, perhaps more confidently one can talk about the speed with which the writings could be supplied to the readers, thanks to not only the by then commonplace printing press but also the emergence of effective postal system. As such, a travelogue that appeared in regular instalments days after the actual events was bound to draw attention. The accounts from different Muslim countries reaching wider audiences and covering a broad array of information on social, economic, political, as well as religious life in other Muslim countries helped the emergence of a global Muslim public opinion. The newspapers and journals never sold too much and the level of literacy was low. Hardly any newspaper was founded to make money. The journals and newspapers were read aloud by one who could to the others who listened. And from there the word spread around in its most traditional and enduring way, from mouth to ear. The nineteenth-century form of travelogues in the Muslim world played a role in the emergence of a global community of Muslims or the Muslim world in its modern reincarnation.

The letters by Dr Ansari were not meant to be a travelogue. His purpose was different from the numerous European, American, and Muslim travellers who wrote about their experiences. He did not intend to give practical advice to future travellers. He did not mean to 'convey the wonders of the new civilization' he encountered. Nor did he seek 'to offer, often quite self-consciously, a critique of [his] own society'.[9] Yet he became part of a re-imagination of the world fashioned in the nineteenth century by Muslim travellers who had become essential agents for increasing awareness about other Muslims living beyond their borders in faraway lands. The numbers that the *Comrade* sold really did not matter too much. It may be safe to assume that the primary motive of Dr Ansari for writing regularly was a sense of accountability to the people who sent him to Turkey on an important mission and entrusted a cadre of people to help do a job. Nowhere is there a sign that Dr Ansari wrote to become a famous politician or to shape the public opinion in a certain direction. His political ambitions all became manifest long after his return from the Balkan mission. He also could not have entertained a literary ambition, and as eloquent as his prose was, its strength was in its professional, even ascetic, clarity of communication. He feigned no pretensions to being a literary travel writer. Yet, I assume he must have read and been influenced by the travelogues of other fellow Muslims who wrote about their travels to the Ottoman Turkey.

One does not know whether he actually read earlier travelogues about Turkey such as the one by Shibli Numani. Yet, one does see Numani being in the circle of Maulana Mohammad Ali and Dr Mukhtar Ahmad Ansari already at the time the Medical Mission left India towards Turkey. In fact, the first letter presented in this book explains how Numani was among the ones who were present at the farewell of the Mission in mid-December 1912. Numani was actually reported as reading a poem that touched the crowds that came to see off their heroes. Not the usual form that heroes are depicted in classical dramas and myths. They did not bear weapons, display muscle. They were instead doctors, male nurses, ambulance bearers, and young students and volunteers from around British India who would travel to another country. It would be normal for Dr Ansari to feel the burden on his shoulders and seek refuge in transparency and regular coordination and feedback with the organizer and home support for the overall Mission to Turkey. Given their personal acquaintance, one can surmise that Ansari did read or listened to accounts of Numani's 1892 travels in İstanbul and that he might have consciously or unconsciously mirrored several of the focal enquiries in Numani's travelogue. In fact, irrespective of whether or not he read Numani's or anyone else's travelogue, his letters did address many of the issues of interest and concern to the Indian Muslims back home and invoke keywords that were of significance to them. These included the questions such as how magnificent was the leader of the Muslim world, how much of the old grandeur of the empire was now visible, what were the estimable and objectionable traits and characteristics of the Turkish people, how much was their suffering, and how did the Ottoman society deal with some of the difficulties and tensions associated with European modernity that Indian and other Muslims too confronted. People yearned for clarity, for truth, for reaffirmation, for relief, and for lessons. Ansari letters may not have been intended or even drafted as the usual travelogues. Yet, these letters gave glimpses on all those points, whether intentionally or by chance.

The argument can be sharpened further by taking a closer and comparative look at two travelogues about Ottoman Turkey, written in similar or at least not too far apart periods. These are Allama Shibli Numani's *Safarnama-yi Rum, Misr o Sham* published in Lahore in 1894 and the letters-cum-travelogue written by Mukhtar Ahmad Ansari and published in 1912–13 in Delhi. One can also throw into the fold Munshi Mahbub Alam's *Safarnama-yi Yurop, Bilad-i Rum, Sham o Misr* published again in Lahore in 1908.[10] Several emphases of the first Urdu travelogue of the new genre written by Shibli Numani to describe the Ottoman Empire chime with those of the Alam's travelogue and Ansari letters written close to two decades later.

Among these emphases that Numani's travelogue and Ansari letters shared was the criticism of the European orientalist accounts of the Ottoman Empire and society. Numani wrote that insofar as the Ottoman Empire was concerned, '[t]he circle of writers is very extensive in Europe and therefore it includes all kinds of people—biased and honest, shallow and deep. But in talking about the Turks, all difference of degrees disappears and the same sound comes out of every instrument.'[11] In this regard, one can argue that the travelogues of Muslim travellers in the Muslim world and in the Ottoman Empire came to mean more than an exploration. The main source of news and commentary for the Urdu press on Turkey continued to be the English language press. Thus notes Adeeb, 'English prejudices for or against the Ottomans were, therefore, an essential ingredient in Indian Muslim evaluations of the Ottoman Empire.'[12] Nonetheless, the travelogues became part of the Indian Muslim written media's growing protest and rebellion against the dominant discourses that were concocted and instilled by the imperial powers and their civil societies as well as proxies in colonized lands. After making direct observations regarding the two hospitals in İstanbul, Dr Ansari abandoned his inherently diplomatic tone and punctuated that

[f]rom what follows, when describing the hospitals at Hadimköy, Gnifer and Yesilköy, you would see that not only the general press of Europe was full of a series of calumnies and false reports about the Turkish organization, but even the medical Press was affected by this religious bigotry and fanaticism, and stated facts about the medical organization which on examination one finds altogether incorrect and exaggerated.

Similarly Mahbub Alam from Lahore had also argued that

contrary to what European authors say, 'Turkish blood' has remained 'pure' after all the centuries of empire; or that there are so many dogs in Istanbul because the Turks are kindhearted and considerate; or that Ottoman officials are not corrupt and that he never saw anyone take a bribe, but that they often bend rules out of kindness and a sense of hospitality towards foreigners. Indeed, the politeness, hospitality, and decency of the Turks are a constant preoccupation.[13]

In fact, in a way, the Muslim travelogues became a rebellion against constant misinformation and what the diplomatic and reserved Dr Ansari would call a 'tissue of malignant lies' which always vilified, demonized, ridiculed, and patronized the Muslims and non-whites. Only Muslims could do bad things because they were bad people was the simple logic that permeated even the most sophisticated minds. The most notorious examples include acquiescence of the otherwise brilliant historian Arnold Toynbee to draft British war-propaganda material to be used against the Turks. His oeuvres included the *Blue Book*, which made it look like that after five centuries of peaceful living together, when Armenians not only preserved their community and faith but in fact became the closest and most trusted of all the various Ottoman communities, the Turks grew tired and attacked them unilaterally. As frivolous as this argument was, surprisingly the mud stuck. Like Mahbub Alam and Dr Ansari, Mushir Hosain Kidwai is yet another example of those who rebelled: 'The record of the Turks is clean from the stain of such butcheries as have been committed in the Congo, or in British Colonies over indentured labourers, or in German Africa to enrich the European capitalists and profiteers.'

He would reason:

> Even such Powers as England, which were in a position to appreciate the difficulties of governing countries with so mixed a population, blamed the Turks for not introducing a constitutional system of government. The British statesmen who failed to manage the government of two small islands, and could not concede Home Rule to one of them simply because it contained people professing two different branches of one religion, demanded of the Turks to ignore the diversity of race, religion and language in their Empire and to concede constitutional government at once. The British Government, who are not even now prepared to give Home Rule to India, on the plea that it is populated by peoples professing two different religions— Hinduism and Islam—demand autonomy, even independence, for different portions of the Ottoman Empire. Is that reasonable?[14]

The power of those words was hidden in their truth and therefore the wartime propaganda and incitation of violence was employed relentlessly by the western powers that were intent on destroying the Ottomans. The only Muslim power that had the audacity to stay on its two feet at the apex of the age of imperialism and colonialism could not have been also the only empire to appear clean from the vile of empires. The rest is another story which is yet to be researched and written in all its dimensions and free of the geopolitical, ideological, and religious zeal that has kept distorting the accounts.

Another emphasis that the Numani and Ansari travelogues shared pertained to the modernization or degree of modernity of the contemporary Ottoman Turkey. The Ottoman experience with modernity, along with that of Khedival Egypt, was closely followed. The former was perhaps more important than the latter because the Ottomans were a much weighty polity than Egypt, although Egypt's deep-rooted intellectual influence over the Arab world cannot be denied. The Ottoman experience was also important because the Ottoman process was more indigenous than that of Egypt's, which copied Ottoman Sultan Selim III's reforms, which were undercut by his assassination. However, the rebellious

Ottoman Pasha Muhammad Ali of Kavala could not fulfil his dream of building a modern empire in place of the Ottoman and Egypt fell under British control. Coming from the Aligarh College, which embodied Indian Muslim's modernization process, Shibli's attention to how the Muslim world in general and the Ottoman Turks in particular addressed the issue of modernization must be considered natural. He would make a point of noting that the dress of the men was European and even the dress of the religious *ulema* was under European influence. Yet Numani, a modernist himself, was not convinced that modernity brought happiness to the Ottoman Turks. As glorious as the empire was even during its decline, most of the Muslims were not actively engaged in industry and trade. The European parts of İstanbul were prosperous and the Muslim parts were poor and chaotic. And, that '[t]he old and new civilizations are in a state of conflict, and no synthesis of values has emerged. Conservative minded people appear to be unaware of the swift passage of time, and the progressives hardly practise what they preach.'[15] The later travelogue by Mahbub Alam about his travels in 1900 marked İstanbul's modernity more vividly.

> In Istanbul, even south of the Golden Horn, he constantly notic-
> es differences from India and which he chalks to the influence of
> Europe: European dress, eating with knife and fork while sitting in
> chairs, but also such things as written menus in restaurants, or the
> procedure in a barber's shop. The images are multifaceted and chan-
> nelled through his own experience and his own position as a racially
> marked member of a colonized society.[16]

Again in terms of gauging and contrasting modernity, Shibli's writing also included 'a survey of modern education followed by detailed descriptions of selected institutions; an account of the libraries of İstanbul and their holdings; and a brief introduction to modern Ottoman letters and printing and publishing'.[17] He regard-ed his favourable observations as a refutation of the European argu-ments that Ottomans were essentially a reactionary and fanatical polity and society. Similarly, Dr Ansari also paid significant atten-tion to the Ottoman institutions and reserved considerable space in his letters to describing and comparing them to European and indeed Indian ones. Thus, Ansari's characterization of Haydarpasa

Hospital and the Military Medical College underscores the examples of Ottoman institutional modernity as well as refutation of European characterizations. Thus, Dr Ansari in his letter dated 11 January provides a detailed account of his observations in the two medical establishments:

In the afternoon twelve members of the Mission went with me to Haydarpasa a place across the Boğaziçi in Üsküdar, the Asiatic portion of Istanbul. We went there in a boat and saw on our landing there the magnificent railway station which is the terminus of the line running between Istanbul and Aleppo. I have not seen any railway station either in Europe or in India which can come anywhere near it. We visited the Military Medical College and Hospital. Aziz Pasha, the chief of the hospital, was exceedingly courteous and took us round this magnificent hospital where we saw 1,000 Turkish soldiers being nursed and looked after. The wards were clean, paved with glazed tiles, and furnished with modern iron beds. The sheets, pillow cases and towels were clean; the blankets were thick and warm; and altogether there was nothing lacking to make the patients comfortable and cheerful during their stay in the hospital. All the patients in this building were medical cases and numbered 1,000. This hospital would compare favourably with any European hospital, and it was certainly much cleaner than the hospitals one sees in France and Italy. The building itself is very stately and, being situated on the shores of the Boğaziçi, commands a beautiful view with plenty of pure ozonic air and sunshine. The next building, which is made of solid stone with very fine carvings, was the Army Medical College itself. At present this is also used for patients numbering 650 to 750. The building across the road facing it is devoted entirely to surgical cases. The entire interior of this building, the floor, walls and ceiling of the corridors and the wards are tiled with glazed tiles. There are small wards for one or two patients and large wards for 100 patients. The arrangements here were absolutely perfect. Everything was scrupulously clean, and I can assure you there are not many places in London, Berlin, Vienna or Paris which can boast of a hospital like this. The hospital has a most modern operating theatre and X-Ray department, and a staff of surgeons, assistant surgeons, sisters and nurses who are quite up-to-date. I was shown a patient who had an operation performed on his head following a bullet wound and the result was ideal. I was told on enquiry that the staff consisted of teachers and professors of European fame, and they turned out 100 to 120 army medical men every year.

In addition to the educational and other institutions in the context of modernity, the travelogue by Numani would devote a special attention to the public position of women which he observed in Turkey. The role of women in the society and their education is directly reflective of any society's encounter with modernity. Numani thus wrote:

> The thing that is most valuable and worthy of description in the culture and progress of the Turks is the education and the social life of the women. The two large nations of the world, i.e., European and Asiatic, are at the extremes in this question and therefore the condition of both is objectionable. The Turks have adopted a middle path that combines the good of both and is devoid of the ills of either. Turkish women are educated, but they are not given instruction in shamelessness, show unnecessary independence and dance (and that too with unrelated men). They veil, but they are not ignorant, nor like an animal in human shape, locked up in the prison of the house and unaware of the world.[18]

Khaled Adeep notes that Numani's 'assessment of women's education is telling, for it encapsulates the anxieties of his audience back in India'.[19] Ansari, however, abstained from making comparisons with India in this regard. Nonetheless, he made a point of the education and refinement of the wife of a former Ottoman consul general he encountered in Egypt, stating, 'We were then introduced to Madame Noureddin Bey, wife of a former Consul-General in Bombay and now P.S. to the Khedive, who was acting as the matron in charge of the women refugees. She is a Turkish lady of education and refinement and spoke French most fluently.' On the other hand, Ansari does refer to the clothing of the women he encountered on the streets in İstanbul stating, 'The women are seen going about in the streets freely with a "charchef" which is generally made of silk and covers the entire body and face. But the outline of the face can often be made out even through the thick black veil.' A Turkish woman Dr Ansari got to know in İstanbul appeared to have made a very positive impression on him. This was Halide Edip Adıvar, a Turkish novelist, columnist, intellectual, and political activist. Dr Ansari wrote to the editor of the *Comrade* recommending her as a columnist:

She belongs to the Party of Union and Progress and is a very active worker, not only politically, but in almost every sphere of activity, for the benefit of Turkey. She used to write almost daily in the Tunin when the paper was being published, and has written to many of the leading French and German papers as well as in the Manchester Guardian and for the Jeune Turc. She is considered one of the leading lights of the Party of Union and Progress, a silent, though very effective, power working behind the scenes. I considered myself very fortunate in having met her as she will be very useful. I have persuaded her to become a contributor to the Comrade as soon as she returns from the German Hospital where she has been advised to go for a rest cure, having worked very hard during the war in helping the organizations for the sick and wounded and the widows and orphans. She hoped one day very soon, after this crisis was over, to visit India and deliver a series of lectures in different Muhammadan centres to give correct ideas about Turkey and her people to the Muhammadan public in India. Unfortunately I have not been able to see her again, but I hope to do so before our hospital is established in Ömerli. I think Madame Saleh [Halide Edip] will be an additional attraction as a contributor for the Comrade, if any attraction is necessary at all.

Halide Edip did not become a contributor to the *Comrade* but in 1935, Dr Ansari as chancellor of the Jamia Millia Islamia invited her to Delhi to give lectures on Turkey, which he described as an inheritor of a great culture and one of the great melting pots of the world. Halide Edip's Delhi lectures were published by the Jamia Millia Islamia under the title of *Conflict between East and West*, with a generous introduction by Dr Ansari about her:

[S]he is one of those in whose life two ways of thought, two methods of social organisation came into conflict. Her early years were spent in a typically Eastern household; her education and the problems of her time brought her face to face with the West. It would have been easy for her, like so many educated women of the East, to deny her own culture and assert the actual if not moral right to accept what standards she liked. It may also have been possible to take refuge behind self-adulatory prejudices and close her eyes to the new duties and responsibilities. But rather than live out her life, with an inner futility masked by cultural accomplishments and fine manners, or a social and moral atrophy decked out in the guise of ancient and established virtue, she flung herself into the thick of the fight, and has emerged victorious. She has grasped the fundamental values of the West, freedom, organisation, efficient social co-operation; and her active life of service and guidance has made her treasure all the more highly the pearls of great price, which, we are told, may be found only in the East inner quietude, spiritual harmony, the realisation of a unity beneath all diversity, a love beyond all hatred.

These lines told volumes about not only the great admiration he held for Halide Edip and the Turkish nation, but also about the effortlessly reconciliatory tone Dr Ansari took throughout his life with respect to relations and tensions between European modernity and the Muslim world. He successfully mitigated this tension while steadfastly remaining on the side of modernity.

The three travelogues also characteristically touched upon the observations about the traits and characteristics that defined the host society writ large. Numani devoted 'a large section to the "morals, etiquette and the way of life" of the Turks, which he characterizes as the epitome of hospitality and generosity, without "useless grandeur".'[20] Ansari too makes direct observations on Turkish hospitality in favourable terms. During his tours of the country side Ansari reported his encounter with a villager as 'a very touching and pleasing little incident'. As Ansari was taking snapshots of the snow-covered Toros mountain range and the green valleys, he was accosted by a farmer returning from the field. The villager asked Ansari where he came from and on learning Ansari's country and religion, 'he looked so immensely pleased that kissed my hands and invited me to a cup of tea in his cottage'. Ansari characterizes this meeting as an 'example of that true fraternity which is only practiced in Islam though preached by many other religions'. Ansari was to comment that the villager's hospitality was real and genuine, and he wrote that he would 'never forget the happiness that cup of tea gave me and my host. It was the best cup I ever had in my life'. In a separate note Ansari mentions 'great hospitality and that essentially Turkish courtesy which has earned the Turks the deserving epithet of "the gentleman of Europe".' In a letter dated 12 January, Ansari makes another reference to the hospitality of the Turks he met at the warzone:

Horses were brought for us to ride, but our Manager declined (Let us not be said through any fear) to ride such a very short distance as the Red Crescent Hospital, in spite of the Mud Atlantic. The Turks are very polite people and to please the guests would even face the prospects of a mud-bath rather than refuse a request. We walked, or rather swam, in the mud.

In a similar vein, the Medical Mission's chance encounter with a house bearing the name of Fethi Bey, the hero of the Turkish–Italian War of 1912 in Tripoli, also receives broad treatment in the letter dated 3 May written by another member of the Mission, Ghulam Ahmad. Ghulam Ahmad mentions that while he and two fellow members of the Mission were touring the battle fields close to their hospital tent, they came across the house of Fethi Bey. They handed a name card to the soldier standing outside the house:

He took our card at once and came with an invitation from his master to enter the house. But when we looked at our boots which were not exactly as they wear them in Bond Street, you can imagine our hesitation in entering an immaculately clean house with a polished wooden floor. As we walked through the hall we left big lumps of mud behind us which the servant swept away, only to do it over again when anyone of us passed the hall again. Our host showed us great hospitality and that essentially Turkish courtesy which has earned the Turks the deserving epithet of 'the gentleman of Europe'. We vaguely hinted about some hotel where we could spend the night, but our host would not hear of it, although the poor man possessed only two beds in the house and searched all over the village to procure some more beddings in which he did not succeed. Nevertheless he was rather suspicious of us and made enquiries about us and wrote profuse notes and dispatched them, I think, to the authorities ... The dinner was a sumptuous affair consisting of seven courses, all of us eating from the same plate in the good old Turkish fashion, the only incongruous element being the use of knives and forks. We were afforded a beautiful view of the lake in the moonlight through the powerful field glasses which these officers gave us. As bed time approached Hafizji began to wonder whether his highly scented stockings might not have the effect of an emetic and spoil the evening's dinner. My own fears and tribulations were not small when I thought of the hundreds of thousands of my pet 'colonists' whom I had nourished on my own life-blood, and now that they were fattened and sleek the agony of losing them in this house was great, indeed. There was a regular tug-of-war as bed time, the host wasting to give us the beds and sleeping himself on the Ottoman; but we were three to one and at last prevailed on him to sleep in one of the beds.

An aspect of Numani's travelogue was the fascination with the persona of the sultan caliph and the almost besotted characterization of an encounter with this most revered leader. In the case of Numani, an audience with the sultan caliph did not occur. Instead, Numani managed to get into the Hamidiye mosque in Istanbul to meet Abdulhamid II and was present in the mosque when the caliph arrived among the cheering crowd. Numani wrote about the emotional response he could not help give when the second *hutba* was read by the muezzin at the mosque: 'Tears continuously flowed from my eyes and for a long time, words of prayer continued to issue uncontrollably from my tongue.'[21] One would find similar ecstatic characterization, albeit characteristically less poetical, in Ansari's audience with the sultan caliph who would characterize this meeting as the 'greatest event of our stay in Turkey'. While Ansari was luckier in obtaining an audience, Numani also secured a decoration of the Mecidiye Order during his audience with the Grand Vizier Gazi Osman Pasha.

Both Ansari and Numani made a point of liaising with the other foreigners present in İstanbul. Dr Ansari, in fact, started his stay with a visit to the British Ambassador in İstanbul and then visited with the Iranian Ambassador. More notably, he made a call to a number of officials including the prime minister; the ministers of interior, finance, and foreign Affairs; and not to mention, several generals. He met local dignitaries also during his travels in central and southern Turkey. He appeared to have displayed significant energy in getting to know key personalities and liaising in support of his Mission. Dr Ansari's report about his audience with Prime Minister Mahmud Şevket Pasha shortly before his assassination read as follows in his letter dated 22 February:

Mahmud Şevket Pasha received me most courteously, and shook hands with me in a most cordial manner. I explained to him the feelings of the Muslims of India at the great crisis which Turkey was going through and the hopes they now centred in him and his Cabinet for saving Turkey and the whole Islamic world from disgrace and utter loss of prestige. He was very brief in his reply, but his words were pregnant and sincere. He said, among other things, that the Muslims of India had been very generous in their help towards the relief of the wounded and the sick, and that the Turks would never forget their kindness and help at such a time. After reading the Turkish translation of your letters and cable he was very pleased, and made enquiries about you and all that you have done in organizing the All-India Medical Mission and the Red Crescent Fund for the relief of the wounded soldiers and the refugees. He promised to send your telegram to his Imperial Majesty the Sultan, and said that I will have the receipt sent to me in due course of time for the three drafts I had given him from you. I asked him about the war to which he replied that they were ready for it, but he was not sure of the Balkan Confederacy. As regards Adrianople, he said that the garrison had enough provision for two months. In the end, he promised a private presentation of all the Members of the All-India Medical Mission to His Majesty the Sultan, and expressed a desire to see them himself.

One would not miss the ambassadorial tone in his reporting and the sympathy and respect he apparently felt for the Ottoman grand vizier. This kind of close interaction with the sultan and prime minister ensured that the Medical Mission led by Dr Ansari was visible both in İstanbul but also back in Delhi, both among the Indian Muslim readership of the *Comrade* but presumably also among the ever watchful British authorities wary of the Indian sympathies for Turkey. Shibli Numani too had spent time with foreigners and locals in İstanbul, probably more so given the demands of the extant duties of Ansari as a medical doctor during war. Numani in this context spent much time in the company of provincial Arabs in İstanbul. He, in fact, seems to have befriended a Syrian Arab right on the ship towards İstanbul. These contacts should be expected to play some role in shaping the optic of both Ansari and Numani.

Last but not least, both travelogues mention touristic sites of interest to broader audiences. Numani mentions his stopover in the western port city of İzmir and mentions that there were over

'300 mosques, several being of great size and splendour. The water-front boulevard was flanked with hotels, restaurants, theatres, dancing halls and the trading premises of the Christians. At night, the "corniche" took on the atmosphere of a fair, with crowds of people in the streets and music and song emerging from all directions.' This Aegean port would be where the Greek invasion at the end of the First World War would begin and end. The first bullet of the Turkish war of liberation would be fired in this city by a journalist. However, the Greek army would burn the entire city to ashes once defeat became evident as they were fleeing back into the depths of the Aegean Sea. The same fate of being burnt down would be shared by many other Balkan cities, wiping away the Ottoman Turkish past and leaving no cultural artefacts. Numani also referred to the unique natural beauty of İstanbul and stated that the city contained

> 500 mosques, 171 baths, 324 caravanserais or khans, as well as those for schools, colleges, printing presses, libraries, dervish lodges, etc. Nu'mani is much impressed by the cafes of Istanbul, some of which have imposing edifices. Tea, coffee, juices and other comestibles are served round the clock, and newspapers brought in for the convenience of clients. He comments that it is a pity that Indians do not have a taste for such cafes, and prefer to assemble for sittings at the house of a friend.[22]

Dr Ansari's travel to Konya contains details about the Mevlana Celaleddin Rumi's *dargah* and mosque in the city. However, he was no less elaborate of his account of the Topkapı Palace in İstanbul, the seat of Ottoman power until the nineteenth century. He starts by setting out the items of particular interest to the Muslim readers and moves on to markers of European fascinations about the Ottoman royal lives. Thus, about items of particular interest to the Muslim audience, he wrote:

> The next building which is built in pure Saracenic style is the Khirka-i Shariff tomb. In this shrine are placed the Prophet's mantle, the javelin and the sword. The Sanjak Sheriff the sacred standard of the Prophet is also kept here closely guarded. The place where those holy relies are deposited is a square hall with a central place shut from public gaze by beautifully worked green curtains. The marble

screens surrounding this hall gave us a glimpse of the central shrine. In this buildings are also kept a carpet of Syyedena Abu Bakr and four copies of the original Quran arranged by Syyedena Osman. The Quran of Syyedena Osman when he was murdered is also presented here, with blood stains on its pages. Syyedena Ömer's arms and turban are also deposited here. This shrine is opened only once a year on the 15th of Ramazan for the procession of the Khirka-i-Shariff. In the lobbies surrounding this central hall are kept some historical aims. The sword of Sultan Mohamed the Conqueror and the guns used in his time are to be seen here. A beautiful specimen of calligraphy executed by Sultan Mahmud II is hung to the lobby. Baghdad Kiosk built by Sultan Murad IV in true imitation of a Kiosk he had seen in Baghdad, is a wonderful piece of pure Saracenic white architecture. Built of spotless white marble, it commands an extensive view of the beautiful blue Boğaziçi and the limpid, mobile waters of the Sea of Marmara. Here the Sultan retires when he visits the Khirka-i- Shariff Jame on the 15th of Ramazan. On the entrance to the central hall is executed following couplet in mother-o- pearl: 'Let the door of happiness be open for you always in this Dargah; Because I am witness that there is no other God but Allah.' The walls of the kiosk are artistically decorated with blue tile, and the interior of the dome is covered with deer-skins wrought with most artistic floral designs and perfect tughras. The doors, dewans and sofas are inlaid with mother-o-pearl and are of the rarest and choicest kind, and give an idea of the life of the period of Khalifa Haroon-ul-Rashid.

These descriptions must have fascinated the Muslim readers back in India who marvelled at the unique wealth of Muslim heritage that was at display and protection in İstanbul, the half a millennial seat of the Islamic caliphate. References to the personal belongings of the Holy Prophet and three of the most revered early caliphs and companions of the Prophet, Abu Bakr, Osman, and Ömer, were bound to generate excitement among most of the Indian Muslims. On the other hand, the absence of references to the Zulfiqar sword of the Holy Prophet handed over to the fourth Caliph Ali ibn Taleb and other items of interest to the Shia Muslims may be noted. One would assume these to be on display even at the time.

Dr Ansari's description of the Topkapı Palace in İstanbul then makes a shift towards the account of the harem or the private chambers of the sultan and his extended family and staff:

We were shown the golden corridor and the staircase leading to the Harem where, after the murder of Sultan Murad, the janissaries rushed to kill all the royal princes, but they were turned back by the coolness and presence of mind of the Sultan's wife, who threw buckets of glowing charcoal on their faces. The window through which the Sultana made Sultan Mahmud jump out is adjoining this staircase, also the room where he was proclaimed Sultan in the very teeth of the revolt of the Janissaries. There were secret ladders, hidden passages leading from one building to another. In fact all those contrivances which were necessary in those days when the palace intrigues and plots were the rule of the day. In passing out of the Harem we were shown the place where the chief of the eunuchs used to punish the offenders. On the gate could be seen the dried scalp of one of the eunuchs hung by Sultan Mahmud. A secret balcony which we entered from the Harem overlooked the hall, where the discussions of Vozara and Vokals used to take place. In this balcony the Sultan used to sit and over hear all the discussions without being seen. The building on the extreme right with yellow domes is the remains of the Byzantine palace, used as the sweet kitchen in the time of Sultan Selim, where he had hidden himself from the Janissaries.[23]

Dr Ansari's 'teetotal' treatment of his tour avoids the usual European fantasies about the harem of the sultan and instead remains focused on the palace intrigues, a safer aspect of the European fascination with the Ottoman royal life.

Khaleed Adeeb argues that 'although he was loath to admit it, Shiblī could never shake off a sense of foreignness in Istanbul'.[24] This he attributes mainly to his lack of knowledge of the Turkish language. The language issue appears to have affected the Indian Medical Mission some two decades later. Numani, in his three months, made some attempt to learn the Turkish language by hiring a tutor. His tutor did not accept money from Numani after he learned that Numani intended to learn Turkish only for scholarly reasons. While Dr Ansari appears to have made no attempt to learn the language, both Numani and Ansari ultimately resolved their language problems by hiring interpreters. No doubt, aggravated by the similar language barrier which the Indian Medical Mission experienced in Ottoman Turkey, Ansari too remained an outsider to the society amidst which he spent six months and with whom he forged emotional bonds. Yet, Numani, Alam, as well as Ansari and his colleagues did learn intimately about the Turkish society. They came to appreciate the perceptions, aspirations, challenges, and the extant state of Turkish society and polity through direct contacts with both the leaders and the people of the country. Through his letters, Dr Ansari provided an unintended travelogue to the Indian masses, who were eager to follow the events and also learn about their beloved Ottoman Empire and the brave Turkish people whose struggles they had come to admire.

The letters also provided a diary and a storyline for the Indian Muslims to monitor what their representatives, heroes of Islamic duty, were experiencing day by day amongst the embattled Turkish nation. The following chapter will reconstruct the story of the Indian Medical Mission to the Balkan Wars from the beginning until the end as reported by Dr Ansari to the Indian Muslims a hundred years ago.

Notes

1. Jan Fleischhauer, 'Germany's Best-Loved Cowboy: The Fantastical World of Cult Novelist Karl May', *Der Spiegel* 13 (26 March 2012).

2. See http://www.amazon.com/Oriental-Odyssey-III-Adventures-Kurdistan/dp/0971816425 (accessed on 1 May 2013).

3. Richard Rorty and Gianni Vattimo, *The Future of Religion*, edited by Santiago Zabala (New York: Columbia University Press, 2005), p. 72.

4. Bernard Lewis, *The Muslim Discovery of Europe* (New York: W. W. Norton, 1982), p. 80.

5. For an extensive study of the issue, see Roxanne L. Euben, *Journeys to the Other Shore: Muslim and Western Travelers in Search of Knowledge* (Princeton: Princeton University Press, 2006). See also Nabil Matar, *In the Lands of the Christians: Arabic Travel Writing in the Seventeenth Century* (London: Routledge, 2003); Nabil Matar, *Turks, Moors and Englishmen in the Age of Discovery* (New York: Columbia University Press, 1999); Tarif Khalidi, 'Islamic Views of the West in the Middle Ages', *Studies in Interreligious Dialogue* 5, no. 1 (1995), pp. 31–42.

6. Nabil Matar, *In the Lands of the Christians: Arabic Travel Writing in the Seventeenth Century* (London: Routledge, 2003), pp. xxv–xxviii.

7. Kemal Karpat, *Türk Dış Politikası Tarihi* (İstanbul: Timaş, 2012), p. 17.

8. Syed Tanwir Wasti, 'Two Muslim Travelogues: To and From Istanbul', *Middle Eastern Studies* 27, no. 3 (1991), p. 457.

9. Khaleed Adeeb, 'Pan-Islamism in Practice: The Rhetoric of Islamic Unity and Its Uses', in Elisabeth Özdalga, ed., *Late Ottoman Society: The Intellectual Legacy* (New York: Routledge Curzon, 2005), p. 208.

10. For the analysis of Numani's travelogue, I rely on Khaleed Adeeb and Syed Tanvir Wasti's separate studies; on Adeep again for Alam's travelogue.

11. Adeeb, 'Pan-Islamism in Practice', p. 211.

12. Adeeb, 'Pan-Islamism in Practice', p. 211.

13. Adeeb, 'Pan-Islamism in Practice', p. 213.

14. Syed Tanvir Wasti, 'Mushir Hosain Kidwai and the Ottoman', *Middle Eastern Studies* 30, no. 2 (April 1994), p. 255.

15. Wasti, 'Two Muslim Travelogues', p. 467.

16. Adeeb, 'Pan-Islamism in Practice', p. 213.

17. Adeeb, 'Pan-Islamism in Practice', p. 211.

18. Quoted in Adeeb, 'Pan-Islamism in Practice', p. 212 from *Allāma Shiblī Nu'mānī, Safarnāma-yi Rūm, Misr o Shām*, edited by Muhammad Riyāz (Lahore: Maqbūl Akaidamī, 1988 [orig. 1894]), p. 19.

19. Adeeb, 'Pan-Islamism in Practice', p. 212.

20. Adeeb, 'Pan-Islamism in Practice', p. 212.

21. Adeeb, 'Pan-Islamism in Practice', p. 212.

22. Wasti, 'Two Muslim Travelogues', p. 468.

23. Dr Ansari's letters dated 12 July 1913.

24. Adeeb, 'Pan-Islamism in Practice', p. 212.

6

The Indian Medical Mission
in Turkey

Members of the Mission and Their Turkish Contacts

The story of the Indian Medical Mission to Turkey in 1912–13
brings together a cast of remarkable personalities. Dr Ansari's letters involve the reader directly with these extraordinary people.
Each of them deserves a separate study, and several of them have
indeed been subject to such targeted rigorous analyses. These
extraordinary men include Dr Ahmad Mukhtar Ansari, the leader
of the medical team on the ground in Turkey; Maulana Mohammad
Ali Jauhar, the leading patron of the Mission and its interface with
the Muslim community in India as editor of the *Comrade*; Enver
Pasha, the controversial and yet inspirational leader of the Young
Turks; and Dr Besim Ömer Pasha, revolutionary obstetrician
and public-health leader as well as the Indian Medical Mission's
chief interlocutor in Turkey as vice-president of the Turkish Red
Crescent.

The *Comrade* in its 28 December 1912 issue published the
list of members of the Medical Mission dispatched to Turkey.
The doctors included Dr Mukhtar Ahmad Ansari from Delhi,
Dr Ali Azhar H. Fyzee from Bombay, Dr S. Muhammad Naim
Ansari from Jaunpure, and Dr Mahmud-ullah and Dr Shamsul

Barry from Calcutta. The head-dresser was Ghulam Ahmad Khan, BSC. Other dressers included M. Nurul Hasan from Meerut; Mohammad Chiraguddin from Delhi; Syed Tawangar Hussain from Pundri, District Karnal; Hamid Rasule from Chhupra, Behar; Abdul Waheed Khan from Mirzapore; and Husain Raza Beg from Ghaziabad. The male nurses and ambulance bearers included Abdur Rahman Siddiqi from Surat, who was also the manager of the Mission; Qazi Bashir-uddin Ahmed from Meerut; Shuaib Quraishi from Aligarh; Mohammed Abdul Aziz Ansari from Yusufpure of District Ghazipore; Khaliquz Zaman from Lucknow; Mansoor Ali Amethi from District Lucknow; Yusuf Ansari from Gangoh of District Sharanpore; Abdur Rahman from Peshawar; Syed Ismail Hussain Shirazi from Sirajganj of Bengal; and Tafazzul Husain from Delhi. The composition remained more or less the same throughout the course of the Mission, although some changes did occur. The author of one of the few accounts of the Mission, Syed Tanvir Wasti, writes that after the Indian Medical Mission set up the field hospital in Ömerli, Dr Abdur Rahman Bihari and Dr Raza Haider joined the Mission from London; four others, Aale Imran, and Hasan Abid Jafri from England; and Mirza Abdul Qayyum from India also joined. In addition to these Indian Muslims, an Egyptian physician, Dr Fouad, was also recruited by the Mission.[1] However, among those counted by Wasti, Dr Ansari seems to acknowledge particularly Dr Fouad. Dr Ansari does none-theless mention that Dr Shamsul Barry had to return due to his illness. Although not part of the medical team, Zafar Ali Khan appears in several instances in the letters.

While some of them have been the subject of biographical stud-ies, overall there is a need to study the ensuing careers of the members of the Mission. We know that several of them went on to assume important roles in independent India and Pakistan. Chaudhry Khaliquzzaman, who later became the President of the Pakistan Muslim League, wrote that Shuaib Quraishi, Rahman Siddiqi, and he were constant visitors to Delhi to meet Maulana Mohammad Ali and Dr Ansari to discuss politics. During his later studies, Khaliquzzaman shared a room at the Sahib Bagh boarding house with Aziz Ansari, who studied law and became a notable lawyer in India. One would wish to include, in this book, a long biography of Mirza Abdul Qayyum, who was martyred fighting bravely for the Ottoman army during the First World War. About Abdurrahman Peshawari, who remained in Turkey after the Medical Mission left, we know a tad more. He fought as an Ottoman officer in the First World War, including at the Kut al Amara battles in 1915–16. He was awarded with the Turkish Medal of Independence. His story is mentioned by Halide Edip Adıvar, the fiery Turkish revolutionary and talented public orator and author, in *Inside India*, her book about her visit to India in 1936 to deliver lectures, when she stayed with Dr Ansari and also visited with the family of Abdurrahman Peshawari. She tells us that 'Abdurrahman [Qureshi of] Peshawar after fighting at different fronts in the Great War, joined the Turkish Nationalist struggle at Ankara in 1920 and worked with the writer at the headquarters'.[2] Syed Tanvir Wasti, in fact, notes with reference to the biographical book by A. S. Shahjahanpuri that Peshawari was also a member of a diplomatic delegation sent by the Turks to Germany in 1916.[3] More notably, he reportedly joined Mustafa Kemal Atatürk in Amasya in 1919, as Mustafa Kemal Pasha was holding his historic tour to organize the Turkish war of liberation against the foreign forces that occupied Turkey after the defeat of the Ottomans in the First World War. In 1923, Atatürk was to dispatch Peshawari as envoy to Kabul. Peshawari thus came to be tightly incorporated into the Turkish ruling party. His developing career would come to a sudden halt in 1925, when he was murdered in İstanbul by an unknown person or persons. Halide Edip remarked that '[n]either the motive for this ugly crime nor the criminals have been brought to light'.[4] Peshawari was 'like a younger brother' to Foreign Minister Rauf Orbay and shared his house. Ironically, and indeed sadly, perhaps this more than anything else resulted in his untimely death. Accordingly, Khaliquzzaman argued that 'someone who wanted to play foul with the life of Rauf Bey mistaking Rahman for him is suspected to have killed him'.[5] Halide Edip would lament that Abdurrahman Peshawari 'was a brave and able officer, and a lovable person'. I would add that he also appears as an extraordinary man.

Dr Ansari, through his letters, brought to his audience several Turkish personalities that are not less noteworthy. Among them, two particularly stand out. One is the immediate counterpart of the Mission in Turkey, namely Dr Besim Akalın, who is mentioned and praised repeatedly in Dr Ansari's letters. Another name of national and indeed international fame is the fiery soldier and politician Enver Pasha. Some biographical sketches on these two personalities may help put the references to them in perspective.

Starting with the latter, Dr Ansari in his letter to Mohammad Ali Jauhar describes Enver Bey with the following sympathetic and insightful words:

> He came to visit us in the hospital where we are staying. He is only a young man of about 35, exceedingly handsome, with most expressive eyes full of determination. His demeanour was that of a very strong man, chastened with hardships and sufferings. It was quiet and yet characteristic, modest and yet commanding respect. A man who is born to command and to elicit implicit faith and admiration from those who work under him.

Enver Bey, at that time, was already among the key leaders of the Young Turk Movement, which toppled Sultan Abdulhamid in 1908 and was soon to stage another coup, when the Medical Mission was in Turkey.

Enver Bey was a product of his times but was perhaps a character who would have left his mark on any epoch that he would have lived in. He was born in the same year, 1881, as the great Mustafa Kemal Atatürk and became a major figure in Turkish history before Mustafa Kemal. At the turn of the twentieth century, when he was in his mid-twenties, he was called a hero of freedom—this was only six years after he had completed his military training in 1902, coming second in his class at the Mekteb-i Harbiye Şahane or the Royal War College. By his mid-thirties, in 1913, he became one of the most powerful men in the Ottoman Empire as a member of the triumvirate leading the Young Turks, as the Committee of Union and Progress is better known. He soon accumulated even more power by marrying into the royal family and leading the war effort during the First World War as the war minister. Şuhnaz Yılmaz rightly points out: 'There are few characters in Turkish history whose rise and fall have been as rapid and as dramatic as those of

Enver Pasa.'[6] And his fall and death were as dramatic as his rise and reign.

Enver Bey's early military career in the Balkans as part of the Third Army in Macedonia was to shape his career as a military officer and a political activist. The Third Army at the time was conducting operations against militia bands that were, in fact, composed of Bulgarian, Greek, and Albanian nationalists trained and equipped by the Balkan governments. He was recognized soon as a talented and courageous military officer well versed in such warfare that would be needed against non-regular but nonetheless well-organized forces. His experience in the Balkans would prove most useful in setting up non-regular Arab units that shattered the aspirations of the Italian army in 1911 for a rapid victory after their unexpected assault in Libya. He emerged as a military leader commanding a strong dedication among the soldiers and officers he led. His charisma was to stay with him until he died on the battlefield in Central Asia, fighting a cause that was already lost.

Even more important were the political opinions he developed during his early tenure in Macedonia about the predicaments of the Ottoman Empire and how to resolve them. According to Enver Bey, the reason for the strength of the insurgency in the Balkans was the corrupt rule of Sultan Abdulhamid II. Not buying into the pan-Islamist rationale, he observed that the Balkan peoples were not fully alienated from the Ottoman Empire, their state for the preceding many centuries, and thought that return to constitutionalism would assuage the majority of them. Yet the constitution of 1876 was suspended by Abdulhamid II in 1877 and the sultan employed his iron hand, not bound by the constitution. His reassignment in Monastir brought Enver Bey into direct contact with the then secretive organization of the Committee of Union and Progress. The committee was established in 1906 upon the foundations of the Young Turk Movement which was already in full swing since 1878. The Young Turks were originally a pro-reform network of open and secret associations of progressive military cadets and university students. Their intellectual base was articulated through the journals published in Paris, emphasizing reform and education of the Ottoman masses in order to replace

Abdulhamid II's despotism with the rule of the intellectuals. The formation of the Committee of Union and Progress followed up on the split within the movement that occurred in 1902 and provided the Young Turks with a revolutionary organizational vanguard. At the nucleus of the committee was the Ottoman Freedom Society that was inaugurated in Selanik by Mehmed Talat, which went on to recruit like-minded activists from the Third Army where Enver as well as Mustafa Kemal were also serving. Among the committee members, Enver proved most useful by utilizing his organizational skills to put together an effective resistance to the İstanbul government and the sultan. The committee appealed to the sultan to restore the parliament and the constitution. Abdulhamid's efforts to suppress the resistance culminated in a dirty war of assassinations and a chase between the sultan's agents and the committee's activists. Enver's escape into Macedonian hills in June 1908 settled him on a point of no return. A month later the Committee of Union and Progress was to assassinate the commander of the Ottoman forces in Monastir. Arguably, the committee seemed to command the support of Turks in the Balkans, which were concerned by the rumours of an agreement between the British and the Russians on ending the Ottoman rule as well as of an imminent Austrian–Hungarian assault on Albania. Thus came the first Young Turk Revolution in July 1908. Yielding to fierce opposition, the sultan restored the constitution and Enver consequently rose to popular acclaim. He turned into a hero overnight, seizing the imagination of the people. Yılmaz writes, 'Owing to his significant role in the restoration of the constitution, Enver's fame kept increasing: his pictures appeared everywhere, babies were named after him and even his moustache style known as "Enver bıyığı" became very fashionable.'[7] After the revolution, Enver did not take an active portfolio in the government in İstanbul and was instead sent as a military attaché to Berlin, where he developed an admiration for the German war machine. In Berlin, he forged strong links with Germany that were to remain with him during his following fateful years in high politics and war.

One of most controversial roles he played was in bringing the Ottoman Empire into the First World War on the side of Germany against Britain, France, and Russia. Most historians attribute this to his admiration for Germany, developed during his tenure in Berlin. However, the fact of the matter appears to be that the anti-British conviction was already entrenched within the Committee of Union and Progress long before the Great War. As Hasan Ünal documents,

> From the perusal of these CUP [Committee of Union and Progress] publications from 1902 onwards, two principal observations may be made. First, the CUP exhibited a marked hostility and suspicion towards all the Great Powers and a strong resentment of their interference in Ottoman affairs. Second, even at this stage before its assumption of power, the CUP manifested no special sympathy, as alleged, towards the Constitutional Powers, Britain and France. On the contrary, anti-British statements outnumber statements against any other Power.[8]

The committee was, however, mindful of the significant influence and means that the British Embassy in İstanbul employed and sought to appease and deal with the British Empire. Enver took active part in the negotiations with the British and grew inexorably more aversive to British policies against the Ottoman Empire. As the British policy to protect the Ottomans against the Russian Empire waned, the German economic influence, including through the construction of the Berlin–Baghdad railway, as well as its military influence, through the dominant role it undertook in the modernization of the Ottoman armies, grew exponentially. So much so that as Dr Ansari and his team were leaving Turkey to return to India, the Ottoman Empire was appointing a German general, Liman von Sanders, as the chief of staff of the Ottoman armies. The committee did make an effort to counterbalance the German influence by asking Britain to upgrade its navy. The ill fate of this move turned into a nail in the coffin of a Turkish–British alliance. The Ottomans ordered two dreadnoughts to be built by Britain and raised the funds through the money collected largely by the people on the streets. However, Britain took a fateful and ill-omened decision to confiscate the two ships. Both Turkish and Indian streets were to burst into outrage upon the announcement made to that effect by the First Lord of the Admiralty Winston Churchill. There was only one road to take for İstanbul after that, and the Ottoman

Empire joined and lost the First World War under Enver's lead as war minister on the side of Germany.

From then on, it was a watershed not only for the Committee of Union and Progress but also for Enver Pasha. Having lost the war, he fled İstanbul on the German torpedo boat U-67 towards Crimea. In July 1919, a special court martial in British-occupied İstanbul condemned him in absentia to death for taking the country to war. He ended up in London where he opportunistically pledged support to the Bolsheviks against Britain and to Britain against the Russians. The British refused but the Bolsheviks showered him with support. The plan of the organization he led, called Muslim Revolutionary Society, was twofold: 'direction of the Muslim revolutionary movement in India and elsewhere aimed at the overthrow of British rule, and extension of this movement into North Africa to upset the French and Spanish regimes'.[9] At the Baku Congress of the Eastern Peoples, he 'declared himself head of a "revolutionary organization of Morocco, Algiers, Tunisia, Tripoli, Egypt, Arabia and India" which might unite Muslim peoples outside Turkey on Pan-Islamic lines'.[10]

It can be assumed, however, that the real object of both the Russians and Enver Pasha and his associates was the replacement of Mustafa Kemal as the leader of the Turkish revolutionary movement. The Bolsheviks entertained the hope that Enver would help them spread communism in Turkey and shift the country into the Soviet orbit. But the triumph of the Turkish liberation war and the consolidation of the Ankara government disrupted Enver's as well as Bolshevik plans. Changing tack, in a bid to court the new government in Turkey, the Russians subverted Enver's plans to overthrow Mustafa Kemal. Historian Salahi Sonyel writes that the Russians

carried out a very skilfully conceived plan to prevent Enver from succeeding in his attempt to upset Ankara. They organized a kind of revolt against him in the Batum area, ostensibly by the Caucasian nationalists. The scheme was carried out with such skill that Enver was thoroughly puzzled, and found he could not cope with the situation. Seeing all his plans destroyed, he left for Moscow, and his partisans dispersed. The Bolsheviks gave him a good reception, and told him that his failure was due to incomplete organization, and promised to help him again.[11]

They then sent him to help quell an uprising in Tadjikistan by Muslim insurgents in Central Asia. However, once in Turkestan, he was persuaded instead to join the 'Basmaji' rebels and lead their forces against the Russians. He was killed at the age of 41 by the Russians during that war in 1922, one year before the modern Republic of Turkey was declared as an independent, sovereign state with its capital in Ankara.

Indian Muslims had followed Enver closely and revered him as a courageous Muslim soldier, the son-in-law of the caliph, striving to save the Ottoman Empire from extinction. Dr Ansari also regarded him very highly. In his letter detailing the coup led by Enver on 23 January 1913, he could not hide his excitement. He wrote that Enver

> rode on a horse with a few soldiers to Bab-i-Aalee and, on being challenged by the sentinel at the entrance, he said he had come to save Turkey, and made a brief but touching speech, which moved the soldiers so much that they all joined him, and he marched into the room where the Cabinet had assembled to do the work of selling their country to their enemies.

The controversy around Enver's stormy and ultimately flawed political career, short as it was, is never likely to end.

The other significant protagonist in the story of the Indian Medical Mission, Besim Ömer Akalın (Basim Omar Pasha), is a less controversial figure, whose lifetime challenges and achievements have been significant.

On 10 April 1912, the largest floating vessel in the world sailed from Southampton with over 2,200 passengers aboard, including some of the wealthiest people in the world. The ship sailed first to Cherbourg in France and then off to the North Atlantic towards New York. The list of passengers aboard *Titanic*, which was to sink on that maiden voyage, included an Ottoman gynaecologist, who was travelling to the United States to attend a medical conference in New York. His name appeared among the 1,513 persons who died in the biggest maritime accident in history. But, in fact, the extraordinarily heavy rains in France in the April of 1912 delayed this passenger's train to Cherbourg and he missed the trip by four hours. As upset as he should have been on that day, Besim Ömer

Pasha, after hearing the news of the sinking of the *Titanic* told journalists that having survived the disaster, he was not afraid of any accident ever after.[12] This doctor, who was saved by fate, ended up being one of the small numbers of people whose bust was erected at his workplace, the Haseki Hospital, even as he was still alive.

This is the same Dr Besim Ömer Pasha who would meet the Indian Medical Mission in İstanbul eight odd months later as the members of the Mission sailed into the city aboard *SS Romania*. The reception was led by the Inspector General of the Ottoman Red Crescent Sociey Mehmet Ali Bey, and included the guard of honour and band. Dr Besim Ömer Pasha as the vice president of the Red Crescent would assist the Mission during their stay in Turkey. Mukhtar Ahmad Ansari's letters leave no ambiguity as to the deep respect and sympathy the two medical men held towards each other. Thus, Dr Ansari wrote in one instance:

> The Pasha is a very eminent surgeon and Gynaecologist of European fame and the real backbone of the Red Crescent movement in Turkey. He made a speech in Turkish, which was translated to us by Saleh Effendi in Urdu, welcoming us in the name of the Croissant Rouge and the Turkish nation and thanking us for the Islamic love and brotherhood which we had shown in coming here for their help and succour. He said that the Croissant Rouge was yet an infant and that its foster-father was India. In reply to his speech I thanked him heartily on behalf of the Mission and pointed to him that this infant which was brought to life by the famous accoucheur (himself) had soon under his skilled care become a vigorous and lusty child proving itself most useful to its mother Turkey in time of her need.

Dr Besim Ömer Pasha was born in 1862 in İstanbul as the son of an Ottoman parliamentarian. He completed his early education in Macedonia and returned to İstanbul to continue his military studies. He finished medical school and was appointed to serve briefly as a military doctor in the Balkans, until he contracted typhoid at the Greek border. Dr Besim Ömer then proceeded to France in order specialize in obstetrics, ultimately becoming the founding father of obstetrics as a medical science in Turkey.

Dr Besim Ömer's career would reach a fork soon after he returned from France to Turkey in 1891. As a professor of obstetrics, he wanted to establish a birth clinic in İstanbul. The Orthodoxy of the time would not permit such an institution as the belief was that only illegitimate children could be brought to life outside the comfort and discretion of one's own house. He nonetheless established a secret clinic, the first birth clinic in the Ottoman Empire, close to the school of medicine in İstanbul in 1892. He and his students persevered against criticism and consolidated the clinic. This became another turning point in his life as Besim Ömer Pasha started a vigorous public education campaign to rid the society of ignorance on health issues and superstition. Thus, as much as obstetrics, Dr Besim Ömer has also become synonymous with preventive medicine in Turkey including dietary advice. One of the several studies he published in this regard was a detailed account of the benefits of grape.

At the same time, this relentless physician also took an active part in improving the institutionalization of health services, both as an educator and as an administrator. Perhaps one of his particularly valuable achievements in the field of health services was the establishment of a nursing course at the conference hall of the Dar-ul Fünun Academy in 1913–14. Nursing was one area where he merged his legacies in public education and health institutionalization. At a time when no such courses were available, Dr Ömer argued strongly that nursing was a distinct discipline requiring specific training as the task involved much more than keeping the patient warm and clean. One particular challenge at the time was to recruit women for the nursing profession which required dealing with male bodies. Besim Ömer convinced well-to-do young women of İstanbul to attend his courses. This was a revolutionary move, which meant that a significant number of workers could enter the profession.

The need for nursing services became brazenly obvious and acute during both the 1911 Trablus war against the Italians and the Balkan Wars. During the Balkan Wars, an attempt was made to rectify the shortfall in nurses by running newspaper advertisements for recruiting voluntary personnel. However, those who responded to these advertisements had little training in nursing and were acting mostly as good Samaritans.[13] Although Dr Ansari, in his letters, gives full credit to how at least one main hospital in İstanbul had nursed the patients, the shortage of qualified nurses caused significant loss of life during these two wars. After these wars, the courses provided by Besim Ömer Pasha not only provided a fresh supply of qualified personnel but also laid the basis for institution-alized training schools for nurses as of 1925. The immediate bene-fit was already achieved during the First World War in which some 300 graduates of Dr Ömer's nursing course took employment in treating the wounded soldiers.[14] Turkish sources are full of praise for the very successful service rendered by the Turkish nurses in the First World War, including at the famous Gallipoli battle.

Dr Besim Ömer lived comfortably after the First World War and served in the most distinguished fashion until his passing away in 1943, some six years after Dr Mukhtar Ahmad Ansari. After the Turkish Republic was established, he took on the surname of Akalın (or White Forehead, if one is to translate literally from Turkish). The Turkish poet Yahya Kemal Bayatlı was to write in his memoirs that Dr Besim Ömer Akalın truly had the head of a physician. One can only guess what the poet meant by those words. Yet knowing Dr Besim Ömer Pasha's remarkable achieve-ments in public medicine, one is inclined not to dispute.

The Journey to İstanbul

More than a month into heavy fighting in the Balkans, Dr Ansari was reporting by end November 1912 that their 'mission of mercy' was ready to deploy to Turkey. He assembled 'eight fully qualified medical men, five with European qualifications and three hold-ing Indian Degrees and Diplomas'. Three of these doctors were to join the Mission in İstanbul from London. Additionally, there were eight dressers and nine male nurses to travel from India with the Mission. One of the male nurses would also take over the task of the manager and accountant of the Mission. Dr Ansari pointed out particularly that 'we could take many more male nurses if we wanted, but we find nine are ample for all our requirements'. Chaudhry Khaliquzzaman, in his memoirs, would recall years lat-er that he was recruited into the Mission in Aligarh while playing tennis:

I was playing tennis in front of my room, bare-headed, bare-footed, my hair all dishevelled, I heard Rahman [Siddiqui] calling me, accompanied by a well-dressed, handsome gentleman standing by his side. I was introduced ... to Dr. Ansari. I expressed my joy and admiration for him for having undertaken the responsibility of leading the Medical Mission. He told me that he had come to Aligarh to find some young men to go with him to help his discharge his duties ... By the evening I had made up my mind to join the Mission.[15]

Several others were to join the Mission from the Aligarh College. But in his letters, Mukhtar Ahmad Ansari proudly noted that

ours is a truly All India Medical Mission, as we have got representatives from every province of India. It is very gratifying to notice that the men who have joined the Mission are from the cultured middle and higher classes, representing the flower of Mohammadan youth, who are fully alive to the responsibilities and nature of the work with which they are entrusted. I have the fullest confidence that all the men will do their duty to the best of their abilities and prove worthy of the trust which their co-religionists have placed in them by sending them as their representatives in the Mission.

As several members of the Mission did not have prior medical or paramedic training, Dr Ansari was to train members of the Mission on daily routines during the journey aboard the ships.

The uniforms of the Mission were selected with particular attention and purpose by Dr Ansari. While he goes into details as to what every member of the team was supplied with, he makes a particular note of the Jodhpur-breeches which 'have been selected not only from the point of view of comfort and utility, but also to impart to the mission uniform a distinctively Indian character'. The Mission members would also wear a badge on the left arm with a red crescent and two silver crescents, one on either side, with an inscription in Arabic that read 'The Indian Medical Mission'. The only distinction between the doctors and the dressers was the brown leather belt with pouches that would be worn by the doctors.

Dr Ansari decided not to carry the medical supplies and instruments from India to Turkey. Instead he sent a list to the Indian Muslim jurist and political leader Syed Ameer Ali in London, 'giving him full particulars of the quality of instruments, appliances, dressings, disinfectants, tinned provisions and other invalid foods to be sent straight to the Constantinople, as to reach there before us'. The list that Dr Ansari sent to Ameer Ali was 'based on the one prepared by the great English experts for field hospitals in the South African war, only minor differences being made owing to difference in climate, and season of the year'. Ameer Ali was, however, requested to consult expert opinion in London to select the best and cheapest material in the market. The purpose for ordering the equipment and supplies from London was to allow team members to travel light with only their own personal luggage. However, the team nonetheless appears to have carried some bandages, dressings, disinfectants, and minor surgical instruments that were donated by a company from Calcutta.

At that stage, the team was ready to deploy but waiting for their passports. Dr Ansari was reporting that they had heard rumours that the Government of India, the term used at the time to refer to the British Empire's representatives in India, would not permit the Mission to proceed to Turkey. But he quickly refuted these rumours and stated instead that the viceroy had promised to request the British Ambassador in İstanbul and agent-general in Cairo to assist the Mission. The later memoirs of Chaudry Khaliquzzaman also collaborates the support received from the British authorities. He relates, for instance, that the members of the Mission were received by the British Viceroy Lord Harding just before they departed from Bombay.[16]

The journey from the United Provinces to the port of Bombay was nothing short of a triumphal procession. Thus, Wasti writes, 'A huge crowd of well-wishers saw the train off from Lucknow with poems, prayers and tears; the venerable Shibli Nu'mani was there at the station, and Maulana Mohamed Ali himself was to escort the Mission by train to Bombay. A similar reception took place along the train's route to Bombay at Bhopal.'[17]

The Mission left Bombay with a hearty farewell aboard the Italian vessel *Sardegna* on 15 December 1912. The ship also carried Her Highness the Maharani Holkar of Indore and her suite of ladies going to Europe. They were to pass through Aden and reach Suez on the morning of 26 December. From there on, the

Mission took the railway route to Alexandria through Ismailiya and Banha. The Mission received much consideration and support from the Egyptian officials and people: 'The Customs Officer who was an Egyptian gentleman showed his appreciation and sympathy and only opened a box or two probably in order to swear he had gone through the formality. A small crowd of Egyptians had gathered there and they were very enthusiastic and showed us every courtesy and consideration.'[18] That said, the trip from Suez to Alexandria also had its challenges. In addition to the expensive freight charges and food at the hotel, Dr Ansari writes that '[t]he journey from Ismalia to Benha was a little more cramped though the scenery around made up for the discomfort in the train. The change at Benha was accomplished under stress of time and a jabbering crowd of porters who wanted "Bakhsheesh" [tip] from every single member of the Mission.' The final stretch of the train ride was from Banha to Alexandria on the same day. The train was 'most congested but full of very sympathetic Egyptians and Turks'. The Mission almost had its luggage sent to Cairo instead of Alexandria but was saved by the intervention of Dr Ansari and the British captain who was assigned by the occupation forces in Egypt to assist the Mission. After touring the city to inspect the alternatives, the Mission decided to check in at the eighteenth-century seaside Hotel Metropole at a discounted rate.

The next morning in Alexandria, the Medical Mission had the opportunity to meet the Turkish refugees from the Balkan Wars sheltered at a Khedival palace at Ras-el-Tin. They were told of

> the atrocities perpetrated by the Servians in throwing always from the windows the Turkish sick and wounded, there to die of cold, starvation and disease … a good many other inhuman deed done by the Balkan armies during their occupations of Salonica and Kavalla amongst them the murder of the weak and innocent women and children, the insults and injuries to the women, the spoliation, burning and looting of their hearths and homes and the unspeakable miseries caused to these innocent non-combatants.[19]

These depictions, writes Dr Ansari, went straight to the hearts of the Indian Medical Mission and reinforced their determination to help the wounded in the war.

In Alexandria wherever the Mission went, they were met with cheering crowds. Their departure from the docks, this time aboard *SS Romania* en route to İstanbul, was another spectacular event. Dr Ansari wrote:

> There were banners bearing the Red Crescent carried by the crowds, and burning speeches were made by several persons denouncing the atrocities of the Balkan armies and a poem in Arabic was read by a gentleman in our honour. Then began the loud, lusty and continuous cheering from the crowds who continuously kept it up until our boat was out of sight. And not being content with that, several boats full of people followed our steamer for a long distance cheering us and singing Arabic songs.

The Mission arrived in Piraeus on 29 December and toured Athens before it embarked on the last stretch of its voyage to İstanbul the same day. Dr Ansari gives an eloquent account of their passage from the Turkish straits where he underscores, 'There is no doubt that the entrance to the Straits is well fortified and would smash up any fleet which tried to enter into it.' This message was to be ignored at great cost to the British imperial navy and the assembly of forces collaged from around the empire including India almost two years later in 1915. Much more than a quarter of a million young lives were lost in an ill-conceived campaign in a meaningless war that resolved nothing and culminated in more wars, and decided by a polity whose interests, perceived or real, were alien to the troops they put together from Rajasthan, Brisbane, or Wellington, if not Liverpool. Given the large number of desertions and defections from the troops of the Indian units, insult was added to injury by combining them into joint units with the English forces, where they could be monitored more closely and even led to death in frontal units. Such is the tragedy of empires and their wars. Today a citadel towers over the Turkish straits as a remembrance for the Gallipoli wars, not as a reminder of the hard-won victory in Turkey's war of liberation, itself an inspiration for Indian independence, or as a demonstration of anger against the lives incinerated in pursuit of imperial hegemony and as a consequence of elite folly, but rather as a token of reconciliation and peace. Every year, thousands from around the former British Empire assemble in Gallipoli to mark a war which had dubious aims and little impact on the larger First World War. On that occasion they read the historic magnanimous words of Mustafa Kemal Atatürk engraved at the Anzac cove:

> Those heroes that shed their blood and lost their lives. You are now living in the soil of a friendly country therefore rest in peace. There is no difference between the Johnnies and the Mehmets to us where they lie side by side here in this country of ours. You, the mothers, who sent their sons from faraway countries wipe away your tears; your sons are now lying in our bosom and are in peace. After having lost their lives on this land they have become our sons as well.

Wars, whether cold or active, are marked by information operations that involve distortion or concoction of information in order to shape the public and enemy perceptions in the desired direction. One of Dr Ansari's letters contains an example of the incidence of such information operations when he talks about the Turkish navy's *Mecidiye* warship. Thus, Dr Ansari writes, 'The boat "Medjidiyeh" which was reported to have been struck by a torpedo from a Greek boat and sunk was there in a very good condition.' Dr Ansari also reported that although taken individually, the Turkish fleet appeared in best working condition, he was not impressed by the overall strength of the Ottoman fleet. During the passage through the Turkish Straits, two doctors boarded the ship to escort the Mission. The Mission reached İstanbul early in the 'dull, cloudy and misty morning' of 30 December 1912. Dr Ansari was poetic in describing the approach to İstanbul:

> About 6:15 we could clearly discern the shadowy outlines of the minarets and domes, the old fortresses and the new buildings along the shores of the Bosporus. There by Stamboul in its proud but sad dignity, and the feelings it aroused in one's mind were difficult to analyze. Those hills and old forts now crumbling down had seen the advent of the mighty Turks, the fall of the Byzantine Empire and the rise and glory of the Osmanli. Now, alas! The time had come when they were watching the gradual dismemberment of their Empire and the Decadence of Moslem rule.

The Mission found a large crowd of Turkish people joined by a guard of honour and military band waiting for them. The reception party was led by Colonel Mehmet Bey, the inspector general of the Croissant Rouge:

> We formed a line walking in twos, and as we came down with Colonel Mehemet Ali Bey, the Guard of Honour gave us a salute and the band played the Turkish National Anthem. That was the first and would probably be the only place for representatives from India to be honoured with a salute. You could imagine how much we all appreciated this and felt the honour bestowed on us. In one action our eternal brother-hood was sealed.

The same morning, the Mission met with Besim Ömer Pasha for breakfast at the Kadırga Hospital, where the Mission was to stay until it was deployed to the border. Besim Ömer Pasha was to call the Ottoman Red Crescent organization yet an infant and that 'its foster-father was India'.

Initial Days in İstanbul

Anxiously waiting for the designation of a site to set up the field hospital, members of the Indian Medical Mission toured İstanbul. It was during this initial tour that Dr Ansari seems to have developed the idea that a relief fund for the Turkish refugees from the Balkans would be very useful. After seeing a crowd of women in ragged and torn clothes who were 'refugees from the different Turkish villages now in possession of the Balkan Confederacy', he wrote,

> The Government is very good to them. They are clothed, housed, and fed by the Municipal Funds and are provided with money when they are sent to the provinces in Asia Minor. However, on making inquiries, I felt sure in my mind that, an organized relief fund to help those sufferers from the war would greatly mitigate their suffering and materially help them to start in life.

The same day the Mission was able to meet the minister of foreign affairs and the chief of staff of the ministry of war. The latter suggested a place for the field hospital. In one day, Dr Ansari reported blithely, they were able to make progress. The other Indian medical team in town was the Bombay Mission which was headquartered in the University College of Sciences (Dar-ul Fünun) and, although having arrived earlier, could not yet start working as their equipment had not arrived from India.

During their tour of the various medical facilities in İstanbul, Dr Ansari and his team appears to have been particularly impressed by the Haydarpasa railway station and the Military Medical Hospital adjacent to it. He wrote:

> We went there in a boat and saw on our landing there the magnificent railway station which is the terminus of the line running between Constantinople and Aleppo. I have not seen any railway station either in Europe or in India which can come anywhere near it. We visited the Military Medical College and Hospital ... The wards were clean, paved with glazed tiles, and furnished with modern iron beds. The sheets, pillow cases and towels were clean; the blankets were thick and warm; and altogether there was nothing lacking to make the patients comfortable and cheerful during their stay in the hospital. All the patients in this building were medical cases and numbered 1,000. This hospital would compare favorably with any European hospital, and it was certainly much cleaner than the hospitals one seen in France and Italy.

Regarding the Army Medical College too, Dr Ansari was most openly appreciative: 'The arrangements here were absolutely perfect. Everything was scrupulously clean, and I can assure you there are not many places in London, Berlin, Vienna or Paris which can boast of a hospital like this.'

It was against this background that the Indian representatives seem to have lost their patience about the false propaganda or 'tissue of malignant lies', as Dr Ansari called them, about the Ottomans that was to become a major hallmark of the Balkan Wars and the First World War:

> From what follows, when describing the hospitals at Hademkui, Gnifer and San Stefano, you would see that not only the general press of Europe was full of a series of calumnies and false reports about the Turkish organization, but even the medical Press was affected by this religious bigotry and fanaticism, and stated facts

about the medical organization which on examination one finds altogether incorrect and exaggerated. I do not mean by this that there is no room for assistance in this present unusual situation. It is bound to affect even the best organized country.

Dr Ansari goes further in his letter to underscore that

[i]t may be of interest, by way of comparison, to mention here that the results of the German Red Cross Hospitals, the British Red Crescent Hospital sent by Mr. Amir Ali and the French Red Cross Hospitals have been very unsatisfactory, whether due to the lack of skill or interest of the doctors sent in these Missions. In fact there is a feeling here, no doubt erroneous, owing to their bad results that these men deliberately maimed and dismembered the patients when a conservative treatment would have saved the lives and limbs of many of the patients placed under their treatment.

As Azmi Özcan showed, the controversy about the performance of British and other foreign medical missions and the accusations about their alleged wilful mistreatment of the wounded Ottoman soldiers continued. The reports about the distribution of Bibles and anti-Turkish pamphlets at the British relief camps in Turkey aggravated the Indian Muslims even further.[20]

Setting Up the Ömerli Field Hospital

On 12 January, Dr Ansari, accompanied by the manager of the Mission Abdur Rahman Siddiqui, carried out the initial exploration of the region around Hadımköy where the field hospital was to be set up. He reported several other field hospitals including two belonging to Egyptian Red Crescent working in good condition. In İstanbul, the site was designated as Sancak Tepe. However, the Generals in the field after consultations decided to change the site instead to Ömerli, 'which is behind the lines of defence and yet not so bitterly cold or damp as Sanjaktapa. There is also a plentiful supply of good water at Ömerli which is not found at Sanjaktapa.' The site for the tents was under the shelter of a hill facing the Ömerli railway station and separated from the railway line by a small stream. 'There is a natural spring with a plentiful supply of drinking water by the side of our camp, and with a bridge across the stream the camp will be a minute from the railway station', wrote Dr Ansari, openly appreciative of the venue selected for the hospital. Upon their return to İstanbul, Dr Ansari and the Mission members decided to field the hospital by 25 January 1913.

In a whimsical note, Dr Ansari reported that the setting up of the hospital tent proved challenging. First, with the help of soldiers, the Mission had to make a small bridge over a stream that separated the railway line from the hospital site. None of the members of the Mission had previous experience in pitching a tent, and it took a great deal of effort, time, and discussion to set up the first tent: 'By the end of the evening we succeeded only in pitching up one double-tent and a bill tent. Next day we succeeded in putting up three double-tents, one single tent, the operation tent and the remaining two bill tents: a mixed shower of rain and sleet prevented us from putting up the last tent.' But he quickly added in his letter to Mohammed Ali:

> It would have done your heart a lot of good if you had seen the members of your Mission working in the teeth of a most bitterly cold wind and the mud almost knee-deep. Here at least there was no distinction between the doctor and the dresser, everyone hammering the pegs, fixing the poles or spreading the canvas and doing the work like real enthusiasts.

To aid the Mission, 100 soldiers were sent, yet to no avail as the inclement weather did not allow further work. The country was at a war against a ruthlessly hostile coalition of countries who approached the capital city by a few tens of kilometres only. It was a wonder that anything was working at all.

However, the team managed to put things in place one day before the hostilities resumed, resolving a shortage in tents by purchasing them locally from a British firm in İstanbul. The Mission was to let go of two of its members even before the fighting began due to illness. Thus, Dr Barry and Husain Reza Beg would return to India ahead of the rest of the members of the Medical Mission.

Ansari Contemplating Relief Work on Migrants

Dr Ansari's letter of 20 January reveals that he continued to develop the idea of helping the Turkish refugees from the Balkans even as he was preparing to deploy the first field hospital in Ömerli. Not only that he was thinking about it, but also Maulana Mohammad Ali seemed on board from this early stage onwards. In fact, the idea of splitting the Mission into two appears to have come from Mohammad Ali. Thus writes Dr Ansari:

> The mission can very easily be divided into two units, one working at the Ömerli Hospital and the other either in the front (in case of war) or in Anatolia where most of the emigrants have been sent. In the latter condition, which seems to me most likely, our work would be just as useful as in the case of war. The section in Anatolia would have a house rented for the purpose for the hospital and dispensary. And the chief feature of the work of this section would be house to house visits not only to treat the patients there and to supply them with the necessary medicines in their homes, but also to furnish them with food and necessary clothing, and when the bread winners are cured, to help them with a small sum and start them on their work. I think this would be a far greater work than half a dozen field-hospitals.

The plan was for the Mission to work in cooperation with the Ottoman Red Crescent for the migrants' relief work but to retain own register and employees.

The Language Issue Is Resolved

As the Mission was nearing its deployment to Ömerli, the letters revealed certain weariness on the part of Dr Ansari. He wrote, 'I cannot tell you what difficulties are placed in our way here even in arranging a small matter. Our things have all arrived last week, and in any other country but Turkey everything would have been arranged in a day or two.' A point underscored in both Mukhtar Ansari's letters and Chaudry Khaliquzzaman's memoirs were the initial difficulties in communication. This appears to have started even before the ship carrying the Mission docked in İstanbul. The medical doctors who were sent to Dardanelles to escort the

Mission did not speak English or Urdu. Dr Ansari recorded this encounter, which he still believed was most useful, as '[i]t was most amusing to see our attempts to make him understand our meaning as he knows only French and Turkish.' Khaliquzzaman also noted with reference to their early days in İstanbul that '[n]ot knowing the Turkish language we felt very awkward in meeting people and talking to them in broken phrases, composed of English, Urdu and a few words of Persian and Arabic'.[21] In order to resolve this persisting problem, Dr Ansari decided to hire an Egyptian physician Dr Fuad Bey as both a doctor and interpreter, in addition to two Indian nationals who spoke Turkish fairly well. Although Dr Ansari does not disclose the names of these two Indian youths, he mentions by name a third person, an Egyptian youth then studying at the Mercantile Naval School in Turkey by the name of Mahmood Mazhar, who joined the Mission as a volunteer without pay.

The Young Turk Coup D'état

Having determined the final location for the first field hospital and explored the region, Dr Ansari and Abdur Rahman Siddiqui returned to İstanbul from Ömerli on the afternoon of 23 January 1913, only to find the city in upheaval. Dr Ansari writes:

> As I drove past the sublime Porte I saw some five to eight hundred soldiers standing inside the enclosure of Bab-i-Aalee, and a crowd at the balcony of Bab-i-Aalee, along the steps, the road, the gate-way and the entire public thoroughfare. This was the memorable day on which the coup of the Party of Union and Progress was carried out in order to catch the Cabinet of Kiamil Pasha red-handed in the very set of signing the reply to the Note of the Powers ceding Adrianople.[22]

The Committee of Union and Progress, the Young Turks, had been forced out of power in July 1912, shortly before the Balkan Wars which began in October. The committee was already losing face due to the Italian–Turkish War and the uprising in Albania. A small secretive group that named themselves 'Saviour Officers' (Halaskar Zabıtan) led the opposition to the committee and forced them out of government in July 1912. The ensuing government of

Ahmed Muhtar Pasha too was not able to cling on to power and resigned 21 days after its formation in the face of the defeats in the Balkan Wars. The new grand vizier was Mehmed Kamil Pasha who would, for all intents and purposes, govern the Ottoman Empire and take the country to the London Conference during the armistice. A large segment of the people was distressed about the poor conduct of the Ottoman armies against the Balkan confederacy and put the blame on the War Minister Nazım Pasha. The committee suspected that the Ottoman government would cede Edirne to Bulgaria at the negotiation table rather than continue the war. The European powers were already pushing in that direction. To forestall that outcome, on the morning of 23 January 1913, some five years after their first putsch in 1908, the committee seized the initiative. The rest is found in Dr Ansari's personal account from what he gathered of the day:

Enver Bey had ridden on a horse all night from Gallipoli and, reaching Constantinople on the morning of 23rd, made all the necessary arrangements, placing his men in the different cafes and houses in the vicinity of Bab-i-Aalee. He rode on a horse with a few soldiers to Bab-i-Aalee and, on being challenged by the sentinel at the entrance, he said he had come to save Turkey, and made a brief but touching speech, which moved the soldiers so much that they all joined him, and he marched into the room where the Cabinet had assembled to do the work of selling their country to their enemies. He entered this room accompanied by another army officer, Najef Bey, and demanded the resignation of the Cabinet from the Grand Vizier. He held the form of the resignation and asked for their signature, which was meekly complied with by Kiamil Pasha and a few others. But Nazim Pasha got up in a rage and ordered his A.-D.-C. to get these intruders arrested by the gendarme. Shots were exchanged in which Nazim Pasha, his A.-D.-C. Najef Bey and two other were killed, but the remaining Ministers were kept under guard. Enver Bey then processed to the Sultan's palace and got the Imperial iradeh appointing Mahmood Shevket Pasha as the Prime Minister and entrusting him with the formation of a new Cabinet.

The Grand Vizier Kamil Pasha, held at gunpoint by Enver Pasha, attempted to write in his resignation letter that he was yielding office upon the suggestion of the military forces. However, Enver

Pasha had him add that the resignation was upon the suggestion of the people and the military. As the drama was unfolding within the prime ministry (Bab-1 Ali), a certain crowd was cheering outside in favour of Enver Pasha and Talat Pasha. Dr Ansari writes:

The crowd was waiting for the arrival of Enver Bey, and the appearance of a motor car with Enver Bey, Talat Bey, and Mahmud Şevket Pasha was the signal for a tremendous outburst from the crowd outside Bab-i-Ali. Enver Bey was the hero of the moment, and the crowd carried him shoulder high to the Bab-i-Ali. He was embraced and kissed until he was nearly smothered. Then the Grand Vizier, according to the ancient custom, made a short speech to the crowd in which he expressed the hope that he would receive their cooperation and help in the difficult task of government at such a critical time. The crowd cheered him very heartily. The party then entered the Bab-i-Ali, followed by the great crowd in which some of the members of the Mission were also included. They entered every room and also saw the chair in which Nazim Pasha had been killed. Very soon after the streets were quiet and no external sign of such a great revolution was obvious even in the streets round the Bab-i-Ali.

This point, the voluntary evacuation of the crowd without further fuss and the rapid return to normalcy on the streets, seems to have astonished the Medical Mission. Dr Ansari reflected:

It struck an outsider as a very extraordinary thing that events of such great moment should be enacted in such a quiet manner without any obvious change in the daily life of the Turks. Is it possible that the Turks have got inured to these vicissitudes and take them with a philosophical calm, unthinkable by us Indians to whom such events are extraordinary and unusual? Or, is it they have grown indifferent and callous and take any sudden change in their government with the indifference of an absolutely lifeless and spiritless people?

He wrote that his own answer was the former.

Dr Ansari explains that after the coup, the German, Austrian–Hungarian, and Russian attitudes towards the Ottomans had changed towards more being supportive. He noted, however, that only England and France remained reticent. He argued that '[i]t is obvious that the Young Turks have saved the prestige of Turkey and mean to die honourably, if death must come. It is impossible even for an adversary to abstain from admiring their pluck, although it still remains to be seen whether this pluck is going to save Turkey.' He nonetheless asserted that '[w]e wish to God that Turkey would declare war again, and regain a moral and territorial victory over her toes'. As we will see, the war would indeed resume. Edirne would be lost and then regained.

The Gallipoli Expedition and the Çanakkale Hospital

The government of Mahmud Şevket Pasha supported by the Young Turks staged the Bab-ı Ali coup on 23 January with the pretext that the government they toppled would cede Edirne to the Balkan powers. Instead, they developed a proposal that would divide the larger province of Edirne, with the city itself remaining in Turkish hands. One could only speculate as to what would have happened if the Bulgarians had accepted the deal. The fact is they rejected it and the next phase of the First Balkan War began on 3 February, right after the Balkan League denounced the armistice. A critical object of this phase was the capture of Edirne from the Turks. The city was already cut off from the rest of the country and was not receiving any replenishment. The Balkan occupation army had already swept by Edirne all the way to the outskirts of the capital İstanbul. The new government planned to ease the pressure on the fortress city. Enver Pasha was to personally lead this campaign to clear the Gallipoli peninsula and connect with amphibious forces. It was an ambitious plan which could have not only saved Edirne but also helped encircle the occupation forces targeting İstanbul from behind. But it was a campaign against an enemy force that fielded twice as many guns.

As planning was under way, medical units were also being recruited for the Gallipoli campaign. The exact location was at first not known. Dr Ansari wrote: 'I have had to divide the Mission into two units: one remains in Ömerli—under Dr Naim, and the other is going under me to an unknown destination with Enver Bey's attacking army.' Beasim Ömer Pasha sent an urgent telegram to Ömerli in order to summon Dr Ansari to İstanbul in a hasty fashion. This was both to discuss the treasury bonds and to send a part of the Mission to Gallipoli. Dr Ansari was jubilant: 'This news ought to immensely please you', he wrote, 'as ours is the only Mission out of the seven which had applied which has been given this great honour and distinction of accompanying Enver Bey.'

The Medical Mission sailed with the amphibious forces aboard the boat *Cambridge* leaving İstanbul on 18 February with some 300 packages of medical material. They landed successfully in Şarköy the next day. A smaller group selected from members of the Mission then marched with the advancing Ottoman army. The initial expectations about the course of the war were most positive. Dr Ansari wrote that '[t]he Ottoman army has driven the Bulgars all along the line so far. They are near Adrianople now, and the relief of the fortress is expected daily'. To that Maulana Mohammad Ali responded in the *Comrade* as follows:

> The landing of the expeditionary column of 60 thousands of all arms under the command of Enver Bey was reported by Reuters long ago and later on the expedition was declared to have failed. We cannot, however, believe that a column of 60 thousands, after effecting a successful landing, would 'fail' without fighting a battle and even encountering the enemy.

Nonetheless, in addition to being outgunned, the Ottoman forces were also facing another and apparently equally daunting challenge. In Dr Ansari's words, the Ottomans 'had not only to fight against the soldiers of the Balkan Confederacy and the resources of the whole of Europe, but the forces of Nature seem to be working against them'. He would add that '[a]fter the re-commencement of the war the Turks have had several successes and advanced several kilometres specially along Tchataldja, but the weather prevents them from taking any offensive at present'. This was a weather the likes of which the Indian Medical Mission had never seen before: 'Here the wind seems to blow from every direction all at once, and the flakes of snow pour down so thick that it is impossible to see more than few yards ahead. It seems like a mixture of snow, fog and cyclone. In a few minutes exposure the hands, feet, nose and ears become numb and lifeless.' Under these circumstances, the campaign bogged down and, for all intents and purposes, failed to either relieve Edirne or to circle the enemy. But the Indian team was impressed nonetheless: 'Anyone who has seen the soldiers which compose the present Turkish army, as I have had several occasions of seeing in the hospitals, would not doubt that the Anatolian soldiers are about the only soldiers whose spirit would remain undaunted in spite of the severest winter and the greatest hardships that any army could be exposed to.' Enver Pasha personally advised Dr Ansari to set up the hospital not on the field, as the weather was too cold to keep wounded soldiers in tents, but in the town of Çanakkale. In that hospital, they were to treat 171 inpatients and 101 outpatients in the month of March 1913. More than half the patients that were brought to the Çanakkale hospital during the Gallipoli campaign 'were in the extreme stage of exhaustion due to exposure to cold and disease, some of them dying a few minutes after their arrival in the hospital'.[23]

The Fall of Edirne

One of the most fateful moments of the Balkan Wars was the fall of Edirne after the heroic resistance spanning few months. Dr Ansari suggested that '[i]n well informed circles in Constantinople the fall of Adrianople was known to be imminent a week or two days before the actual occurrence'. The major fighting that caused thousands of lives was, in fact, strategically unnecessary and inconsequential. The city was already bypassed with Balkan forces, who had reached long before and threatened the borders of İstanbul. The city was cut off from logistical reinforcements. It would face an inescapable starvation had the siege continued. There was no hope of lifting the siege anytime soon either by the Turkish forces incarcerated in the fortress city or by the Ottoman forces further east. However, the general public was inconsolable. Following the fall of Edirne, the bulk of the fighting shifted again to Çatalca where the Ottoman forces were pressing hard against the Bulgarian army. It appeared that the bravery of Şükrü Pasha and his men in Edirne ignited the will of the Ottoman army and with the successes in Silivri battles, Dr Ansari reported, the spirit of the army was splendid. The fighting on this front compelled Dr Ansari to return to the Ömerli hospital from Çanakkale and reassume the lead as Dr Naim had to return to India because of his illness.

Turkish Inspiration for the Permanent Red Crescent Society in India

At the turn of the twentieth century, internationalist movements were in their infancy and among them the Red Cross movement was the one that led the way. The International Red Cross and Red Crescent movements were founded by the Geneva Convention on 22 August 1864 in order to treat the wounded during the wars. Although the Ottoman government ratified the convention on 5 July 1865, the actual formation of the society was delayed until the 1877–8 Russo-Ottoman War. The establishment of the Ottoman Red Crescent in 1877 was to be celebrated by Gustave Moynier, the president of the International Committee of Red Cross, as a turning point in history on the grounds that this was the first time that the Islamic world was integrated into an institution shaped by the Christian world. However, the Red Crescent Society was dissolved after the Russo-Ottoman War and re-established on 20 April 1911 during the 1911 Turkish -Italian war in Libya. The 1912–13 Balkan Wars were perhaps the biggest challenge faced by the organization soon after its re-institution, one which the Red Crescent Society braved with flying colours, with significant help from the Indian Muslims. In fact, the assistance to the Ottomans and indeed to the Ottoman Red Crescent (Croissant Rouge) had already started during the 1911 war against Italy. It was against that background that the vice president of the Red Crescent Society underlined at his reception of the Indian Medical Mission that 'the Croissant Rouge was yet an infant and that its foster-father was India'. The categorization of the Indian assistance as the 'foster father' became even truer in the course of the Balkan Wars. The foreign donations constituted a very significant part of the assets of the Red Crescent Society. When the mobilization for the Balkan Wars was announced in September 1912, the Red Crescent Society owned more than 70,000 Ottoman liras. The donations from the Ottoman citizens as well as foreigners exceeded every expectation by reaching 350,000 Ottoman liras. Out of this total amount, 230,000 came from Muslim countries. However, with donations equivalent to nearly 200,000 Ottoman liras, Indian Muslims alone accounted for more than the domestic and other foreign assistance put together.[24] Having learned of the figures announced in the Ottoman Red Crescent Society's first ever annual report,[25] Mohammad Ali rejoiced in the *Comrade* dated 29 May 1913 that '[i]t is, indeed, gratifying to learn that the contribution of India to the Ottoman Red Crescent Society not only exceed the contributions of every other country, but that they exceed the contribution of all the other countries of the world put together, including Turkey!' He also added that 'not all the contributions of a country like Egypt were sent to the Ottoman Red Crescent Society, nor is the entire contribution of India represented by the amount sent to the Ottoman Red Crescent Society'. Dr Ansari was to suggest that '[i]t would gladden the generous Indian Mussalmans to learn that they stand first in the aid rendered to the Ottoman Red Crescent. This is the most convincing proof that the Indian Musssalman has the largest heart although he has the shortest purse'.

While the Indian Muslims were massing up such generous assistance to their brethren in Turkey, India itself had no such permanent structure to avail of to extend the much-needed assistance to vast numbers of people afflicted frequently by various calamities. Thus, towards the end of the tenure of the Indian Medical Mission in Turkey, Dr Ansari developed the idea of establishing a permanent Red Crescent Society in Delhi. The idea seems to have come out of his close interactions with the Ottoman Red Crescent Society, the work of which the Indian team appreciated immensely. The Red Crescent Society provided a model for the Indian team to witness first-hand. Thus, a fortnight after the Mission's arrival in İstanbul, Dr Ansari wrote:

> I am convinced after thorough and searching investigation that this is the only organization worthy of support from India where every penny is used to good purpose and Dr. Muhammad Husain and myself have thought it necessary to sign a telegram sent by Bessim

Omar Pasha to the different papers in India for publication in order to direct all the money to the Croissant Rouge and prevent its going to quarters where one cannot find anything about the money.

In a more detailed report, Dr Ansari was to renew his admiration for the work of the Red Crescent Society, stating:

> We have gathered every possible information regarding their work and have come to the conclusion that, although they are by no means very quick in their undertakings or prompt in their organization, they have done a vast amount of work during this war … We have visited their stores and their work room where the ladies sew linen, under clothing, stockings, etc. etc. for the patients and the emigrants, we have also seen for ourselves the manner in which clothes, blankets and other necessary articles are distributed to the different sections of the emigrant population encamped round about Constantinople. And, although we have not been able to visit the food camps, we know on good authority that good, wholesome and sufficient food is cooked and supplied twice daily to the emigrants … For this work they have divided Stamboul in to various sections or areas, each area being worked by one local team who prepares a list of the different families of the emigrants with their needs. The Central Office sends one of its members with food, clothing, bedding, etc. according to the requirement to be distributed in the presence of this member and marked off in the registers.

The success of the Ottoman Red Crescent Society in both medical and relief work convinced Dr Ansari of the utility of such an organization also for peacetime functions in response to civil disasters including epidemics.

Accordingly, as he was preparing to draw close the Mission to return to India in end May, Dr Ansari wrote:

> At first I was thinking of handing over all our tents and equipments to the Ottoman Red Crescent, but I have changed my mind now. I mean to bring back to India everything that would be necessary to look after fifty patients. This would from the nucleus of the permanent Red Crescent Society at Delhi. Considering the innumerable claims on the generosity of the poor Musalmaans of India this is hardly a fit time to expect a great deal of support from them for

establishing a permanent Red Crescent Society. But if we possess the necessary equipment a great deal of useful and humane work could be done in India with the help of only a small sum. For instance; a very small unit of two doctors, one compounder and three or four dressers, with equipment for twenty-five beds, could be sent out to combat dreadful epidemics like cholera, plague etc., which break out in India and carry off so many thousands of people every year.

Dr Ansari argued that the Red Crescent 'could also undertake with greater success than Government officials inoculation against plague, typhoid, etc. It could do a great deal of ambulance work and treatment of accidents, etc., by sending out units during big fairs like the Nauchandi in Meerut, the Numaiha at Aligarh, the Magh Mela in Allahabad, or the Sonepur fair in Behar'. All said, 'the most useful service of the permanent Red Crescent would be when it would go out with the Hajis to Mecca', wrote Dr Ansari, underscoring a need that was felt by the large number of Indian Muslims who went on pilgrimage every year. As such, the Ottoman Red Crescent Society inspired the Indian Red Crescent alongside the Egyptian and Afghan societies, which were also inspired by the Ottoman experience.

Demand for Turkish Orphans in India

On 20 May, Dr Ansari wrote to Mohammad Ali Jauhar that he was getting letters from private individuals requesting him to bring some Turkish orphans to India. He commented that he had no doubt these people were actuated by the most human desire to help in bringing up these poor, homeless, fatherless children. Yet, he wrote, it was impossible to accede to their wishes, as these orphans were at once sent to the government orphanages and cannot be secured. Nonetheless, in a subsequent letter, he was to report that he had 'seen and selected six boys and four girls, their ages varying from six to nine years to be dispatched to India'. However, 'owing to the necessity of getting the final permission of Djemil Pasha, Chief of the Municipality', Dr Ansari was unable to bring these orphaned children with the Mission to India, although they would 'follow in a week or two together with two Turkish ladies, the widow and the daughter of a Turkish officer, who have been left destitute and absolutely unprovided for'. He reported that 'those ladies come from a respectable family and know French, Arabic and Turkish perfectly and are expert on needle work'. One can presume that Mohammad Ali too asked for these orphans to be brought to India, since Dr Ansari wrote, 'As arranged with you, the ladies services will be utilized as teachers in your family or in a girl's school. I have left Haji Abdullah, an Indian, who worked as interpreter in our Chanak Kila Hospital, to accompany them to India.' Apparently, Dr Ansari was 'forced for want of time to leave the question of the orphans half-finished in the hands of' the Manager of the Mission. There is no record as to whether these ten children and the accompanying two ladies did actually travel to India.

Resettlement of the Balkan Refugees

Dr Ansari and the members of the Medical Mission came across the plight of the Turkish refugees expelled from various Balkan countries during their travel to İstanbul when they stopped in Alexandria. As they were travelling through the city, they began noticing the refugees sheltered in one of the Khedival palaces in Alexandria, Ras-el-Tin Palace. The Mission visited the palace and was taken around the inoculation department and the dispensary. They saw about 1,000 Turkish refugees of all ages and were met by a deputation of the notables amongst the Turkish refugees. The Chief Medical Officer Dr Himmat addressed the Mission in English and described to them 'some of the most touching and pathetic scenes which his rescuing party had beheld at Kavalla', in today's Greece. He used terms such as 'atrocities', 'inhuman deeds' or 'unspeakable miseries' to characterize the treatment of innocent non-combatants by the Balkan armies during the occupation of Salonica and Kavalla.

Dr Ansari wrote further that '[t]he description of these refugees reaching the shelter of the Khedival yacht which brought them to Egypt was specially touching and pathetic how they described it as the "ship of safety" how they kissed the very steps which took them to the boat with tearful gratitude'. These and many scenes depicted by Dr Himmat, wrote Dr Ansari, 'went straight to our hearts and made us even more determined to do all that lay in our power to lessen the sufferings sympathize with and soothe the bleeding hearts of our fellow-Moslems in Turkey'. During their stay at the Ras al-Tin Palace, the Mission also heard a Turkish journalist by the name of Djafar Effendizadeh Omar Sirat, who was also among the group of notable refugees, make a speech with tearful eyes in which he expressed gratitude and appreciation on behalf of the Turkish refugees and gave the Mission the fullest assurance that there would be thousands of Turks like him awaiting most anxiously their arrival amongst them. This initial encounter with the refugees not only clenched their will to fulfil their mission of mercy but it also seems to have set the stage for the subsequent emphasis by Dr Ansari to construct villages for the resettlement of the refugees.

The Mission caught further glimpses of the refugees from various Turkish villages that came under the possession of the Balkan Confederacy 'in very ragged and torn clothes, looking the very picture of misery and helplessness awaiting food and clothes'. Dr Ansari observed that the 'Government is very good to them. They are clothed, housed, and fed by the Municipal Funds and are provided with money when they are sent to the provinces in Asia Minor.' The Ottoman Red Crescent and several other charities were also engaged to provide relief. However, when he enquired further, he wrote, 'I felt sure in my mind that, an organized relief fund to help those sufferers from the war would greatly mitigate their suffering and materially help them to start in life.' Although the issue of providing relief to not only the wounded soldiers but also the refugees apparently did come up, and two cheques were provided at Dr Ansari's meeting with the Grand Vizier Mahmud Şevket Paşa soon after the coup in January, Dr Ansari next mentioned refugees in April.

Towards the end of the First Balkan War, when the two hospitals transitioned from treating those wounded in battles to providing care to the sick, the work on resettling the refugees (muhajirs) from the Balkans gained priority in Dr Ansari's eyes. Thus, by 14 April 1913, Dr Ansari relayed his intention to make a tour in Anatolia and İzmir with Zafar Ali Khan, as a representative of the Ottoman Red Crescent, to select a suitable place for the 'colonization' of the Turkish refugees from the Balkans. His intention was to form a reliable organization into which he would be able to insert some half a dozen members of the Mission to play a practical role in the resettlement work by staying for some time in Turkey. He thought retaining these members of the Mission at a moderate monthly pay would be required for the smooth functioning of the construction work. However, the resettlement plans required new funds which Dr Ansari estimated to be in the environs of 20,000–30,000 pounds in order to build a model village, with 100 to 150 houses containing as many families. That would relieve 1,000 to 1,500 emigrants, a small number given the scores of families uprooted from their homes, but it would nonetheless 'sow the seed of greater things in future', wrote Dr Ansari. It is not clear what was meant by greater things but one idea was the establishment of an international Muslim cooperative league, with one million shares to be sold to the Muslims of Turkey, India, Egypt, Morocco, Persia, and other Muslim countries. The object of this cooperative society would be to foster Muslim industries and to encourage industrial development in Turkey.

In his letter dated 6 May 1913, Dr Ansari gave details of the meeting of the Indo-Ottoman Colonisation Society, which discussed under the chairmanship of Dr Esad Pasha on 2 May the government scheme for colonization. At the meeting, Dr Esad Pasha was asked to ascertain from the government the various tracts of land at its disposal, their irrigation facilities, their proximity to railways and the sea, the condition of labour, and the nature of soil. The relevant information to be compiled would help a select committee with an agricultural expert in its tour of inspection in Anatolia. The final scheme, with the plans of the village and cottages, would be submitted to the Ottoman government after the return of the committee. Another decision was for the Ottoman and Indian committees to work together, having a common advisory council, but separate executives. Before the month of May expired, two more meetings of the Indo-Ottoman Colonisation Society were held, and a constitution was drawn up for presentation to the Minister of the Interior Talat Pasha for approval. The government presented a list of lands in Anatolia at its disposal and which it could grant for resettlement purposes.

The list contained lands in Ankara, Adana, Bursa, and Konya. The approval for the Society for the Colonization of the Macedonian Refugees soon came and a committee of four persons was dispatched to choose the site for the colonization of the village with due regard to sanitary, agricultural, and economic conditions. The committee consisted of Zafar Ali Khan; Agah Bey, representing the Ottoman Red Crescent; Saleh Bey, an agricultural expect; Dr Ahmed Fuad, joint secretary; and Mukhtar Ahmad Ansari, secretary. The itinerary would start with Ankara and move on to Konya and thence to Adana. The exact location of the two villages would be decided upon after the completion of the tour. A synopsis of Dr Ansari's exploratory tour in Anatolia and the selection of the two sites are provided in the ensuing chapter. Dr Ansari was, however, not able to see the beginning of the work on the resettlement. The literature appears vague about what exactly was built after the team left. More research is needed in this regard.

Azmi Özcan notes that work did indeed start and, thanks to the campaigns led by the *Comrade* and *Zamindar*, funds continued to pour in all the way until the end of the First World War. More refugees poured in after the Mission departed from Turkey particularly during First World War, which started soon after. The Ottoman Red Crescent and the government made herculean efforts to resettle big numbers of refugees and it seems possible to conclude that the groundwork done by the Indian Medical Mission and the funds extended by the Indian Muslims were most helpful in that regard.

Travels in Anatolia

The letters that describe the visits that started from İstanbul's magnificent Haydarpasa railway station on 28 May 1913 display such an avid eye for the beauty and uniqueness of the region that even after 100 years, they can still be read with delight. As Dr Ansari travelled eastward towards Ankara, then an ancient small town yet to be made the bustling capital of a modern democracy commanding a G-20 economy, he set eyes on the Moda district where the 'deep blue sea of Marmora here dips towards Islands forming the gulf of that name and the Principio islands with their red soil and modern red tiled villas make a contrast picture worthy of sight'. He notices the factory of the town of Hereke, where world-renowned 'fazes, silk cloths, rugs, carpets and many other goods were manufactured and worked by purely Turkish capital'. He observes that '[t]he most striking was the fact that only women were seen working in the fields: probably the male population was all drained by the army'. He witnesses beyond İzmit that '[t]he mountain tops, the valleys and the plains are all covered with groves of olive trees. Cultivation is done everywhere as far as the eye could reach. Neat little houses and villas could be seen here and there peeping through the green foliage. Nature is seen here in its greatest profusion and makes it an ideal spot of beauty.' Near Sapanca, Dr Ansari sees

> several little villages of the Caucasian refugees along the shores of the lake; they could be seen working in the fields in their picturesque costumes. To those who have seen the Swiss mountains, this part of the Turkish dominions would appear equally enchanting if not superior. There are beautiful fruit gardens and orchards all along the shores the lake and some of the best grapes are grown in this district.

As his train steams onwards, he lays on Eskisehir, the old city, and notes the region's historicity:

> It was in the vicinity of this town that the Saljuks had granted a free land to Toghral for his services in helping their army which was about to be defeated by the hosts of Tamerlane. The little village of Qarajah Hissar where Osman, the founder of the present dynasty, raised the flag of independence first is nearby and a monument marks the place where Osman made his declaration.

Only Ankara, which receives its name from the slate-grey colour of the rocks on which it is built, seems not to have impressed Dr Ansari visually: 'Indeed this part of the country presented the most desolate and depressing view. Here and there were some low-lying marshy plains, but even in these parts nothing but rank grass and reeds grow.' Yet, again historicity seems to have caught up with Dr Ansari as he remarked that Ankara is 'situated on the southern side of a hill and dates back to the time of the Romans. In the times of the Seljuks this city was besieged by the conquering hosts of Tamerlane and would have been lost if it had not been for the timely help of Toghral and his well-trained horsemen.' In Ankara, Dr Ansari had, on the other hand, only words of appreciation for the educational establishments which he visited.

Of all the places Dr Ansari visited outside İstanbul, Konya seems to have influenced him particularly. He devoted a separate and rather detailed section to the visit to the shrine of the great Sufi teacher and saint Rumi. He also reported the warm reception accorded by the Governor of Konya Ali Rıza Bey, who encouraged the visiting delegation to establish the village for the refugees in his province. Dr Ansari saw a bustling city with a government scheme to canalize and irrigate half a million acres of land, a hire-purchase scheme to provide modern agricultural implements to the farmers, a large magazine operated by the *maulvis* (Mevlevis), and a two-year-old yet already profitable Muslim Bank, which he relayed in delight. As he wrote, 'These signs of commercial and economic activities amongst the Musalmans of Konia gave us great heart and hopes for the real consolidation of the Ottoman Empire. It must be mentioned that all this is the result of the activity of the Party of Union and Progress in Konia.' Another point he saw fit to report was how a Colonel Surtis showed utter distrust in the Turkish people by distributing aid to the refugees in Konya through a foreign missionary institution in preference to the Ottoman peoples. The committee decided to mark down a site in Chomra as a possible location for a resettlement village, on an artificial hillock about four miles from the railway line, close to an ancient Roman town then called Binbir Kilise.

A cooperative governor awaited the committee also in Adana. Dr Ansari appears to have been impressed by the agricultural scheme around the Adana region. He wrote:

Indeed all the agricultural operation here are carried on in the most modern and up-to-date manner with the least amount of labour. It makes one wonder could some of the Indian journals have the audacity to call Turkey the most backward country, when they must know that in India agriculture is still being carried on in the most primitive condition without the least improvement in the methods of agriculture for the last 150 years. I assure you, Adana, could give many lessons to most up-to-date agricultural districts in India.

Another site was selected at the Adana province, close to the sea. Dr Ansari appeared impressed by the tomb of the Abbaside Caliph Mamun-ul-Rashid, 'that elegant, cultured Abbasside monarch, who died in this vicinity where he had come on a political mission, and was buried at Tarsus'. He wrote:

The Tomb of one of the greatest of the Arabian Monarch, the grandeur of whose court is still recounted in many an Arabic poem, is simple to the extreme and devoid of any of those paraphernalia which mark the last resting place of the great monarchs. It was his express will that this should be so, as simplicity was the key-note of the private life of this monarch and that of his father, the great Harun-ul-Rashid.

On Dr Ansari's way back to İstanbul, the Grand Vizier Mahmud Şevket Paşa, which the Mission revered most highly, was assassinated. At any rate, time was too short before his scheduled departure from İstanbul back towards India. Dr Ansari was to leave before the resettlement work was to begin. He left behind a few men to look after the project.

His travelogue-like dispatches from the inspection visits to parts of Anatolia awakened Dr Ansari to the value and the promise of the land. He seems to have become aware of the stakes that were involved. As he wrote: 'Many empires have risen, reached their zenith, decayed and disappeared, before the very eyes of these unchanging mountains and rocks. It makes one wonder what fate awaits the only remaining Moslem State which now holds this historical place under its sway.'

Audience with the Ottoman Sultan and Caliph

On 17 June 1913 Sultan Mehmed Resad V received the members of the Indian Medical Mission, which Dr Ansari was to recount as the 'greatest event of their stay in Turkey'. The team, accompanied by

Besim Ömer Pasha, was taken to the royal Yıldız Palace in İstanbul in a carriage and was first treated to some refreshments and then ushered into an audience with the sultan. Besim Ömer Pasha presented Dr Ansari to the sultan and, in turn, Dr Ansari presented his team one by one to the sultan, who graciously bowed as each member was presented. After the introductions, the sultan expressed his appreciation for the Mission's assistance to the Ottoman soldiers during the Balkan Wars. Dr Ansari wrote later that 'His Majesty was visibly touched as he spoke these words; he invoked God's blessing on the members of the Mission for their work of mercy so asked us to convey to the Muslims of India the eternal gratitude of His Majesty and the Ottoman nation.' The audience with the Ottoman sultan, wrote Dr Ansari, was a distinction that all members of the Medical Mission were naturally proud of because 'for a Mussalman it is a great honour to kiss the robes of the Khalifat-ul-Muslimeen'.

The Mission Leaves Turkey

Dr Ansari reported that the Ömerli hospital was closed on 22 May followed by the other one in Çanakkale two days later. Before their closing, the hospitals had started to extend outpatient medical services and even 'feeding daily 70 women and children refugees at Kala-i-Sultanieh and 30 at Hindia (Ömerli)'. Before their closing, the minister of interior paid a visit to the Kadırga Hospital to meet with the members of the Indian Medical Mission. He extended the appreciation and gratitude of the Turkish government. Dr Ansari wrote: 'The scenes of leave-taking as Hindia, and Sanjak Tepe, from General Izzet Pasha and Abdus Salam Pasha, were most touching and will ever remain in our memory.' The Mission decided to send materials for 50 beds back to India while storing the rest with the Red Crescent. Their medical mission thus coming to an end, the Indian Medical Mission left Turkey on 19 July 1913 aboard a Romanian vessel with great pomp as they were received at the İstanbul docks. Dr Ansari reports in his letter published in the *Comrade* on 29 July that the Minister of the Interior Talat Bey led the procession to bid farewell to the departing Indian medical team. Several other dignitaries also joined the ceremony including Emin Pasha, the head of the army medical department, Besim Ömer Pasha with all the members of the central committee of the Ottoman Red Crescent, Dr Esed Pasha, president of the sanitary department of İstanbul and president of the Indo-Ottoman Colonization Society and many other *anjuman*s and societies, Maulana Sheikh Abdul Aziz Chawish, principal of the Medina University, and many other Egyptian and Ottoman personalities. Dr Ansari reported that large numbers were present to see the Mission off but does not offer estimates about the number of the attendant crowd. The minister, in his 'short and touching' speech, bid the Indian team farewell and expressed gratitude on behalf of the Ottoman government and the Ottoman people. He stated that the Balkan Wars had caused them much sorrow and entailed great sufferings, but the sympathy and the great help of the Muslims of India and the presence of the Indian Mission had consoled the nation and had made them forget their great trouble. Talat Bey underscored that the Ottomans would never forget this brotherly help rendered by the Muslims of India. After the minister kissed and embraced every member of the Mission and said that he was leaving them to the care of God, all present followed his example. Dr Ansari wrote that the Mission departed with tearful eyes and sorrowful hearts, feeling that they were leaving their home and family in Turkey, only to go to another home and family in India. The team was overwhelmed by the touching expressions of fraternal regard and brotherly feelings exhibited by their Ottoman brothers.

Not all members of the Mission returned to India together with Dr Ansari. Dr Mahmudullah, Hamid Rusul, and Tafazzul Husain stayed in İstanbul to go to Hajj, and Abdul Rahman Pashawari remained for health reasons. He was later to join the Ottoman army during First World War. Messrs Shoaib, Khaliquzzaman, Manzoor, Ghulam Ahmad, and the general manager Abdur Rahman Siddiqui opted to return after a month, whereas Maulvi Mohammad Sharif and Mirza Abdul Qayum would stay on to look after the refugees and colonization work. Dr Raza Khan returned to Edinburgh. The remaining members of the Mission including Dr Fyzee, Dr Rahman, Bashiruddin Ahmad, Nurul Hasan, Abdul Aziz Ansari, Mohammad-Uddin, Yusuf Ansari, Sherazee Chiraguddin, and Tawangar Husafe returned to India with Dr Ansari. They were to be accorded a hero's welcome in Bombay and Delhi, where some

30,000 people amassed in decorated streets, throwing garlands at the members of the Mission and chanting the name of Dr Ansari, the hero of 'Islamic duty'.

Notes

1. Syed Tanvir Wasti, 'The Indian Red Crescent Mission to the Balkan Wars', *Middle Eastern Studies* 45, no. 3 (May 2009), p. 397.

2. Halide Edip Adivar, *Inside India* (London: George Allen & Unwin, 1937), p. 130n1.

3. Wasti, 'The Indian Red Crescent Mission to the Balkan Wars', p. 399. The biographical book on Peshawari in Urdu that Wasti refers to is A. S. Shahjahanpuri, *Ghazi Abdurrahman Peshawari Shaheed* (Karachi: North Western Hotel, 1979).

4. Adivar, *Inside India*, p. 130n1.

5. Chaudhry Khaliquzzaman, *Pathway to Pakistan* (Lahore: Longmans Green and Co, 1961), p. 25.

6. Şuhnaz Yılmaz, 'An Ottoman Warrior Abroad: Enver Paşa as an Expatriate', *Middle Eastern Studies* 35, no. 4, Seventy-Five Years of the Turkish Republic (October 1999), p. 40.

7. Yılmaz, 'An Ottoman Warrior Abroad', p. 42.

8. Hasan Ünal, 'Young Turk Assessments of International Politics, 1906–9', *Middle Eastern Studies* 32, no. 2 (April 1996), p. 31.

9. Salahi R. Sonyel, 'Mustafa Kemal and Enver in Conflict, 1919–22', *Middle Eastern Studies* 25, no. 4 (October 1989), p. 508.

10. Glenda Fraser, 'Enver Pasha's Bid for Turkestan: 1920–1922', *Canadian Journal of History* XXII (August 1988), p. 198.

11. Sonyel, 'Mustafa Kemal and Enver in Conflict', p. 513.

12. See http://www.turknostalji.com/haber/titanik-faciasindan-kurtulan-turk-381.html (accessed on 7 November 2012).

13. Nur Sari and Zühal Özaydın, 'Dr. Besim Ömer Paşa ve Kadin Hastabakici Eğitiminin Nedenleri (II)', *Sendrom* (Mayis 1992), p. 73.

14. Hale Tosun, 'İstanbul'da Kurulan Cumhuriyetin İlk Milli Hemşirelik Okulu: Kizilay Hemşirelik Okulu', *Maltepe Üniversitesi Hemşirelik Bilim ve Sanat Dergisi, Sempozyum Özel Sayisi* (2010), p. 126.

15. Chaudhry Khaliquzzaman, *Pathway to Pakistan* (Lahore: Longmans Green and Co. 1961), p. 21.

16. Khaliquzzaman, *Pathway to Pakistan*, p. 21.

17. Wasti, 'The Indian Red Crescent Mission to the Balkan Wars', p. 396.

18. Dr Ansari's letter dated 30 December 1912.

19. Dr Ansari's letter dated 30 December 1912.

20. Azmi Özcan, *Pan-Islamism: Indian Muslims, the Ottomans and Britain, 1877–1924* (Leiden: E.J. Brill, 1997), p. 152.

21. Khaliquzzaman, *Pathway to Pakistan*, p. 21.

22. Dr Ansari wrote that the authorities in İstanbul censured his message about the coup, deleting five names and several words from his original telegram.

23. Dr Ansari reported nine deaths.

24. The data is compiled based on the Society's documentation by Hüsnü Ada in '[t]he First Ottoman Civil Society Organization in the Service of the Ottoman State: The Case of the Ottoman Red Crescent (Osmanli Hilal-i Ahmer Cemiyeti)', unpublished Master's thesis, Sabanci University, September 2004.

25. Dr Ansari made a point in passing in his letter dated 20 January that he induced the Ottoman Red Crescent Society 'to publish an account of their work in the form of a booklet and also the total amount of money received from India up to the present time', which the Society responded to by publishing its first ever Annual Report in mid-1913.

7

The Indian Medical Mission
in Hindsight

In spite of the rather significant visibility that the Indian Medical
Mission led by Dr Ansari enjoyed at its time in 1912–13, later
studies on the period tended to either completely overlook their
effort or mentioned it only in passing. There are indeed very
scanty accounts of the Mission. One of the dedicated studies of
the enterprise was provided by Syed Tanwir Wasti in an article.
It provides useful information on the background, composition,
and activities of the Mission. There is also useful information
on some of the members of the Mission and their careers after
the Mission was terminated. However, there is no data on the
number of patients treated by the Mission and the nature of their
wounds. Wasti correctly places the Mission in the context of
the Indian Muslims' heightened political sensitivities in support
of the Ottoman sultan caliph, yet he does not make an attempt
to trace the influence of the Mission on either Indian politics or
relations between Turkish and Indian Muslims. The question thus
remains as to what was the actual impact of the Indian Medical
Mission. To answer that one must perhaps first refine and focus
the question. The impact of the Mission can be explored by break-
ing the analysis into more focused parts, involving areas in which

the Mission could have been expected to exercise influence. The primary purpose and objective of the Mission was, of course, to provide the Ottoman Turks with medical assistance. Therefore, its scorecard should be reviewed foremost with reference to the contributions it made to the struggling Ottomans in terms of treating their wounded. Although it did not initially figure prominently among its objectives, after witnessing the situation on the ground, Dr Ansari's Mission also set out to help address the problem of refugees. Thus, its success in tackling the difficult task of providing housing to the Turkish refugees expelled from the Balkans needs to be brought under limelight. This is intrinsically related to one of the two Muslim internationalist projects which the Mission started during its tenure in Turkey, namely the International Muslim Cooperative League. The other internationalist project not directly related to addressing the hardships caused by the Balkan Wars, namely establishing an international Muslim college in the name of Medina University, could deserve a separate assessment. However, it is important to recognize that the Mission was not only a medical or humanitarian endeavour. It was also a pan-Islamic endeavour, with political significance back home in India. Hence, a separate lens could be brought on the influence or meaning the Indian Medical Mission had on popular perceptions at home. Related to that vantage point would be a look at their inputs towards the popularization of the movement against British rule starting to gather pace in India.

In the ensuing paragraphs, I will take a bite into this analysis, bringing in not only the letters by Dr Ansari but also other accounts of the Mission. One should, however, acknowledge upfront that further research is needed to provide a fuller account of the impact the Mission has directly or indirectly made in each of these categories of analysis.

Impact on the Ottoman Army and Society

The Indian Medical Mission led by Dr Mukhtar Ansari arrived in İstanbul when the worst of the fighting in the First Balkan War was already over. The actual fighting began with the Montenegrin attack on 19 October 1912 and continued until the armistice in Çatalca on 3 December. The Greeks did not observe armistice and continued fighting, notably around Yanina.

Edirne was under siege and the Bulgarian army was stopped at Çatalca, about 60 kilometres from the Dolmabahçe Palace of the Ottoman sultan caliph in downtown İstanbul. The Ömerli field hospital set up by the Indian Medical Mission was close to 20 kilometres from the Çatalca front. The second phase of fighting would take place between 3 February and 30 May. It was during this phase that part of the Indian Medical Team would be taken to the actual warfront. In February 1913, Enver Bey would personally ask for the Indian Medical Mission to support the Turkish forces raiding the Bulgarian occupation forces in Çanakkale. When in Bolayır two armies came head to head with intense artillery fire, the Indian medical team was in safe distance but nonetheless part of the action. The Ottoman plan to clear the Gallipoli Peninsula and to link up with Ottoman forces landing at Şarköy failed and a stalemate developed, with the Bulgarian army stuck in Çatalca and not being able to move forward, and the Ottoman forces not being able to push back or defend territories in the western Balkans including Macedonia. Close to 150,000 lives were lost, and even greater numbers of civilians killed, maimed, raped, and expelled from their homes, forced into a long march to safety. When a forced march was imposed in 1915 on parts of the Armenian population residing close to the Russian warfront, it was cried foul. The Indian medical team did not directly experience the atrocities against the Turkish populations in the Balkans. It did not suffer with the attacked populations, such as in Edirne during its siege by the Bulgarian army. Yet, it witnessed the state of the incoming refugees and felt their pain nonetheless. One can argue that as much as the naturally positive disposition of the team members towards their co-religionists in Turkey, it was these personal observations of the Balkan refugees that solidified the resolve of the Indian team. This is acknowledged, in fact, by Dr Ansari. In his letter dated 30 December, he wrote about meeting around 1,000 Turkish refugees of all ages and a deputation of the notables amongst the Turkish refugees. He related the reports of the atrocities perpetrated against the Turkish residents in the Balkans. He recounts that the sick and wounded were thrown off the trains and that the non-combatants, including women and children, were murdered. Dr Ansari referred to the report he received describing 'these refugees reaching the shelter of the Khedival yacht which brought them to Egypt [being] specially touching and pathetic how they described it as the "ship of safety", how they kissed the very steps which took them to the boat with tearful gratitude'. As a consequence, Dr Ansari wrote, 'These and many scenes depicted by him [the medical officer-in-charge Dr. Himmat] you could well imagine went straight to our hearts and made us even more determined to do all that lay in our power to lessen the sufferings sympathize with and soothe the bleeding hearts of our fellow-Moslems in Turkey.' Dr Ansari was to hear similar scenes and stories throughout the Medical Mission's tenure in Turkey. The emphasis that the team laid in the resettlement of the Balkan refugees was a direct consequence of the plight of the refugees directly observed by the Indian team.

Contrary to their expectations and the reports coming through the media, the Indian Medical Mission encountered a state that was still functioning in full vigor. The refugees were in a wretched condition but there was an organized effort in place to provide and care for them. The problems that existed could easily be attributed to the ongoing war, which would have challenged the governance capacities of any nation. The team was met at the İstanbul harbour by Ottoman authorities and ushered into the Kadırga hospital where they would stay until an appropriate venue was allocated for them to deploy their field hospital. All the incoming foreign medical teams were joined by the Ottoman Red Crescent or Military Medical Corps and deployed to where they were most needed. Dr Ansari referred to the efficiency of the Ottoman Red Crescent and asked Mohammad Ali to channel all aid through this organization. In 1913 the Ottoman Empire was not a defunct state but rather was working in full swing, although very much in need of assistance given the nature of the sustained onslaught for very many decades thereto. This alone shows the existence of a working organization and arrangements to welcome foreign teams and provide orderly Ottoman state assistance to their deployment where they were needed. The ability to receive assistance requires an absorption capacity which is particularly needed in times of calamity and even to date remains wanting in most disaster and war zone environments around the world. In this regard, there is little doubt as to the nature and magnitude of the disaster at hand. Medical historian Özaydın notes: 'The problem of the wounded, the outbreak of cholera and the refugees who were left out in the open during the cold winter started a chain of disasters. There were so many wounded and sick in İstanbul that, including bar-racks and police stations, many government buildings were turned into hospitals, and mosques were given to the refugees.'[1] Under these circumstances, the Military Medical Corps and the Ottoman Red Crescent had been able to set up a working scheme to absorb the very welcome medical and humanitarian assistance offered by the 'Red Cross from Germany, America, Belgium, France, Holland, England, Sweden, Romania and Russia together with the Red Crescent that had been formed in Romania, England, Egypt and India'.[2]

Dr Ansari's travels in Turkey also confirmed the existence of a functioning state, albeit strained by the refugee flows and eco-nomic difficulties. In this context, Dr Ansari devoted considerable space to the educational institutions he encountered in Ankara in his letter dated 26 June, written aboard the ship en route back to India. Ankara would later become the capital of the modern Republic of Turkey. Dr Ansari, however, appeared unimpressed by the rocky landscape on which the city was built. Thus, he wrote:

In spite of the depressing general appearance of the town, signs are not wanting of sincere efforts on the part of the unionist Government to improve the conditions of the people. Directly after the Consultation the Government opened primary schools, one girls' school, one higher primary school and one secondary school where free education is given. Recently the efforts of Nihat Bey, the delegate for the Party of Union and Progress, have brought into exis-tence an up-to-date primary school on the latest model. There is a secondary school where all the modern sciences are taught and a Darul-Moallimin preparing teachers for primary schools. Under the able guidance of Maulana Huseyin and his staff, this school is doing splendid work. A visit to the different classes in the school con-vinced as that the teaching here is very sound and practical ... Our visit to the school of industry and the agricultural college proved highly satisfactory. The latter institution has been working for the last there and a half, years and consists of a staff of eight teachers. There are forty boarders who are fed, clothed and taught free of any charges (thirty-five Muslims and five Christians). The classroom, library, scientific laboratory, zoological and geological museums were up to date and most complete. We saw here the rearing of silk-worms and the preparation of butter, cheese, etc. in the cow-shed attached to the college. This dairy-farm was kept most scrupulously clean, the diet, the quantity of milk, the amount of butter, etc. being all noted on a chart in each shed. Attached to this institution was also a shed where six fine Arab stallions were kept for covering mares. Sabah was the most perfect specimen of an Arab horse it had been my lot to set eyes on. The experimental farm attached to the college covers an area of 1,000 acres, where all the modern, up-to-date agricultural implements and methods were being used. A very large poultry-farm is also attached to this institution. We had a very splendid lunch given [to] us here by the Director of the College.

Dr Ansari's admiration in his observations and encounters with the Ottoman officials in Konya also attest to the functioning state of the Ottoman polity even during the Balkan Wars, shortly before the empire's final and decisive war, namely the First World War. In his letter dated 26 January, Dr Ansari related his observations in the following words:

I must mention here that the Ottoman Government has canalized and completed the irrigation of half a million acres of land in Konya. It was arranged that we should go next day with Nadir Bey and Dr. Besim Bey to inspect this canalised land ... We then visited the Government depot where a large number of modern agricultural implements were exhibited and sold to the farmers on hire-purchase system. There was also a German mart for agricultural implements. But the thing which delighted us most was our visit to a large magazine started by the Maulvis [Mevlevis or the members of the Rumi dargah] where every kind of article from finest silk down to ordinary broom was sold by these Maulvis themselves. The next most pleasing visit was to the 'Moslem' Bank which has been started for the last two years with a capital of £T [Turkish currency] 70,000. The Manager, Ahmed Hazne Bey, told us that the last year's net profits were £T 8,000, a tidy little sum which speaks volumes for the management of the

Bank. This year they were going to undertake the electric installation in the town and as electric tramway which the Manager of the Bank hoped would bring larger profits to the shareholders. Their new building situated in the principal street of the town was almost complete, and they hoped to transfer the Bank there within a month. These signs of commercial and economic activities amongst the Muslims of Konya gave us great heart and hopes for the real consolidation of the Ottoman Empire. It must be mentioned that all this is the result of the activity of the Party of Union and progress in Konya.

An interesting point Dr Ansari reported in the same letter pertained to the deep distrust the missionary activities created in the Konya province: 'The Vali [Governor] asked us if we belonged to the same society which Colonel Surtis represented. On being informed in the negative he spoke to us of the utter distrust shown by the colonel in the Turkish people by distributing aid to the refugees in Konya through a foreign missionary institution in preference to the Ottoman peoples.' Dr Ansari would similarly voice admiration for the infrastructure built by the Ottoman government in the Konya province in central Turkey:

Next morning we started with Nadir Bey and Dr. Besim Bey to Çumra where the staff of irrigation engineers have their headquarters. The source of the water is a very large like in the Karadağ Mountains some ten miles distant. The water is diverted into a river, the Çarsamba Çayi, from which by means of dams and sluicegates the flow of water is maintained into the primary canals and thence into the secondary and tertiary systems. The irrigation scheme, which was started more than four years ago, has now been completed and supplies an areas of half a million acres.

It was at this location that Dr Ansari and his colleagues would decide to set up a settlement for the Turkish refugees from the Balkans. His observations about other parts of central and southern Turkey confirmed those in Ankara. Thus, for Erzin in southern Turkey, he wrote:

The population of this vilayet is 450,000, out of which there are 80,000 Armenians. But the curious fact was that in spite of the richness and fertility of the land and the wealth of the farmers the revenue derived by the Government was only half a million pounds. The chief cultivation in the vilayet was wheat and other serials, but recently cotton growing is being carried on an extensive scale although the quality of the cotton is inferior to that produced in Egypt and India. Fruits of all kinds are grown here in abundance and are shipped at Mersin to Europe. Some of the finest apricots and plums I have ever tasted in my life were given to us by Dr. Refik Bey, Chief of the Sanitary Department here. We visited the secondary school, which has 180 boarders and is one of the finest institutions of the kind. The school of industry here is a very extensive institution with a large carpentry department, a smithy with an iron forge attached to it. I saw several engines being repaired here and a large number of ploughs, sheaving machines and other agricultural implements. They have a printing press where every description of printing was being taught to the students and the local bi-weekly paper, Ceyhan, was printed here. The agricultural college is the most up-to-date institution, has a staff of twenty teachers and over 200 students and has been doing splendid work for the fast five years. Some very important experiments on cotton growing are at present being carried on in this institution, the results of which are expected to be of greatest economic importance to the vilayet. The orphanage which is constructed to accommodate 300 inmates is very well governed and looked after. Most of the children there, numbering 140 altogether, were Armenians.

Dr Ansari's admiration reached a climax when he compared his observations in Turkey with India in his letter dated 26 July. He wrote:

Our train passing through the fertile valley of Ceyhan, where as far as the eyes could reach nothing but cultivated fields could be seen. This was the reaping season for the wheat crop. The reaping was done by means of the modern machinery driven by a horse, which cuts the corn and collects it in sheaves at the rate of 20 acres a day. In other place [sic] one saw grain being cropped and separated from straw and husk by engine-driven machinery. Indeed all the agricultural operation here are carried on in the most modern and up-to-date manner with the least amount of labour. It makes one wonder could some of the Indian journals have the audacity to call Turkey the most backward country, when they must know that in India agriculture is still being carried on in the most primitive condition without the least improvement in the methods of agriculture for the last 150 years. I assure you, Adana, could give many lessons to most up-to-date agricultural districts in India.

However, Dr Ansari also voiced criticisms when he encountered shortcomings. He was critical of certain roads and more notably of the Ottoman finance authorities who had not proceeded as quickly as Dr Ansari thought was necessary in issuing bonds for sale in India. In one instance, about a couple weeks after the medical team arrived in İstanbul, Dr Ansari appeared to have lost his nerve about the red tape he encountered. Thus, on 20 January he wrote in exasperation that the Mission encountered difficulties in fulfilling even small chores and complained that only in Turkey it would take a week instead of a day or two to arrange for the dispatch of their equipment to the field hospital in Ömerli.

In another rare outburst of anguish, Dr Ansari wrote on 3 March:

> One cannot help feeling that the Turks have got absolutely no business capacity, and in arranging the issue of Bonds on such favourable terms they are not as prompt as they might be. That money is most urgently needed by them at present is most obvious to all, and at such a critical state in the life of their country they should be lacking in energy and zeal to expedite the issue of Bonds shows a great weakness and explains a great deal why they have failed so miserably.

The critical tone would, however, remain extremely rare, with letters displaying greater admiration as he experienced and learned more of the country.

What may be regarded as conspicuous by its absence was the work on addressing the most tragic and pressing of the problems encountered by the Ottoman army and society, namely the widespread epidemics of cholera and other diseases. Dr Ansari's letters provide no account of any work done to address the epidemics. This is conspicuous for two reasons. First, epidemics, especially cholera, had made a major impact in the Balkan Wars. Shortly after the outbreak of the First Balkan War, epidemics of cholera, typhoid, and dysentery broke out in the region. The contagion was exacerbated by the difficulties in maintaining sanitary discipline in war zones as well as shortage of medical personnel. It was spread around by the civilians displaced by fighting and hostile Balkan armies. The toll taken by cholera and other epidemics were reported to reach tens of thousands. The diseases affected both the soldiers and the refugee populations. The epidemics seemingly had direct impact on the war-fighting capability of the Ottoman army. The grave situation in this regard has been thoroughly documented by Turkish and non-Turkish studies and the press of the day, including in India. For instance, a French correspondent was reporting that patients suffering from cholera were being transported to Red Crescent hospitals and to Yesilköy in large groups.[3] Second, the Indian Medical Mission was aware of the scourge of epidemics rampant in the region even before they departed India towards Turkey. In fact, the topic of the cholera epidemic during the Balkan Wars and the potential role of the Indian Medical Mission seem to have been given the centre stage by the British Viceroy immediately before the departure of the Mission from Delhi. Thus, receiving Dr Ansari and other members of the Indian Medical Mission on the day of their departure from Delhi, the British Viceroy 'expressed the hope that the Indian Medical Mission would prove even more useful than other medical missions and field-hospitals, as cholera being particularly an Asiatic epidemic Indian doctors were far more qualified to deal with it than European doctors'.[4] In response 'Dr. Ansari informed His Excellency that he was taking with him special cholera outfit ... of which Dr. Ansari had had extensive practical experience during the last outbreak in Delhi, having had to deal with about fifty cases daily and succeeded in curing 80 percent, in spite of having been called in generally very late'.[5] However, it must have been the choice of the Ottoman authorities and not that of the Mission that they were deployed in Ömerli and Çanakkale and not other venues where they could have partaken in efforts to treat epidemics. And the team did not report encountering epidemics in their tour of central and southern Turkey, the sole exception being syphilis in Ankara which was 'twice as common amongst the Christians and Jews as amongst the Muslims'.[6] The team did not seem to offer any advice on addressing the disease, although they reported that a separate wing was established for this purpose by the hospital they visited in the city.

Every single life saved is a success story in its own right. That aside, the overall numbers of patients that the Indian Medical Mission treated can be considered as relatively limited when compared to the overall dead and wounded. Thus, Dr Ansari reported in his letter dated 7 April 1913 that for the month of March '[t] here were 171 in-patients and 101 out-patients'. For the months of February and March, the total number of inpatients in both hospitals was 177 and outpatients 140. At the Çanakkale field hospital directed by Dr Abdur Rahman, 9 wounded patients died while 78 were cured. On 20 April, he reported that at Çanakkale '[t]he total number of patients up-to-date has reached 292, the number of patients at this moment in the hospital being 108. The number of out-patients since my last letter has reached 102.'[7] Dr Ansari was happy with the results, indicating that the

> percentage of mortality works out to be 3.3, a figure which speaks for itself and indicates the infinite attention and work which it must have involved to all the staff. And when it would be known that more than half the patients sent to the hospital were in the extreme stage of exhaustion due to exposure to cold and disease, some of them dying a few minutes after their arrival in the hospital, I am confident that all credit should be given to the staff of the Çanakkale Hospital for their splendid work.

However, Dr Ansari appeared particularly proud of the results from the field hospital in Ömerli. Thus, he wrote buoyantly:

> [T]he Ömerli sections of our Mission have beaten all records. Their heroic adherence to their duties, in spite of the bitterest, and the severest winter when their tents were often completely snowed up and their camp was one mass of snow and mud, when the Turk's themselves would not venture out of their houses, has been rewarded with the splendid record of one single death out of a total of 310 patients, which works out to 3 per cent. No amount of words can adequately express their real work and worth. It is by their constant striving to keep up the high ideal that they have secured a reputation which induces the relations of many of the wounded

soldiers to take them straight from Hadimköy and place them in their charge. Such a tribute from the patients and their relations to the honest and good work rendered by the Ömerli Hospital speaks for itself.

In this section, a word on the impact of the Muslim internationalist projects initiated by the Mission may be fitting. Dr Ansari's Mission joined a number of other international medical teams from a diversity of countries, several run by Muslims but also included non-Muslims. These teams became an independent part of an international effort to alleviate Ottoman suffering. The Indian Medical Mission, however, pursued activities that went beyond providing medical relief to the wounded Ottoman soldiers. Two of their pursuits actually pertained to what can be defined as religious internationalist schemes.

A project that Dr Ansari seems to have devoted energy was the establishment of a Muslim University, under the name of Medina University. He reported several ministers and other leading men of Turkey showing keen interest. He wrote:

The Minister of Evkaf [religious endowments] showed great zeal, and wished the University to be started with as much expedition and dispatch as possible. The Nizamnameh [regulation] ... was discussed and sanctioned. Members of the Constitution Committee were appointed, including Mr. Zafar Ali Khan and myself. Shaikh Abdul Aziz Shaweesh, who is the soul of this movement, would probably be appointed Principal of the University.

He asked Mohammad Ali to help prepare a draft for the constitution and curriculum of the Medina University on the lines of the Aligarh University. He also listed a number of personalities in India, including Maulana Shibli Numani, to be consulted to that effect and added that some friends in London and Egypt had also been asked to prepare draft constitutions. Upon the receipt of the three drafts, a constitution committee would draw up the constitution, taking the best and most suitable draft as its basis. In another letter dated 20 May, Dr Ansari related that while waiting for the draft constitutions from India, Egypt, and England, the constitution committee had drawn up a provisional syllabus for the two faculties of divinity and science. According to him, 'the most difficult question would be the finding of suitable professors and assistant professors who would be able to teach the sciences in Arabic'. He expressed the conviction that 'once the university has started on the career even in a modest way, it is sure to pave its way to success'. In his view, 'every Muslim would hail this University as the beginning of the great renaissance in the Islamic world'. While the project was aborted, the intention to establish it can be seen as a manifestation of internationalist and modernist pan-Islamism, aiming at the revival of the fortunes of the Muslim world through education.

Towards the end of the First Balkan War when the two hospitals transitioned from treating wounded soldiers to providing care to the sick, the work on resettling the refugees from the Balkans gained priority in Dr Ansari's eyes. Thus, by 14 April 1913, Dr Ansari relayed his intention to make a tour of the country with Zafar Ali Khan to select a suitable place for the resettlement of the Turkish refugees from the Balkans. His intention was to form a reliable organization into which he would be able to induce some half a dozen members of the Mission to take practical part in the resettlement work by staying for some time in Turkey. However, the resettlement plans required new funds, even to relieve initially 1,000 to 1,500 emigrants, of which only a fraction would nonetheless 'sow the seed of greater things in future', according to Dr Ansari. In this context, Dr Ansari developed the idea of an international Muslim Cooperative League to promote industrial development in Turkey. This idea was indeed approved by the Ottoman government which suggested a number of possible locations in the cities of Ankara, Adana, Bursa, and Konya. The Ottoman government asked the idea to be further elaborated following a fact-finding mission in these cities. A team was set up to explore the suggested plots led by Dr Ansari. The government also approved the formation of a Society for the Colonization of the Macedonian Refugees. Azmi Özcan found evidence that the Comrade and *Zamindar* continued to raise funds all the way until the end of First World War. Although Özcan states that construction work has actually begun, more research is needed on whether resettlement efforts bore any concrete results. Dr Ansari appears to have spent significant time and energy in encouraging İstanbul to issue Ottoman bonds to help garner financial support. The promise of this arrangement, however, seems to have been curtailed by the colonial government's discouragements back in India. While the resettlement activities did not seem to culminate in the building of the colonies, Turkish medical historian Zuhal Özaydın credits the efforts of the Mission and the editor of *Zamindar*, Zafar Ali Khan, with the later establishment of the Foundation to Assist Rumeli [that is, Balkan] Refugees, which she argued 'was a direct result of the suggestion of Muhammed Ali and Zafer Ali'.[8] One must add to this the groundwork done by Dr Ansari and the fellow members of the Indian Medical Mission during their stay in Turkey.

Irrespective of the number of patients healed or the refugees actually settled, the fact of the matter remains that the Ottoman authorities were highly appreciative of the work done by the Indian Medical Mission. This included the sultan caliph himself who unreservedly expressed his gratitude for the sacrifices that the Mission made during their stay in Turkey. Another eloquent official expression of appreciation was voiced at the official farewell dinner hosted in the honour of the Indian medical team by the Ottoman Red Crescent Society. Dr Ansari would write in his letter published in the *Comrade* on 19 July that after 'a most sumptuous meal', the vice president of the society, Besim Ömer Pasha, and several other members of the Red Crescent Society 'made speeches, praising the work of the All-India Medical Mission and thanking the Muslims of India for the generous help they had given to the Ottoman nation in their trial and distress and expressing fervent hopes for a closer and more constant relations between the Muslims of India and Turkey'. Turkish gratitude was also expressed by the Ottoman interior minister during the farewell ceremony at the İstanbul harbour. Thus, Dr Ansari reported in the same letter that after thanking the Indian Muslims for their support, the minister kissed and embraced every member of the Mission. The minister's words had left the members of the Mission with tearful eyes. Dr Ansari added that they felt like they were leaving their home and family in Turkey while going to another home and family back in India.

Impact on the Indian Muslims

As explained in the foregoing chapter, the pan-Islamism of 1913 involved both a shared public opinion and a defensive strategy that was internationalist as well as proto-nationalist in nature. This particular brand of Islamic solidarity emerged around common themes that had generated profound sincerity about the sympathy towards the Turks, the Ottoman anti-imperialist and anti-Christian-supremacist struggle, the concern for the future of the caliphate and the state of the Muslim world, as well as awareness and distaste towards the deliberate and latent reconstruction of Muslim past, and denigration of the Muslim culture. Common themes helped attain public mobilization and thus scale to empower the primary opposition to colonial rule and the emerging nationalist focus, as well as enable the successful use of modernity and modern technology and media. Pan-Islamic solidarity contained the appeal to action to resurrect the dignity of the Muslim nation, both at home and in the rest of the Muslim world. The Indian Medical Mission's categorization as part of a Muslim internationalist framework seems pertinent in a bid to rid the legacy of the Mission of the corruptive formulations of Islamic unity or the pejorative counterpart term of pan-Islam that has held sway to our day and age. Neither the members of the Mission nor those who had organized or materially and morally supported the endeavour entertained a jihadist purpose or perspective that aimed to unite the Muslim world geopolitically through the power of the sword. What had driven them instead was two-fold. First, they wanted to support the power which appeared as the only one that could hold itself against the onslaught of European colonialism and imperialism. Both the relative strength and enduring escape from colonization of the Ottoman Empire and, of course, its direct rule by the sultan caliph factored in a major way in this calculation. A simultaneous, albeit less manifest, purpose was to rally the Indian Muslim community around a common idea and satisfy their urge for action at a historical juncture when their displeasure with the British rule kept surging, yet their cohesion and indeed strength to resist it outright was solidly at bay. For the Indian Muslims, assisting the Turks in their fight meant, latently at least, finding that fighting spirit in themselves. Turks' successes thus became successes of the Indian Muslims. Their unity of purpose in supporting the Ottoman Turks satisfied their elusive quest to find unity of purpose at home. The dignity and pride of the caliph and later the Turkish independence fighters helped mend the self-image of the Muslim world writ large, including its most sizeable part, the Indian Muslims. As such the Indian Medical Mission led by Dr Ansari became a prized vessel of comparison for the Indian Muslims. The letters by Dr Ansari in their eloquent display of the conscientious effort to assist the Turkish effort and the appreciative welcome accorded by the Ottoman authorities and people filled the yearning in the Indian Muslim psyche. These reports ensured that the Medical Mission was a success in the eyes of the very masses that had sponsored the noble endeavour. The efforts of their representatives in Turkey, so deftly reported by Dr Ansari, had given the Indian Muslims a much-needed sense of self-pride. Obviously, their mission to heal the pride of Muslims succeeded not because they managed to sustain the caliphate. This was not their objective and could not be done by a medical mission. They helped heal the pride because the Muslims of India felt proud of their representatives' courage and zeal and their roles in sustaining the enterprise. The Medical Mission resonated with the masses.

In 1913, the British were aware of the growing resentment against their rule and were eager not to provoke it further. Even if they did not yet fear the loss of their empire in India, they needed the acquiescence of the Indians to sustain it in manpower and resource terms. The British authorities, wanting to appear empathetic to their Muslim subjects and unwilling to appear inimical to the Ottomans, chose to support the Indian Medical Mission. The Mission hence sailed to İstanbul via Egypt and Greece under the diplomatic protection of the British Empire. Thus writes Mohammad Ali that the private secretary to the viceroy informed the editor of the *Comrade* on 24 December, when the Mission was already en route to Turkey and one day after the failed assassination attempt on the British Viceroy at Chandni Chowk on 23 December 1912, that the Foreign Office had instructed the Consul General in Cairo and the Ambassador in İstanbul to this effect. A British military officer, Captain H. V. Bagshawe, was sent by General Byng, the commander of the army of occupation at Cairo upon the instruction of Lord Kitchener. Captain Bagshawe accompanied the Mission during their transit through Egpyt and provided useful assistance. The British authorities showed interest also in İstanbul. As the team landed, the Mission met 'a man with a note from the British Ambassador'.[9] After the Mission settled in the Kadırga hospital, the second secretary of the British Embassy paid a visit. However, in Turkey, the Mission did not require the services of the British Embassy as they were from their very landing at the İstanbul port received and attended by the ranking representatives of the Ottoman Red Crescent. Dr Ansari would also pay a visit to the British Ambassador in İstanbul to keep him abreast of the work of the Mission. His letter dated 11 January gave information about his visit with the Ambassador:

> I paid a visit to His Excellency Sir Gerard Lowther, the British Ambassador, accompanied by my cousin, and found him, to my intense pleasure, a perfectly amiable English gentleman. He offered us cigarettes and sat down for over half an hour for what appeared a friendly chat in a private drawing-room. I inquired after Lord Hardinge and was told that he was convalescent and progressing very satisfactorily. It seems Sir Gerard Lowther and Lord Hardinge are personal friends and have spent several years together at the Turkish Embassy. His Excellency was interested in our Mission and inquired about the members of the Mission, our hospital equipment and the place where we were going to fix our hospital. He asked me to always rely on his ready help whenever we were in need of it. After thanking him for his previous kindness and his promise for the future, we returned well satisfied with our visit.

We do not know whether or how often Dr Ansari or any other member of the Medical Mission interacted with the British Embassy after this meeting.

Perhaps more importantly, as part of the British diplomatic protection, the Foreign Office had also informed the belligerents of the composition of the Indian Medical Mission. The information given to the belligerents was 'absolutely necessary', Mohammad Ali Jauhar reports in the *Comrade* dated 11 January, because 'one could not ignore the possibility of a stoppage of the Mission by the Balkan Confederacy on its way to Turkey'. The Mission had a seven-hour stop in Piraeus port of Athens in Greece. Dr Ansari informed the editor of the *Comrade* in his letter dated 30 January that on the morning of the previous day, they arrived in Piraeus after a very shaky voyage. He reported that 'a very searching examination of our passports and our party was made by the Greek port officials. We were advised not to use the Fez to avoid unpleasantness which we followed although I think unnecessarily.' Members of the Mission took the opportunity of the short break in Athens to tour the city. They visited the Acropolis, the Amphitheatre, the stadium, and the museum and drove through the principal streets of the city. Dr Ansari's dispatch from Athens did not elaborate on their impressions of the city or the historical sites they visited. Instead, the letters reported seeing 'young lads and consumptive-looking men dressed in shabby grey uniforms awaiting orders for the front'. At the harbour, they observed 'a hospital ship in which the wounded were brought from Salonika and medical aid is sent to the sick and wounded'. Dr Ansari and his colleagues also 'saw a transport ship just leaving the harbour full of provisions and some soldiers'. From Athens Dr Ansari dispatched telegrams to the president of the Red Crescent Society, the British Ambassador, and their travel agency, informing these parties of the Mission's arrival. As the Indian Medical Mission approached the Turkish straits, the Mission also encountered a fleet whose nationality was 'the point of discussion', although Dr Ansari thought it was probably Greek.

Overall, Dr Ansari was particularly appreciative of the support given by the British authorities and the personal engagement of Viceroy Lord Charles Hardinge. He spared no effort to express his sympathy, never calling into question his or the Indian Medical Mission's loyalties in the eyes of the British authorities. He did not miss civil courtesies and reacted promptly to show his concern to the British officials. The apparent sincerity of the feelings expressed in the telegram sent by Dr Ansari to Lord Hardinge upon the assassination attempt made on the life of the British viceroy in India at Chandni Chowk showcased this point. The Mission learned about the attack in Cairo through an English newspaper on 26 December and immediately sent a telegram to Delhi which read: 'Convey sympathy and deep concern of All India Medical mission to His Excellency. Pray for his speedy recovery and long life.'

The Ansari letters reveal the fact that in 1913 the Indian Muslims' links and allegiance with the British rule were not yet severed. Nonetheless, the strains were naturally there and becoming increasingly apparent. Before an independence-minded political agenda and momentum built up, many learned Indian Muslims, including Dr Mukhtar Ahmad Ansari and the Ali brothers, walked a narrow path between a rock and a hard place. They came across as both loyal and critical of the British colonial patrons. External issues helped them express their frustrations in an extrinsic context. Their sympathy for Turkey and other Muslim causes around the world became a natural and legitimate subject of vocal dissent. Pan-Islamism was first manifest through internationalism before it could be categorized as proto-nationalism. The British authorities appeared highly conscious of what dilemmas the Muslim disenchantment could create for their hold on India. They first responded by playing the Ottoman sympathies against the Indian Muslims and the Ottoman caliph appeared to have obliged in several instances by trying to calm down the Indian Muslim community. Gradually, the gun that the British authorities helped develop turned against them. There developed an Ottoman caliphal discourse and policy that sought influence in India. However, the British also grossly exaggerated the Ottoman and the pan-Islamist influence in the British Raj. One would see that when the Ottoman caliph finally called for a jihad against the British during the First World War, this would create little stir among the Indian Muslims, at least in the beginning. Many Indian Muslims did join the fight against the Ottomans during the war, although British documents reveal that this was neither an easy nor uniform choice for the Indians. The Indian Muslims were to eventually recover and launch a movement of scale unprecedented in its appeal and mobilization at the end of the First World War. Thus, when the Ottomans lost the war alongside the Germans, in 1919 the Khilafat Movement rallied masses in support of the Turks and the Ottoman caliph. Equally significant was their strong support to the Turkish war of liberation from what would prove to be a short-lived invasion of Turkey by a number of imperial powers and their proxies, most notably the Greeks. The development of nationalist and even pro-to-nationalist policy took shape incrementally after the Khilafat Movement lost steam when Turkey abolished the caliphate. While differences of view were relatively more manageable until then, it became too hard to manage after the pull of a common external agenda disappeared. Although disagreements about the future of India and Hindu–Muslim relations were in place long before, after 1924, the Indian Muslims could no longer agree among themselves on these issues. Nationalism became as divisive for them as it was for others in other places.

As their exhilarated reception back in India vividly demonstrated, masses of Indian Muslims, as the sponsors of Dr Ansari's Mission, had been much moved by the laborious and courageous work done in Turkey. Tens of thousands of Muslims, following intently the work, thanks to the detailed and rather regular letters sent by Dr Ansari and published and popularized by Maulana Mohammad Ali, showed their pride with their representatives. The members of the Mission were hailed as heroes who had successfully performed their Islamic duty on behalf of the Indian nation. Their satisfaction catapulted the names of those involved with the Indian Medical Mission to Turkey in 1913 to national fame, preparing them for higher visibility and political roles in India. The Indian Medical Mission was neither the first nor the last of the manifestations of the Indian Muslims' passionate support for Turkey. The story began as early as the mid-nineteenth century and has continued ever since. The Mission kept alive and indeed augmented the existing interests, links, and sympathies with Turkey. Dr Ansari announced later that this aspect was their most important achievement. In turn, it was true that the Indian Medical Mission gave the Turks consolation and a feeling of brotherly and sisterly goodwill during a ghastly episode in their history. The legacy of comparison continues to date with the people of Pakistan, India, and Bangladesh, all of whom continue to entertain strong mutual sympathies towards Turkey and the Turks.

Notes

1. Zühal Özaydın, 'The Indian Muslims Red Crescent Society's Aid to the Ottoman State during the Balkan War in 1912', *Journal of the International Society for the History of Islamic Medicine* 2, no. 8 (October 2003), p. 12.

2. Özaydın, 'The Indian Muslims Red Crescent Society's Aid to the Ottoman State during the Balkan War in 1912', p. 12.

3. Georges Remond, *Bir Fransiz Gazetecinin Balkan İzlenimleri: Mağluplarla Beraber* (İstanbul: Profil Yayincilik, 2007), p. 160.

4. *Comrade*, 21 December 1912.

5. *Comrade*, 21 December 1912.

6. Dr Ansari's letter dated 26 June 1913.

7. Dr Ansari's letter dated 20 April 1913.

8. Özaydın, 'The Indian Muslims Red Crescent Society's Aid to the Ottoman State', p. 13.

9. Dr Ansari's letter dated 1 February 1913.

Epilogue

A notable aspect of the experience of the Indian Medical Mission's six-month labour in Turkey was the closeness with which they interacted with the local political and bureaucratic leaders. Acting as unofficial yet effective representatives of the Indian Muslims, they had their presence known and felt from the sultan downwards in the Ottoman official hierarchy. They had particularly close encounters with some of the people from the Union and Progress Movement, including its key actors such as Enver Bey and Talat Bey. The access given to the Indian team was not limited to the leader of the Mission. A letter sent by Ghulam Ahmad details a trip he made on 12 April with two other members of the Indian hospital in Ömerli hospital to the battle fields. Thus, Ghulam Ahmad in his letter published in *Comrade* on 3 May reports that he, along with Dr Fyzee and Hafiz Muhammad Yusuf Ansari, met Enver Bey in Kale Karası on the outskirts of İstanbul where the British Red Crescent and Ottoman Red Crescent hospitals were also present. He wrote:

We went to Aziz Bey, the commandant, who spoke Persian fluently and hence understood us perfectly. He spoke to us about Langar Shah, an Afghan volunteer, who had fought with Enver Bey in Tripoli and had recently shown marvellous courage and bravery in fighting against the Bulgars at Yalor. He was killed on the 3rd of April in engagement where he rushed with a small number of soldiers in the Bulgar ranks which numbered some six thousand. Aziz Bey is one of the famous officers who had distinguished themselves in Tripoli with Enver Bey's army. We expressed to him our desire to see Enver Bey to whom he took our message. Enver Bey sent for us at once and on seeing us and saying 'Biliyorum' (I know them) the whole aspect of all the officers and men changed towards us like the magic words of Ali Baba, and all the mysteries and secrets were to be shown to us without any further suspicion or questioning.... Enver Bey spoke also very highly of Langar Shah's courage and bravery.... We took a photograph of Enver Bey just before we left him. This place was simply a beehive of activity, every soldier and officer moving with alacrity and determination.

Ghulam Ahmad's letter indicates that they also saw two Pathan soldiers at the Ottoman military camp. From visiting the best-guarded military headquarters to meeting ministers and attending the official meetings of Ottoman institutions, the members of the Indian Medical Mission were granted a warm welcome and a high degree of access in Turkey. While conversing and interacting with the Turks, they must have had a fuller understanding of the country and the aspirations of its people. Despite the language issue always haunting the members of the Indian team, one could expect a learning process to be underway. They functioned as an embassy of the people at a time when India was colonized by a powerful British empire. They successfully represented Indian Muslims in Turkey and learned their ways and circumstances. Back in India, they were accorded rousing reception, bearing resemblance to the show of adoration for the pilgrim on return. The accounts of their Mission in Turkey inspired Indian Muslims and embraced their religious fervour. Dr Ansari, at a meeting organized in Bombay by the Anjuman-i-Islam, gave an account of his Mission's tenure in Turkey and conveyed the feelings of gratitude of the Turks towards Indians. When Dr Ansari mentioned the name of the sultan caliph 'the audience stood up as a mark of respect and offered prayers for the success of the Ottomans'.

The long span of time between the mid-nineteenth century and the 1920s brought the Turks and Indians closer than ever. The Muslims of British India rallied to the support of the beleaguered

Ottoman Empire in every possible way. The Indian Muslims continued to support the Ottoman Empire till its last days and later Turkey as she fought to liberate herself from the short-lived invasion by colonial forces. As Dr Ansari wrote in 1935, 'except that there were Indian Moslems in the British forces in Mesopotamia and Palestine, one may even say that they have been consistent in their friendship and ready to help as far as their position as British subjects allowed them'.[1] Although the Indian Medical Mission was an initiative launched and carried out by the Muslims of India, the Hindus also rallied in its support. The *Ikdam* newspaper in Turkey reported in 1912 that the wealthy Hindus had been competing with the wealthy Muslims in providing aid. It informed its readers that the Maharani of Baroda donated Rs 500 and issued a statement encouraging other Hindu women to follow suit.[2] The motives of the Hindus were obviously not driven by religious affinities. Yet, they too converged with the Muslims, both on the point of unhappiness with the British rule and perhaps in reaction against imperialist dismemberment of a fellow Asian polity.

However, the Indian support came late for both the Indians and the Ottomans. As Mughal–Ottoman diplomacy prevaricated, being bogged down in trivialities such as how to address each other or whose line of blood was superior, Europe transformed itself from a backward region beset with religious wars into an advanced global imperialist force. Europe's great strides in science, economics, warfare techniques, and culture overshadowed the achievements of the Muslims. The three gunpowder empires of the Ottomans, the Safavids, and the Mughals could perhaps muster enough weight to halt the advance of European colonialism as the tide turned after the Europeans began circumnavigating Africa to reach and then dominate and ultimately subjugate the Indian Ocean. It was not possible, however, to define the emerging threat and cooperate against it jointly. Ottomans as the only naval power among them thus lost their influence in the Indian Ocean. The decline of the Ottoman power allowed colonialism to proceed and that too not just in terms of expanding geographically. Rather, colonial powers also pressed ahead with a transformative 'civilizing mission', propelled by religious missionary zeal. Experiencing the comprehensive onslaught, the Muslims nonetheless could not overcome their divisions. Failures to embrace political and social modernity in way that is compatible with their own culture and faith only augmented their suffering. The anguish that exists almost uniformly even today acts as a breeding ground for the extremism that equally hurts the Muslims, adding further insult to their injury.

Therefore, for most of the Muslims around the world, the last century has been a lost time. Time stood still as the Muslims have retained certain lethargy in fulfilling the task of, what Mustafa Kemal Atatürk termed as 'catching up with the contemporary civilization'. Their worries, angers, woes, and divisions have remained more or less the same. The former territories of the Ottoman Empire in the Middle East or West Asia, whichever term is used, reeled under a British–French imposed regional system of nation states and kingdoms, totally alien to the fabric of the region and always unstable. Their experimentations with reform, nationalism, political Islam, and democracy have all suffered either outright failure or significant setbacks. Instability and economic backwardness throughout the Muslim world has been compounded and perpetuated by the massive failure in providing modern education and inculcating secular systems not inimical to religion but reflecting a particular interpretation of it. Particularly, education of the girls has continued to pose an insuperable problem to the Muslim world. At the extreme end, a school for girls run by Turkey in Afghanistan has required constant armed protection. Muslims around the world have voiced similar concerns on a narrow set of foreign policy issues, never being able to converge on policy. Legitimacy deficits continue to haunt governments vis-à-vis their own people in a large segment of the world. Development and governance problems as well as difficulties in embracing modernity obviously are not solely experienced in the Muslim world. This, however, has not changed the fact of Muslim woes. While the world in 2014 looks very different from 1913 in almost every way, the problems of the Muslim world have, in essence, remained not only dire but also overall disappointingly similar in many respects.

Since the Indian Medical Mission returned home and played active roles in the successful Indian independence movement, Indian Muslims were not only divided into three more or less equal parts, divided among Pakistan, India, and later Bangladesh, but also became citizens of mutually antagonistic entities. At the beginning of the twentieth century, the Indian Muslims already seemed as a divided community. They came closest to uniting around a single cause when the news of atrocities against the Balkan Muslims started dominating their newspapers around the late nineteenth century and afterwards. Thus, English-educated liberals, Deobandis, Barelvis, Farang-i Mahalis, the Nadvatu'l-Ulema, the Shias, and others joined hands. Since their deposition from all avenues of prominence in Indian society under the British Raj, their unity of purpose in support of the Ottoman Empire and the sultan caliph transformed them into a force to reckon with, eventually in opposition to the British rule in India. The Indian Medical Mission was a tangible project that rallied Muslims, rich and poor, from all around India to defend what they regarded as the ultimate moral authority, namely the Ottoman sultan, the caliph of the believers. Their pride grew as Dr Ansari's letters published regularly in the *Comrade* and the *Hamdard* provided detailed accounts of the successful tenure of the Mission, which Indian masses supported despite their limited incomes. Other newspapers in India extended strong support to the Mission and its cause. The newspapers in Turkey were also awash with appreciation in their extensive coverage of the assistance received from the Indian Muslims.[3] A characteristic feature of the times was the new-found facility and speed with which news reached the masses. Telegraph lines, railways, steamships, and the vast print media facilitated communication like never before. 'The masses seemed so anxious to have the account of war that the journalists thought it necessary to start fresh papers as the demands suddenly became too numerous', wrote S. M. Naimtullah[4] in 1913.[5] Dr Ansari's letters were not the only means to satisfy the Indians' thirst for news from what would become the penultimate war of the Ottoman Empire. Some Indian newspapers deployed their reporters to Turkey, who covered the events extensively, frequently embellishing their reports with photographs of the Turkish leaders. These leaders became household names, the Muslims' own heroes, who were fighting to defend Islam against what they perceived as an onslaught against their lands and faith. Dr Ansari would write in 1935:

Pan-Islamist sentiment has been one of the Indian Moslem's most sacred and exalted passions. It is because he is helpless, because all his co-religionists are equally helpless, because Western imperialism is aggressive and everywhere successful, that he has become a pan-Islamist. And because Turkey alone of all Moslem countries is free, because, the Turks alone have power to defeat enemies not overwhelmingly strong and the manliness to prefer death to slavery, the imagination of the Indian Moslems converted them into as convinced Pan-Islamists as they themselves, and placed on their shoulders the burden not only of defending their hearth and home, but the honour of Islam and all Moslem peoples as well. The Turks could not, of course, be expected to appreciate this quaint romanticism and chivalry, or endure such oppressive affection. When they declined the honour that had been thrust upon them, the Indian Moslems' dream-world crashed upon their head. They could not think objectively or subjectively. They just could not think and could not believe.

Dr Ansari's time in Turkey, his encounters with the military and political leaders of the day, and his study of the economy, society, organization, schooling, and mindset of the country and its people from İstanbul to Mersin would fall into place in providing a sober look into the new Turkey that rose out of the ashes of the Ottoman Empire. As many of his peers wrestled with the course of Turkish republican experience, Dr Ansari benefited from his insights. Thus, he first refuted the idea that pan-Islamism could have survived the breakaway of the Arab lands from the empire. He wrote:

> [T]he non-Turkish Moslem subjects of the Ottoman Empire were openly and heartlessly treacherous. I cannot here go into the discussion whether their grievances were genuine or manufactured for the purpose, but their attitude would have convinced the most zealous Turkish Pan-Islamist that there was no possibility of co-operation between them and the Turks. The Ottoman Empire is now gone and its non-Turkish Moslem subjects have all got what they wanted or what they deserved, so we may as well admit that the abolition of the Caliphate was a matter of sound policy, for the Caliphate involved the Turks in pretensions which may have given them a certain prestige, but which also exposed them to the jealous wrath of their enemies and the shiftiness of selfish friends.[6]

Dr Ansari then went on to defend the very premise of the Turkish secularism without calling it as such:

> I feel that Indian Moslems should also understand that their perspective is very faulty. They have a tendency, as have all those who are isolated or insular in outlook to identify not only their beliefs, but also their manners and customs, with the prescriptions of their faith. Religion and social life are no doubt inseparable, and a society that altogether overlooks the religious element is sure to drift from one vicious whirlpool to another. But the position of a society that lacks the judgment to distinguish between conservatism and stagnation is equally insecure. Religion is the permanent basis of life, but the true religious spirit does not seek to shackle life in order to preserve a theoretical consistency between fact and belief. It endeavours rather to discover fresh sources of inspiration, which are really nothing more than fresh points of contact between the personality of the founder of a religion and of the follower across the gulf of time and altered social conditions.[7]

The abolition of the caliphate by the Turkish Grand National Assembly on 3 March 1924 forced a change in the ideological outlook of Indian Muslim elites, which also caused a change in the course of the freedom movement in India. As Mohammad Sadiq wrote: 'They came down from the pedestal of abstractions and grappled with the realities of political life. Their pan-Islamic fervour subsided. Rather it was overshadowed by the more urgent, though in no way transitory, issues of the day. In fact, it yielded its place to national consciousness.'[8] As India marched towards independence, eventually Indian Muslims, or most of them, reconciled with the idea of a modern, democratic, secular republic in Turkey and have continued their sympathy towards the Turks. Today residents of New Delhi witness the name of Mustafa Kemal Atatürk as they drive past the official residence of the prime minister of India. Atatürk Avenue also lies in the most prestigious part of the city of Islamabad in Pakistan as well as Dhaka in Bangladesh.

Shortly before the Mission's departure from Suez, aboard an Italian boat on 29 July, members of the Indian Medical Mission encountered the formidable Ottoman destroyer Hamidiye. They spent half an hour on board the warship, meeting with her commandant and sailors. Commandant Hüseyin Rauf Bey, who was 'a young, most handsome and frank Turkish gentleman' received the Mission with 'that genuine and sincere cordiality which the Ottomans have shown us all along'.[9] Rauf Bey told the team that 'he was feeling very much depressed as he had just then received newspapers from home and that their visit had made him happy and enabled him to forget the troubles at home'. The commandant briefed the team about the Hamidiye and her successes in battle and gave 'some interesting photographs of the Hamidiye in actual action and the sinking of the boat Lyres with his autograph on them'.[10] As the Indian team was leaving the Hamidiye, the sailors cheered them while the band was playing the national anthem of the Ottoman Empire, beaten and downtrodden, yet still very much alive.

Khaliquzzaman noted in his memoirs that there was not much time before the members of the Mission had to catch their ship back to India and 'with a heavy heart we left him not knowing whether in our lives we should have any chance to meet him again but as Providence worked, in 1933 Dr Ansari invited him to lecture in the Jamia Millia at Delhi'.[11] After Delhi, Rauf Bey continued his journey to Lucknow to meet Chaudry Khaliquzzaman where he shared his thoughts about developments in Turkey and Mustafa Kemal Atatürk. The commandant of the Hamidiye destroyer Rauf Bey was none other than the future prime minister of the Turkish Republic, Hüseyin Rauf Orbay.

What Khaliquzzaman did not write was that at the time Dr Ansari invited Rauf Orbay to India, the latter was a fugitive from justice in the republic he helped establish. He was convicted due to the thwarted 1926 plot to assassinate Mustafa Kemal Atatürk in İzmir. During the trials, Orbay was in Vienna for medical treatment and refused to return to Turkey, protesting his innocence. He was pardoned soon after but would return only in 1935 and enter politics as a member of the Turkish parliament and ambassador. According to Khaliquzzaman, Rauf Orbay told them in Lucknow that '[i]n spite of his differences with the Ghazi Pasha [that is, Atatürk] he cherished a great respect for him and told [us] that he would never like a hair of his head to be touched'.[12]

Turkish modernity has captured the imagination of the bulging youths in the Muslim and non-Muslim worlds. Many nations look to the Turks as a model for what they can achieve in the course of a few generations. They seek answers to the enduring question of reconciling faith, tradition, democracy, secularism, and modernity by studying the Turkish example. One could speculate that the Turkey of today would have inspired members of the Indian Medical Mission and made them proud. Mustafa Kemal Atatürk or 'Father of the Turks', as the surname reserved for him by the Turkish Parliament suggests, set Turkey on the path where she finds herself today, a rare object of contemporary pride for Muslims around the world.

Notes

1. Azmi Özcan, *Pan-Islamism: Indian Muslims, the Ottomans and Britain, 1877–1924* (Leiden: E.J. Brill, 1997), p. 153.

2. Mukhtar Ahmad Ansari, 'Preface', in Halide Edip Adıvar, *Conflict of East and West in Turkey* (Delhi: Maktaba Jamia Millia Islamia, 1935), p. vii.

3. Serdal Soyluer, 'Balkan Savasi Sirasinda Hintlilerin OsmanlI'ya Yardim Kampanyalarinin Osmanli Basinina Yansimalari', *Sarkiyat Mecmuasi*, Sayi 13 (2008), p. 97.

4. For a detailed account of the coverage of the Mission by the Ottoman press, see Soyluer, 'Balkan Savasi Sirasinda Hintlilerin OsmanlI'ya Yardim Kampanyalarinin Osmanli Basinina Yansimalari', pp. 91–118.

5. S. M. Naimtullah, 'Recent Turkish Events and Moslem India', *Asiatic Quarterly Review* (October 1913), p. 247, quoted in Özcan, *Pan-Islamism*, p. 148.

6. Ansari, 'Preface', in Adıvar, *Conflict of East and West*, p. vii.

7. Ansari, 'Preface', p. x.

8. Mohammad Sadiq, *The Turkish Revolution* (Delhi: MacMillan India, 1997), p. 80.

9. Dr Ansari's letter dated 12 July 1913.

10. Dr Ansari's letter dated 12 July 1913.

11. Chaudhry Khaliquzzaman, *Pathway to Pakistan* (Lahore: Longmans Green and Co, 1961), p. 26.

12. Khaliquzzaman, *Pathway to Pakistan*, p. 26.

Appendix

Letters from Dr M. A. Ansari to Maulana
Mohammad Ali Jauhar

The following pages contain the full text of the letters from Dr Mukhtar Ahmad Ansari to Maulana Mohammad Ali as published in the English-language *Comrade* news journal between November 1912 and July 1913. There is also a selection of other letters dispatched by his fellow team members and published in the *Comrade*.

All the letters are presented as they were published in the *Comrade*. I have made exception to the names of people and places and corrected them as they are spelled in Turkish and thus used internationally today. It should be noted that Turkey had not yet adopted the Latin alphabet at that time, and names were transliterated by Dr Ansari from the Arabic script, which was still in use at the time or sometimes written as it was heard.

Dr Ansari wrote about his final visits around western and central Turkey including to Konya to visit the shrine of Mevlana Celaleddin Rumi. These letters, written aboard the ship carrying the Mission back to India, are placed at the end of the appendix in order to maintain the correct sequence of events. Otherwise letters are provided in the sequence they were published in the *Comrade*. This helps track the events as they were experienced by the Mission. At any rate, the dates are carefully documented throughout this appendix.

The reader is encouraged to delve into the beautiful prose that Dr Ansari has furnished, which is also a valuable primary source in its own right for further research. These letters, published by a journal that was closed down soon after publishing his letters, stood in the library waiting for researchers to bring them to light. They are now provided in this book as a ready reference to illuminate the Indian Medical Mission to the Balkan Wars.

November 1912

Comrade, 30 November 1912

As our arrangements are nearly complete, and we are about to start on our mission of mercy, I feel I must trespass on the courtesy of your columns and give you some idea of the work so far accomplished.

Our list is now complete. We have got eight fully, qualified medical men, five with European qualifications and three holding Indian Degrees and Diplomas. Five of these are proceeding with the Mission from India and three are proceeding straight from London to join us in İstanbul. There are eight dressers and nine male nurses, one of the latter being also the manager and accountant of the Mission. We could take many more male nurses if we wanted, but we find nine are ample for all our requirements. It is worth noting that ours is a truly All India Medical Mission, as we have got representatives from every province of India. It is very gratifying to notice that the men who have joined the Mission are from the cultured middle and higher classes, representing the flower of Mohammadan youth, who are fully alive to the responsibilities and nature of the work with which they are entrusted. I have the fullest confidence that all the men will do their duty to the best of their abilities and prove worthy of the trust which their co-religionists have placed in them by sending them as their representatives in the Mission. I may also say a few words here about the uniform and general equipment of the Mission. Every member of the Mission has been supplied at the cost of the Mission with a khaki semi-military Norfolk-coat made of the warmest woollen material available and two Jodhpur breeches—one plain and one corded. There will be a badge on the left arm with the Red Crescent and two silver crescents, one on either side, on the collar and the coat with a Naskh inscription in Arabic—'Alwad Taiyaba Hinbilad Hind'.

The Jodhpur breeches have been selected not only from the point of view of comfort and utility, but also to impart to the mission uniform a distinctively Indian character. There is also supplied an overcoat, which is also khaki in colour, is made of a very warm material, although very light in weight, allowing perfect freedom in movement. Two Turkish caps and two pairs of brown ammunition boots complete the uniform. No distinction has been made in the uniform of the doctors and dressers except that every doctor will be provided with a brown leather belt with pouches to wear with the Norfolk coat.

Besides the uniform every member of the mission has been advised to furnish himself with the following articles: (1) six flannel shirts (2) six woollen under-vests (3) six woollen under darners (4) six pairs of woollen socks (5) one dozen handkerchiefs (6) three blankets and two pillows (7) six towels (8) brush, comb and a small mirror (9) one woollen undress suit, Indian or English (10) one steel trunk size 30 inches (11) one water proof holdall (12) one Balaclava cap.

As regards the equipment and stores for the field hospital, I have written two long and detailed letters to the Rt. Hon. Mr. Ameer Ali giving him full particulars of the quantity and quality of instruments, appliances, dressings, disinfectants, tinned provisions and other invalid foods to be sent straight to İstanbul, so as to reach there before us. This list has been based on the one prepared by the great English experts for field hospitals in the South African war, only minor differences being made owing to difference in climate, and season of the year. But the Rt. Hon. Mr. Ameer Ali has been given full freedom to consult expert opinion in London in selecting the best and cheapest material in the market. The mission is thus not encumbered with any equipment except the personal luggage of the members. It is worth noting that Thropic Mohamedan firm of Calcutta, Messrs. H. S. Abdul Ghani & co. Wholesale Chemists and Druggists, have very generously offered bandages, dressings, disinfectants and minor surgical instruments, the least value of which would amount to Rs. 1000. It is hoped that other Moslem firms would not lag behind in showing their practical sympathy towards the mission, and would emulate the noble example set by the Calcutta firm.

In the end, I feel it my duty to express the gratitude of the Mission and of the entire community which it represents for the courtesy and readiness which all the Government officials have shown in helping the work of the Mission. Our thanks are also due to all the firms, especially Messrs.

Phelps & Co., Military Tailors, Kashmiri Gate, Delhi, the Railway and Shipping Companies and Messrs, Thomas Cook and Sons, who have given us special concessions and facilities or helped us considerably in hastening our Mission in its departure." After reading this letter our readers will realise that no effort has been spared to complete in detail all the arrangements for the dispatch of the Mission. Those who have been sending funds to us with great liberality and zeal would be glad to learn that the Mission is now almost ready for departure and as soon as the passports are secured, it will leave Delhi for İstanbul.

Our deepest thanks are due to H. E. the Viceroy and the Chief Commissioner of Delhi for the facilities they have so kindly afforded us in the matter of passports. The passports will, we hope, be ready in a day or two and the Mission will sail from Bombay without further delay. We had heard rumours that Government will not permit the Mission to proceed to Turkey; but we are in a position to state that all such rumours are absolutely baseless. As a matter of fact, H. E. the Viceroy has graciously promised to wire to the Secretary of State to request His Majesty's Ambassador at İstanbul and the British Agent-General in Cairo to assist the Mission when it arrives in Turkey and *en route* in Egypt.

M. A. Ansari

30 December 1912

My last letter from Aden had not much news as there was none to give. But this which I am sending from s.s. 'Romania', a day before our arrival at İstanbul, will contain some news which will interest you.

All our lectures and demonstrations were over on the 25th of December. The day before our arrival at Suez. I had arranged them in such a manner that only the revision, should we be disposed to do so, should be done during our voyage in the Mediterranean Sea. Most of the men have availed themselves of the classes, only Abdur Rahman of Peshawar, Qazi Bashiruddin Ahmad and Chiraghuddin have missed nearly half of the lectures owing to their indisposition. I mean however we should be favourably placed to continue the classes for the first three weeks at least thrice weekly in order to make up the deficiency as well as teach them any new matter that may require doing so.

The night before landing at Suez in order to save the uniforms from getting overused and dirty I had thought of going ashore in Mufti. But on second thoughts I asked the men to put on their uniforms and I had every reason to be very glad of having done so, as you will see later.

We reached Suez on the morning of the 26th after the medical inspection was over I found an inquiry that a representative of Thomas Cook was awaiting our party with a launch for us and a tug for our baggage. He had also brought a letter from their office at Alexandria. After our transport Department—Shuaib Quraishy and Abdul Waheed Khan being the foremen—had our baggage removed to the tug, our pasty left s.s. 'Sardegna' after a hearty farewell, in some cases very touching, from the passengers on board, amongst them being also H. H. the Maharani Helkar of Indore and her suite of ladies going to Europe.

Captain H. V. Bagshawe, B. A. M. C. also met us on the launch. He was sent by General Byng the General Officer Commanding the Army of Occupation at Cairo on the instruction of H. E. Lord Kitchener. He had come from the headquarters at Cairo in order to give us assistance at disembarkation and during our journey to Alexandria. He was very courteous and exceedingly agreeable to us and travelled with us by train to Alexandria and was with the party until our boat left the quay at Alexandria. He proved himself of very great use to us. I am going to send a letter to Lord Kitchener and General Byug thanking them for their kindness in giving us such valuable assistance. I will also send a private letter to Dr. Bagshawe.

The Port Medical Officer at Suez was very considerate to us and just had a little soiled linen removed from our holdalls for disinfection. The Customs Officer who was an Egyptian gentleman showed his appreciation and sympathy and only opened a box or two probably in order to swear he had gone through the formality. A small crowd of Egyptians had gathered there and they were very enthusiastic and showed us every courtesy and consideration. Here we were also met by Mr. Abbas M. A. Barry, Government Agent, Army of Occupation, Suez, who accompanied us everywhere and made himself very useful.

The Manager and Shuaib were sent to the port railway station in charge of all the heavy baggage and deck chairs which were registered to go to Alexandria in a van. We found the charges exorbitant and had to pay £6 for the freight. The rest of the party went to a hotel in town, marshalled by a picturesque dragoman, and had their lunch which also proved rather expensive. But it was necessary to fortify ourselves against a long journey by train to Alexandria. The Manager and Shuaib joined the party at the hotel after having arranged about the baggage. There was a large crowd very much interested in us waiting outside the hotel and making all sort of enquiries about us and on learning the object of our Mission the shouts of *Marhaba*[1] were heard over and over again.

Captain Bagshawe brought us an English newspaper through which we learnt the news of the dastardly attack on the life of H. E. the Viceroy and of his having been wounded. The following telegram was dispatched by us at once

26.12.1912. P.S.V. Delhi.
Convey sympathy and deep concern All India Medical Mission
to His Excellency Pray his speedy recovery and long life
Ansari.

The party reached the station at 11:45 and found an immense crowd standing all round our baggage and watching our men. It was very hard work to dispose of all the baggage, the second class carriage being very few. However, we accommodated ourselves and the luggage higgledy-piggledy and made ourselves as comfortable as was possible under the circumstances. The early part of the journey to Ismailia was very dusty. The line passes along the Canal through sandy tracts. This uninteresting part of the journey finished at Ismailia where we changed to another train. Here our transport department did excellent work.

The journey from Ismalia to Benha was a little more cramped though the scenery around made up for the discomfort in the train. The change at Benha was accomplished under stress of time and a jabbering crowd of porters who wanted 'Bakhsheesh'[2] from every single member of the Mission. But our Manager was too cute to let them have more than their due, having previously ascertained form Captain Bagashawe and the Railway Inspector the exact amount payable to the porters. The journey from Benha to Alexandria was accomplished in a most congested train but full of very sympathetic Egyptians and Turks. The men were famished and one gentleman helped himself half a dozen times from a tin of biscuits we were carrying for the whole party until the Manager having discovered his selfishness admonished him mildly and took the tin in his own charge. At last a brilliant idea struck me and I ordered tea baskets for 24 which was highly appreciated by the party, the contents of the baskets and the tea-pots disappearing as if by magic.

It was by the merest chance that Dr. Bagshawe and myself rescued the van containing our registered baggage from being carried to Cairo instead of Alexandria. It would have probably meant a day's delay and a lot of inconvenience if not missing our boat at Alexandria.

During our journey an Egyptian gentleman drew the attention of the Manager to a note in Al-Moayyad about our Mission. It simply mentioned the numbers of our Mission and wished us success in our undertaking. Our train arrived at Alexandria at 8 P.M. Here we were met by Thomas

Cook's agent who took charge of our baggage and had it removed to their van. There was a large crowd of hotel agents at the station, and what with their shouts and with their jostling and pushing it would not have been possible to decide where to stay for the night if we had not followed captain Bagshawe's plan and cleared out of the station with Cook's agent to see a few hotels for ourselves before deciding which we were going to stay in. We had to select a hotel which would be cheap as well as good. We were lucky in having received special concessions at the Hotel Metropole where, owing to the influence of the Egyptian landlord, the Proprietor took us at 6 Shillings per head (inclusive) the ordinary charges being 10/6. The Manager and myself who had come in advance of the party remained in the hotel till the rest of the party arrived there and went round with the hotel Manager who showed us all the rooms. We drew up lists and allotted the rooms to the individual members when they arrived there. Our hotel was situated facing the sea and was very clean, commodious and comfortable.

In the morning Cook's agent had several carriages ready for us and we started to see the Turkish refugees sheltered in one of the Khedival palace in Alexandria, Palace Ras-el-Tin. Dr. Himmat the Medical officer in charge was kind enough to have met one of the party at the railway station and was good enough to send a man in the morning to fetch us to the palace. He had also promised to request H. H. the Khedive to meet us if possible in the palace. We arrived there at 10 o'clock and were met by Dr. Himmat and his staff. He took us round the inoculation department and the dispensary. In the quadrangle of the Palace, we saw about 1,000 Turkish refugees of all ages and we were met here by a deputation of the notables amongst the Turkish refugees. We were taken up to the drawing room of the palace where Dr. Himmat addressed us in English and described to us some of the most touching and pathetic scenes which his rescuing party had beheld at Kavalla. He mentioned particularly the atrocities perpetrated by the Servians[3] in throwing away from the windows the Turkish sick and wounded, there to die of cold, starvation and disease. He mentioned a good many other inhuman deed done by the Balkan armies during their occupations of Salonica and Kavalla amongst them the murder of the weak and innocent women and children the insults and injuries to the women the spoliation burning and looting of their hearths and homes and the unspeakable miseries caused to these innocent non-combatants. The description of these refugees reaching the shelter of the Khedival yacht which brought them to Egypt was specially touching and pathetic— how they described it as the 'ship of safety', how they kissed the very steps which took them to the boat with tearful gratitude. These and many scenes depicted by him, you could well imagine, went straight to our hearts and made us even more determined to do all that lay in our power to lessen the sufferings, to sympathize with and soothe the bleeding hearts of our fellow-Moslems in Turkey. Dr. Himmat assured us we had several hundreds of thousands waiting with forlorn hopes most eagerly for any succour and assistances that a Mission like ours would give to them. He assured us that the work awaiting us there was far more than many Missions like ours would be able to cope with. This news, though it made our hearts very sad, provided us with another justification for our having come all the way to do what we had some tribulations we might find ourselves too late to perform. I made a reply to Dr. Himmat's speech thanking him for the good wishes he had expressed and for the valuable insight which had been given to us by our visit to the Ras-el-Tin and by his speech. Dr. Himmat then announced that H. H. the Khedive was unable, owing to the Friday prayers, to receive us on that day, but His Highness hoped that we would visit Egypt on our return when we would be granted the pleasure and privilege of being presented to him. A Turkish journalist, Djafar Effendizadeh ÖmerSirat, who was also amongst the group of notable refugees made a speech with tearful eyes which we unfortunately could not understand, but which was briefly translated to us by Dr. Himmat. He expressed gratitude and appreciation on behalf of the Turkish refugees and gave us the fullest assurance that there would be thousands of Turks like him awaiting most anxiously our arrival amongst them.

We were then introduced to Madame Noureddin Bey, wife of a former Consul-General in Bombay and now P.S. to the Khedives, who was acting as the matron in charge of the women refugees. She is a Turkish lady of education and refinement and spoke French most fluently. She took us round the female wards and showed us how the Turkish families were housed in the Palace and also the food given to them. Some of the babies were born there.

After saying farewell to Dr. Himmat, Noureddin Bey and Madame Noureddin Bey we drove back through the city and met with a very sympathetic reception from the crowd wherever we passed. Owing to our long stay in the Ras-el-Tin Palace, we had to give up our visit to the sights of the city and we only visited Cook's office for our embarkation tickets and to convert some Circular Notes into gold.

After lunch in the hotel we drove to the docks where we found the gates closed against the crowd. We were admitted as a special favour and on inquiry we were told that the Khedival special was waiting in the dock station ready to leave for Cairo. We arrived at the quay and found a tremendous crowd of Egyptians awaiting us. On the boat Dr. Himmat, in the presence of some 100 Egyptians, made another speech on their behalf in which he praised the Mission and wished them God-speed. A suitable reply was made and after a photograph had been taken our attention was drawn to the lusty shouts of the crowds on land. There were banners bearing the Red Crescent carried by the crowds, and burning speeches were made by several persons denouncing the atrocities of the Balkan armies and a poem in Arabic was read by a gentleman in our honour. Then began the loud, lusty and continuous cheering from the crowds who continuously kept it up until our boat was out of sight. And not being content with that several boats full of people followed our steamer for a long distance cheering us and singing Arabic songs. The following are some of the cheers which they repeated over and over again:

Long live the Indian Mission!	[Yahya Albat Hind.]
Long live Representative of India!	[Yahya Maboos Hind.]
Long live the Heroes and the Warriors!	[Yahya Alahrar Mujahidin.]
Long live the Turkish Nation!	[Yahya Ummah Turkiya.]
Long live the Sultan!	[Yahya Sultan.]
Long live the Khedive!	[Yahya Khedive.]
Long live Islam!	[Yahya Islam.]

Captain Bagshawe waited after saying good bye to us until our boat was out of sight.

On the morning of the 29th, after a very shaky voyage, we arrived at Piraeus, the port for Athens. Here a very searching examination of our passports and our party was made by the Greek port officials. We were advised not to use the Fez to avoid unpleasantness which we followed although I think unnecessarily. As the boat was going to be in harbour for seven hours, we decided to pay a visit under the guidance of Cook's man to all the sights of the Greek capital. We visited the Acropolis, the Amphitheatre, the stadium and the museum and drove through the principal streets of the city. Here we saw young lads and consumptive-looking men dressed in shabby grey uniforms awaiting orders for the front. On our return to our boat we saw a hospital ship in which the wounded were brought from Salonika and medical aid is sent to the sick and wounded. Our boat had already left with the doctors and nurses. We also saw a transport ship just leaving the harbour full of provisions and some soldiers. Whilst we were in Athens we dispatched three telegrams to (1) the President of the Red Crescent Society, (2) the British Ambassador, and (3) cook, informing them of our arrival.

We are already nearing the Dardanelles and in sight of the island of Tenedos (Turkish name, Bozada), where a fleet is at anchor whose nationality is the point of discussion. Some say it is a Greek fleet, others say that the result of the naval engagement a week previous being uncertain, it is impossible to say what fleet may be at anchor.

We are due at İstanbul tomorrow morning. I will let you know in detail any news I may hear during our stay there.

M. A. Ansari

31 December 1912

We have reached İstanbul in all safety. Details by next mail. Great reception. Mohamed Ali Bey (Inspector- General of the Ottoman Red Crescent Society) and Bassim Ömer Pasha (Vice President) saw us. Guard of Honour and Band.

s.s. 'Romania'
Near the Dardanelles[4]
M. A. Ansari

December 1912

Comrade, 1 February 1913

In my last letter I gave you a resume of my doings in İstanbul, but in this one I am going to give you full details which may prove of some interest.

As our boat approached the Straits of Dardanelles we saw three men-o'-war going towards the Aegean Sea some distance from the Isle of Tenedos. These were probably the units of the Hellenic fleet which had engaged the Turkish fleet the day previous in that vicinity. It was a beautiful clear day and the sea was as calm as a lake, the air was transparent and you could see the coast of Europe and Asia converging towards the Dardanelles with little villages dotted here and there along the coast. The approach to the Straits showed steep hills with hidden fortifications. Here and there the muzzles of big guns were to be seen from behind the earth works pointing towards our boat. In some places long flagstaffs pointed to there being an arsenal and some soldiers on duty could be seen walking along. We were told that there were some seventy thousand soldiers stationed there. There is no doubt that the entrance to the

Straits is well fortified and would smash up any fleet which tried to enter into it. Our boat was timed to reach the entrance to the Straits at about 1 P.M., and as we neared the entrance we saw a number of ships all in one line-passing through the Straits. We were told that no boats were allowed before 1 P.M. and after sunset. We soon reached the seaport at the entrance of the Sea of Marmora called Dardanelles, and we could hear from a distance a band playing the Turkish National Anthem. We stopped here only for half an hour and as we proceeded on our journey we saw the Turkish fleet which consisted of 4 gunboats, the 'Medjidiyeh',[5] bearing the Standard of the Admiral, and three torpedo boats. We were also shown the Greek boat which was captured in the beginning of the war. We were not much impressed by the strength of the Turkish fleet although taken individually the boats appeared to be in the best working condition. The Turkish fellow Passengers naturally took great pride in their fleet and thought no end of it. The boat 'Medjidiyeh' which was reported to have been struck by a torpedo from a Greek boat and sunk was there in a very good condition.

Here two Turkish doctors boarded the steamer, one a military doctor and the other Dr. Adani Bey, Member of the Council of the Red Crescent. We got a lot of information from Adani Bey about the working of the Red Crescent Society. He informed us that the most likely places where field-hospitals would be needed should war be declared were at the Dardanelles, Gallipoli and another place on the shores of the Marmora. He gave us a great deal of information about things in general. It was most amusing to see our attempts to make him understand our meaning as he knows only French and Turkish. He also informed us that Enver Bey was in İstanbul and Niazzi Bey was at Scutari[6] and Fethi Bey was in charge of a battalion in the Dardanelles. We passed Gallipoli[7] at about 8 P. M. It was all dark and we could see only the lights on the shore.

Orders had been given to our Transport Department to get all the baggage ready by 6 A. M. At 6:30 we were all ready after a hurried breakfast, groping in the dull cloudy and misty morning to see any landmarks of the Capital of the Turkish Empire. About 6:15 we could clearly discern the shadowy outlines of the minarets and domes, the old fortresses and the new buildings along the shores of the Boğaziçi.[8] There lay İstanbul in its proud but sad dignity, and the feelings it aroused in one's mind were difficult to analyse. Those hills and old forts now crumbling down had seen the advent of the mighty Turks, the fall of the Byzantine Empire and the rise and glory of the Osmanli. Now, alas! The time had come when they were watching the gradual dismemberment of their Empire and the Decadence of Moslem rule.

As the boat approached the quay a large crowd of Turkish people could be seen waiting on the shore. We were met by Colonel Mehemet Ali Bey, the Inspector-General of the Red Crescent, and two military doctors of the rank of Colonel and many other notabilities. The ubiquitous 'Man from Cook's' was there, and we were also met by a man with a note from the British Ambassador. But the Red Crescent with the help of Cook's man took charge of our baggage. We formed a line walking in twos, and as we came down with Colonel Mehemet Ali Bey, the Guard of Honour gave us a salute and the band played the Turkish National Anthem. That was the first and would probably be the only place for representatives from India to be honoured with a salute. You could imagine how much we all appreciated this and felt the honour bestowed on us. In one action our eternal brotherhood was sealed.

We were driven in 8 carriages to the Kadergah Hasta Khaneh[9] (hospital worked under the auspices of the Red Crescent). In the course of our breakfast here Besim Ömer Pasha[10]—the Vice-president of the Red Crescent—arrived with several other notable personages. The Pasha is a very eminent surgeon and Gynaecologist of European fame and the real backbone of the Red Crescent movement in Turkey. He made a speech in Turkish, which was translated to us by Saleh Effendi in Urdu, welcoming us in the name of the Red Crescent and the Turkish nation and thanking us for the Islamic love and brotherhood which we had shown in coming here for their help and succour. He said that the Red Crescent was yet an infant and that its foster-father was India. In reply to his speech I thanked him heartily on behalf of the Mission and pointed to him that this infant which was brought to life by the famous accoucheir (himself) had soon under his skilled care become a vigorous and lusty child proving itself most useful be its mother Turkey in time of her need.

We were taken round the hospital by a Turkish gentleman who is one of the surgeons in the hospital. He showed us some very interesting cases of bullet wounds and gangrene due to cold. Afterwards Baroness Rosen, who is a Belgian lady at present working in this hospital, took us to her wards. It is a hospital with 200 beds comparatively clean and the patients are fairly well looked after. Dr. Sobami Bey, the Director of the Hospital, and the Baroness have shown us every kindness and hospitality and have made us very comfortable. So has Djevdet Bey, the Manager of the Hospital.

Thomas Cook's man could give me no information about our field-hospital, nor could Mr. Mounsey, the Second Secretary of the Embassy, who had called to see us at the hospital. I asked Mr. Mounsey to make inquiries about our field-hospital which was due before our arrival and which would probably be in charge of a storekeeper. I felt very anxious and decided to make inquiries at the British Post Office and Cook's the next day.

M. A. Ansari

1 January 1913

We started after our breakfast with our interpreter for Pera.[11] The streets of İstanbul are made of cobblestones and very badly kept. They are steep and often the gradient is so sharp that one would never imagine that driving in a carriage would be at all possible. But the horses and carriage in İstanbul seem to be made especially for these bad roads and stand the bumps and the sharp turns very well. The houses are built on European models and generally three to four storeys high, with the only difference that all the Muhammadan houses have screens in the front windows. The women are seen going about in the streets freely with a 'charchef' which is generally made of silk and covers the entire body and face. But the outline of the face can often be made out even through the thick black veil. On our way we passed the central municipal buildings where we saw a crowd of women, about 1,000 to 1,500 in number, in very ragged and torn clothes, looking the very picture of misery and helplessness awaiting food and clothes. These, we were told, were the refugees from the different Turkish villages now in possession of the Balkan Confederacy. But the Government is very good to them. They are clothed, housed, and fed by the Municipal Funds and are provided with money when they are sent to the provinces in Asia Minor.

However, on making inquiries, I felt sure in my mind that an organized relief fund to help those sufferers from the war would greatly mitigate their suffering and materially help them to start in life. I have not yet had sufficient time to make a thorough investigation in the matter, but I have been assured by the Croissant Rouge and several other people connected with the different charities that all is being done for them that is possible. On our way to the Galata or New Bridge as it is now called we passed the bureau central of the Red Crescent, the Persian Embassy, the Bureau of Commerce and Industry, the Finance Office and the General Post Office buildings which would be considered first class in any European capital. There are a number of big shops just before you come to the bridge, kept mostly by Armenians, Greeks and Jews. The bridge itself is made of iron and is of modern construction. It spans over the commencement of the Golden Horn and connects İstanbul with Galata and Pera, the European town. There is a toll to be paid by every man who crosses the bridge excepting the military people and the Red Crescent men. Pera is situated on a hill. The streets are narrow and winding although the buildings are mostly made of solid stone and of modern type. Neither Thomas Cook's office nor anyone at the Embassy could be seen, that being the New Year's Day: but we left our cards at the Embassy. We sent the cable to you after considerable discussion with the chief of the staff of the Turkish Telegraph Office, where we had to keep a copy of our Unicode to assure them that our cables were not in any way connected with war news. In the afternoon Colonel Mehemet Ali Bey went with us to the War Office where on inquiry we found that Nazim Pasha had gone to the Grand Vizarate. However, we paid a visit to Found Pasha, his Chief of the Staff, who received us very cordially and gave us coffee and cigarettes after the Turkish fashion. We gave him full details of our Mission and the field-hospital and made urgent request for immediate work. He suggested to us a place near Hadımköy,[12] which is about 15 kilometres from Çatalca,[13] where we could fix our hospital tent and start works as soon as we were ready. We simply jumped at the suggestion and to make the arrangements complete. We went to see the Inspector-General for the Sanitary Department of the War Office, Weiner Pasha, who is the person in charge of field-hospitals. He confirmed the arrangement and told us to proceed to Sanjaktapah[14] as soon as we were ready. We came away well satisfied with the progress we had made so far as we were informed by Dr. Mohamed Husain, the Director of the Bombay Mission, that so far they had not been given any work as their things had not arrived.

Our visit to the Minister of Foreign Affairs, Nuradanghian Bey, was very short and could not have lasted for more than three minutes. He received us in great hurry, read the letter of the Consul-General and talked to Mehemet Ali Bey and our interpreter and then said goodbye.

On our return home we found a letter from Mr. Monsey which he had left in the hospital saying that no trace could be found of our hospital. This news rather upset me and I sent two telegrams at once, one to you and another to Mr. Ameer Ali.

M. A. Ansari

2 January 1913

As this is the rainy season here I found it necessary to provide all the members of the Mission with water proof over-coats and a pair of boots with galoshes. This item came rather expensive and cost us bout CT45, but it was necessary as you would see for yourself. The boots were paid for by the members themselves. We went to Cook's where we were given the bill of lading from Manson & Sons for the goods they had sent by the Messagerie's post—altogether 301 packages. This relieved me of my great anxiety about the cables on the previous evening. There was also a letter from Mr. Ameer Ali and from Dr. Sayeed.

In the afternoon we went to the War Office again and were presented to General Nazim Pasha, who was very nice to us. I told him every detail about our field-hospital arrangements which seem to have pleased him immensely. He said our hospital would prove very useful should war commence. He is a very broad, tall, military looking man of very few words, but genuine and sincere. He offered us coffee and cigarettes and when we were taking leave of him he promised to speak to His Majesty about as before the Selamlik the next day.

We visited the Dar-ul Fünun(the University for Science and Arts) now converted into a hospital under the Red Crescent. The Director of this hospital is a Turkish gentleman who was very hospitable and kind to us. He took our party round to all the wards and showed us the food which was given to the patients. There are altogether over 1,000 soldiers and, although they are over-crowded and the wards are not very clean, they are by no means uncomfortable or badly looked after. The Bombay Medical Mission is quartered here. One of the doctors, Dr. Nazar Han of Bhopal, who was laid up with influenza was about to return to India. We paid him a visit and we met the members of the Bombay Mission.

M. A. Ansari

Kadirgah Hospital, Istanbul, 14 January 1913

I mentioned in my last letter to you an interview with Halide Khanem[15] (Madame Saleh). She belongs to the Party of Union and Progress and is a very active worker, not only politically, but in almost every sphere of activity, for the benefit of Turkey. She used to write almost daily in the Tunin when the paper was being published, and has written to many of the leading French and German papers as well as in the Manchester Guardian and for the Jeune Turc. She is considered one of the leading lights of the Party of Union and Progress, a silent, though very effective, power working behind the scenes. I considered myself very fortunate in having met her as she will be very useful. I have persuaded her to become a contributor to the Comrade as soon as she returns from the German Hospital where she has been advised to go for a rest cure, having worked very hard during the war in helping the organizations for the sick and wounded and the widows and orphans. She hoped one day very soon, after this crisis was over, to visit India and deliver a series of lectures in different Muhammadan centres to give correct ideas about Turkey and her people to the Muhammadan public in India. Unfortunately I have not been able to see her again, but I hope to do so before our hospital is established in Ömerli.[16] I think Madame Saleh will be an additional attraction as a contributor for the *Comrade*, if any attraction is necessary at all.

I have received by the mail copies of letters addressed to you by Mr. Ameer Ali together with a detailed list of all the articles supplied for our field-hospital by Messrs. Maw, Son & Sons. I have already informed you of the receipt of 252 packages; but a further supply was received last Wednesday numbering G9 (?) in all. This brings the total number of packages to 311; and when the remaining 19 packages will be received, the number would come to 330.

M. A. Ansari

January 1913

9 January 1913

Except a visit from Shaikh Abdul Aziz Chawish to our hospital nothing of importance took place on this day. Shaikh Chawish is a very impressive man who chooses every word before uttering it. He talked to us about things in general, mostly weather, and then departed, after giving an invitation to some of the members to be at his house the next day where Enver Bey, Mahmud Shevked Pasha[17] and several other prominent members of the Party of Union and Progress were expected. I could not accept his invitation, but several men from the Mission went to his house and spent a very pleasant afternoon, although they were rather disappointed owing to the absence of the Young Turkish leaders. Dr. Asad Pasha,[18] a very famous Turkish Ophthalmic Surgeon of European reputation, was present at the tea and made some pregnant remarks regarding the condition of Turkey and the Moslem world in general. Our Manager replied and made a great impression on those present by these weighty words! I should have loved to be present there, but I was unavoidably absent.

M. A. Ansari

10 January 1913

Whilst our friends were having tea at Shaikh Chawish's house, I went to see the Persian Ambassador with a few members. His Excellency was very nice to us, gave us some cigarettes and Persian tea and talked to us for quite a long time. He understood English but spoke in Persian. The First Attaché to the Embassy spoke English very fluently, and discussed in a very animated fashion the causes of the gradual decay of Islam. He took the view of Mr. Garvin that the great cause of decay was to be found in the backward conditions of Moslem women both mentally and physically, and the only way to salvation lay in the emancipation of women. His Excellency intelligently followed the discussion and gave his approval to what his Attaché expressed to us. There is no doubt that the events in Turkey and Persia seem to have impressed deeply the mind of all the Moslem world and they are beginning to realise, though, alas! very late, that unless they improve themselves at once they will lose all they possess and be a subject race for ever.

M. A. Ansari

11 January 1913

I paid a visit to His Excellency Sir Gerard Lowther, the British Ambassador, accompanied by my cousin, and found him, to my intense pleasure, a perfectly amiable English gentleman. He offered us cigarettes and sat down for over half an hour for what appeared a friendly chat in a private drawing-room. I inquired after Lord Hardinge and was told that he was convalescent and progressing very satisfactorily. It seems Sir Gerard Lowther and Lord Hardinge are personal friends and have spent several years together at the Turkish Embassy. His Excellency was interested in our Mission and inquired about the members of the Mission, our hospital equipment and the place where we were going to fix our hospital. He asked me to always rely on his ready help whenever we were in need of it. After thanking him for his previous kindness and his promise for the future, we returned well satisfied with our visit.

In the afternoon come twelve members of the Mission went with me to Haider Pasha[19] a place across the Boğaziçi in Scutari, the Asiatic portion of İstanbul. We went there in a boat and saw on our landing there the magnificent railway station which is the terminus of the line running between İstanbul and Aleppo. I have not seen any railway station either in Europe or in India which can come anywhere near it. We visited the Military Medical College and Hospital. Aziz Pasha, the chief of the hospital, was exceedingly courteous and took us round this magnificent hospital where we saw 1,000 Turkish soldiers being nursed and looked after. The words were clean, paved with glazed tiles, and furnished with modern iron beds. The sheets, pillow cases and towels were clean; the blankets were thick and warm; and altogether there was nothing lacking to make the patients comfortable and cheerful during their stay in the hospital. All the patients in this building were medical cases and numbered 1,000. This hospital would compare favourably with any European hospital, and it was certainly much cleaner than the hospitals one had seen in France and Italy. The building itself is very stately and, being situated on the shores of the Boğaziçi, commands a beautiful view with plenty of pure ozonic air and sunshine. The next building, which is made of solid stone with very fine carvings, was the Army Medical College itself. At present this is also used for patients numbering 650 to 750. The building across the road facing it is devoted entirely to surgical cases. The entire interior of this building, the floor, walls and ceiling of the corridors and the words are tiled with glazed tiles. There are small wards for one or two patients and large wards for 100 patients. The arrangements here were absolutely perfect. Everything was scrupulously clean, and I can assure you there are not many places in London, Berlin, Vienna or Paris which can boast of a hospital like this. The hospital has a most modern operating theatre and X-Ray department, and a staff of surgeons, assistant surgeons, sisters and nurses who are quite up-to-date. I was shown a patient who had an operation performed on his head following a bullet wound and the result was ideal. I was told on enquiry that the staff consisted of teachers and professors of European fame, and they turned out 100 to 120 army medical men every year.

From what follows, when describing the hospitals at Hadımköy, Gnifer and San Stefano,[20] you would see that not only the general press of Europe was full of a series of calumnies and false reports about the Turkish organization, but even the medical Press was affected by this religious bigotry and fanaticism, and stated facts about the medical organization which on examination one finds altogether incorrect and exaggerated. I do not mean by this that there is no room for assistance in this present unusual situation. It is bound to affect even the best organized country. But what I maintain is that the assistance needed is not true to the extent that it is represented, nor any more than any other European Power would require at the time of war. The story of the Turkish wounded being left in thousands on the battle-field to die is a tissue of malignant lies which is obvious to even a casual observer who visits the hospitals and sees for himself the number of major operations performed on the patients with results which even the best surgeons of Europe would be proud of. It may be of interest, by way of comparison, to mention here that the results of the German Red Cross Hospitals, the British Red Crescent Hospital sent by Mr. Amir Ali and the French Red Cross Hospitals have been very unsatisfactory, whether due to the lack of skill or interest of the doctors sent in these Missions. In fact there is a feeling here, no doubt erroneous, owing to their bad results that these men deliberately maimed and dismembered the patients when a conservative treatment would have saved the lives and limbs of many of the patients placed under their treatment.

M. A. Ansari

12 January 1913

The Manager and myself left for Hadımköy with Colonel Ali Darwesh Bey of the Red Crescent Society as our guide, philosopher and friend, and our interpreter. Dr. Muhammad Husain also accompanied us with the Manager of his Mission. We left İstanbul at 10.45 am and passed a dozen stations on our way, San Stefano and Ömerli being the important stations. At San Stefano we saw two Egyptian Red Crescent Field-Hospitals. One Ottoman Red Crescent Field-Hospital and one Military Field-Hospital, all in good working order. There were several Red Crescent Field-Hospitals at intervening stations, whose names I don't remember. We were met at several stations by officers of the Red Crescent and the Royal Army Medical Corps who accompanied us to Hadımköy. At Hadımköy General Abdus Salam Pasha, the officer in-charge of the whole of the medical department in this division, met us at the station and salute was given by 100 soldiers awaiting us at the platform. We then proceeded to a house in Hadımköy where we were presented to Ahmad Abuk Pasha, the second Field-Marshal. He is a grand old man with a most impressive personality. He spoke to us in the most eloquent and pregnant words, honest and soothing in his analysis of the causes at work which have brought the present downfall of the Turks. He thought that true Islam was not to be found amongst the Turks: that they had acquired all the vices of the West and lost their real great qualities inherited from Islam which had brought them to this plight. He was very kind and courteous to us and paid us compliments which we thought were out of proportion to our work. General Abdus Salam Pasha and Ahmad Abuk Pasha consulted for some time and then decided to send us to Ömerli which is behind the lines of defence and yet not so bitterly cold or damp as Sanjaktapa. There is also a plentiful supply of good water at Ömerli which is not found at Sanjaktapa. Judging from the sea of mud at Hadımköy, which we were told was much better than at Sanjaktapa, we gratefully acquiesced in their selection of Ömerli and left Ahmad Abuk Pasha to visit the Red Crescent Hospital at Hadımköy.

Horses were brought for us to ride, but our Manager declined (Let us not be said through any fear) to ride such a very short distance as the Red Crescent Hospital, in spite of the Mud Atlantic. The Turks are very polite people and to please the guests would even face the prospects of a mud-bath rather than refuse a request. We walked, or rather swam, in the mud. Our beautiful uniform, boots and breeches and all were forgotten in our anxiety to prevent a fall which was imminent at every footstep as the mud was very slippery here. In one place I had actually to plunge my hand in the mud and just saved myself from a most ignominious fall. My hand was however, ley cold, and yet, I could not put on my gloves owing to the mud. We reached the shelter of the hospital, as you can imagine, with a sigh of relief. After a meal which would be considered regal, we inspected the hospital and found unsatisfactory owing to the mud which, in spite of dry dusting, was quite thick.

At last we got on the horses; Abdur Rahman's being the fleetest. At least that's what he thought. We rode on through hilly tracts full of mud and water until we reached the Army Hospital where Abdus Salam Pasha met us with his staff and took us round the hospital. This is a brick building and accommodates 700 patients. The arrangements here were excellent, most of the cases being medical. They had a splendid pharmacy and a small operating theatre.

Dr. Muhammad Husain took our photographs, after which we started. On outten minutes ride to Ömerli, 'The Roads were hilly and very difficult and with a cold wind blowing against our faces we rode on, our Manager bringing the near, as he insisted on not allowing the horses to run (of course out of consideration for the animals). In his anxiety he rode with ungloved hands which were simply frozen: but how could he possible put on his gloves when once on horse-back? The latter half of our journey to Ömerli was done in pitch dark. The Manager is very proud of his horsemanship in reaching Ömerli safely without a fall. I must say that once or twice he was put to the severest test when Ali Ghalib Bey whipped his horse from behind quite unawares, the horse bolting off suddenly, of course, with Abdur Rahman on the saddle unaided, even to the extent of holding his saddle or putting his arms round the horse's neck. We stayed in a small room in Ömerli and were treated to a sumptuous repast by Dr. Burhan Bey. The next morning we visited the place where our tents are to be pitched. It is under the shelter of a hill facing the Ömerli railway station and separated from the railway line by a small stream. 'There is a natural spring with a plentiful supply of drinking water by the side of our camp, and with a bridge across the stream the camp will be a minute from the railway station. After saying goodbye to Dr. Ali Ghalib Bey, Inspector to the Army, and other medical officers who had accompanied us to Ömerli, we returned last night to İstanbul and explained everything to Besim Ömer Pasha, the Vice-President of the Red Crescent, İstanbul. Owing to the wet weather and the damp soil I have ordered every tent to have wooden floor raised about 2ft. from the ground. This would keep our patients quite dry and prevent cold and damp.

Our transport has been sent to-day to the stores, where all our goods are kept, to separate the tents from the rest of the goods. These will be sent to-morrow and will be ready by Friday or Saturday when all the remaining goods will be sent with a batch from the Mission to get everything ready. We hope by the 25th of this month to be in working older. You would no doubt think us very slow: but I assure you so far as we are concerned not a moment is being lost, but the conditions of transport, etc., make this delay unavoidable.

The Bombay Mission which came a fortnight before us has neither got its tents nor the instruments yet, and I should be very much surprised, if they get their things in a week's time and work by the end of this month.

I will write to you in my next letter about the organization of the Ottoman Red Crescent and the splendid work, medical as well as relief that they are doing. I am convinced after thorough and searching investigation that this is the only organization worthy of support from India where every penny is used to good purpose and Dr. Muhammad Husain and myself have thought it necessary to sign a telegram sent by Besim Ömer Pasha to the different papers in India for publication in order to direct all the money to the Red Crescent and prevent its going to quarters where one cannot find anything about the money.

M. A. Ansari

February 1913

20 January 1913

I received your letter after a long wait, and I assure you it was very welcome. You would have learnt by now about the telegrams which I sent from Suez to the P.S.V. about the horrible outrage on His Excellency.

It must have shocked everybody in India and caused no end of anxiety to the people in Delhi. However, the Viceroy is getting well, and I hope that the culprit would soon be found and punished for this dastardly attempt on the life of Lord Harding.

I have not yet seen the Grand Vizier, nor have I forwarded your cheque to the Sublime Porte. In future I would advise you strongly to send all remittances either to me or to the Red Crescent Ottoman. I am convinced that this is the only institution in this country which has done any good work to lessen the sufferings of the emigrants.

I have thought over your scheme very carefully and think it is not only very sound but most practical. The mission can very easily be divided into two units, one working at the Ömerli Hospital and the other either in the front (in case of war) or in Anatolia where most of the emigrants have been sent. In the latter condition, which seems to me most likely, our work would be just as useful as in the case of war. The section in Anatolia would have a house rented for the purpose for the hospital and dispensary. And the chief feature of the work of this section would be house to house visits not only to treat the patients there and to supply them with the necessary medicines in their homes, but also to furnish them with food and necessary clothing, and when the bread winners are cured, to help them with a small sum and start them on their work. I think this would be a far greater work than half a dozen field-hospitals. Of course, we shall have to have an office in İstanbul, where the Manager and I would work and we shall visit the two hospitals alternately every other week and keep regular registers and accounts of the relief thus undertaken by us.

Both the Manager and myself have visited the Red Crescent and have had long interviews with Besim Ömer Pasha, Vice-President and the real worker in this institution, as well as Mehmet Ali Bey, Inspector-General, and several other men who are doing active work for the Society. We have gathered every possible information regarding their work and have come to the conclusion that, although they are by no means very quick in their undertakings or prompt in their organization, they have done a vast amount of work during this war. We have induced them to publish an account of their work in the form of a booklet and also the total amount of money received from India up to the present time. I think they are going to do it shortly. We have visited their stores and their work room where the ladies sew linen, under clothing, stockings, etc. etc. for the patients and the emigrants, we have also seen for ourselves the manner in which clothes, blankets and other necessary articles are distributed to the different sections of the emigrant population encamped round about İstanbul. And, although we have not been able to visit the food camps, we know on good authority that good, wholesome and sufficient food is cooked and supplied twice daily to the emigrants. There are a certain class of emigrants who have run away from their homes with their horses and cattle and these are supplied with three piastres daily for themselves and the animals. It must also be mentioned that no male members among the emigrants are given any money or clothing unless they are ill as that would be an inducement for indolence. They are sent away to different parts of Anatolia or are supplied with work in İstanbul. For this work they have divided İstanbul in to various sections or areas, each area being worked by one local team who prepares a list of the different families of the emigrants with their needs, The Central Office sends one of its members with food, clothing, bedding, etc. according to the requirement to be distributed in the presence of this member and marked off in the registers. It is interesting to note that nearly all the workers of the Red Crescent, whether they are gentlemen or ladies belong to the party of union and progress, an important section of the organization of the Red Crescent is a bureau which supplies clothing, food and other necessaries to the Turkish prisoners in the hands of the Balkan Confederacy and as much news as is permissible to their relations in Turkey.

Our idea is to work in co-operation with the Red Crescent, although we shall keep our own register and our own employees for the relief work. I would be very glad if you would let me know your opinion about this scheme.

I may mention also that the chief medical officers and managers for the two sections would, in my opinion, be quite capable of directing and managing the affairs of their section. To make matters sure, you would see that I would be myself visiting the two sections every alternate week for doing important operations, auditing their accounts and directing them in other matters.

As regards blankets and clothing I had a long talk with Besim Ömer Pasha, and I think he is right in preferring money to ready-made clothes or blankets as by the time these reach Turkey it would be spring time, the need for blankets would not be so urgent and the clothing will have to be supplied according to the climate Moreover, I don't think that except under-clothing anything else made in India would at all be used by the people here, their clothes are so entirely different.

The great event of the week has been a visit from Enver Bey. He came to visit us in the hospital where we are staying. He is only a young man of about 35, exceedingly handsome, with most expressive eyes full of determination. His demeanour was that of a very strong man, chastened with hardships and sufferings. He was quiet and yet characteristic, modest and yet commanding respect. A man who is born to command and to elicit implicit faith and admiration from those who work under him. He spoke with a certain reserve and expressed his appreciation of our work for his countrymen. It was a thousand pities that the difficulty of the language prevented talking to him at length. After a visit to the wards a group was taken and he departed.

I had another occasion of seeing Madame Halide Edib, who was as interesting as ever. She promised to become a contributor to the *Comrade* as soon as things had settled down in Turkey. We gave a few copies of the *Comrade* for distribution among her friends.

I have had to make some additions in the personnel of the mission, as it was absolutely unavoidable. From the very beginning we had foreseen the necessity of employing interpreters, and our experience has only convinced us of this urgent need. I have secured the services of Dr. Fuad Bey who is the best interpreter (apart from his being a medical man) I have come across in İstanbul. We shall have to pay him a good salary which has not been definitely fixed, but will be between L 6 and L 8 a month. Dr. Fuad knows English and Turkish perfectly and is an Egyptian. I have also secured the services of two dragomen, both Indian, who can speak Turkish fairly well, on a salary of five Medjidiehs which come to about Rs. 12.80 a month. These men will be useful in getting out the history from the patient, and other general work. An Egyptian boy, Mahmood Mazhar, of a respectable family, has joined us as a volunteer without any salary. He has been a student in the Mercantile Naval School and has been a volunteer also. He is willing to serve in any capacity with our Mission. Knowing English and Turkish fairly well, he is a very useful addition to the mission.

I have met Shaikh Abdul Aziz Chawish and found him a very interesting personality: He is full of schemes for reviving the Arabic literature and language.

It is with a great sigh of relief that I am writing to you about the departure of a portion of our equipment to Ömerli in charge of two of our men. I am going there tomorrow with four other men in order to get all the tents pitched and the other arrangements made for camp. I have within three days to return to İstanbul and go back with the remaining articles and the members of the mission. I cannot tell you what difficulties are placed in our way here even in arranging a small matter. Our things have all arrived last week, and in any other country but Turkey everything would have been arranged in a day or two.

M. A. Ansari

Comrade, 15 February 1913

I returned to İstanbul on the afternoon of 23rd January. As I drove past the sublime Porte I saw some five to eight hundred soldiers standing inside the enclosure of Bab-i-Aalee, and a crowd at the balcony of Bab-i-Aalee, along the steps, the road, the gate-way and the entire public thoroughfare. This was the memorable day on which the coup of the Party of Union and Progress was carried out in order to catch the Cabinet of Kiamil Pasha[21] red-handed in the very act of signing the reply to the Note of the Powers ceding Adrianople. Enver Bey had ridden on a horse all night from Gallipoliand, reaching İstanbul on the morning of 23rd, made all the necessary arrangements, placing his men in the different cafes and houses in the vicinity of Bab-i-Aalee. He rode on a horse with a few soldiers to Bab-i-Aalee and, on being challenged by the sentinel at the entrance, he said he had come to save Turkey, and made a brief but touching speech, which moved the soldiers so much that they all joined him, and he marched into the room where the Cabinet had assembled to do the work of selling their country to their enemies. He entered this room accompanied by another army officer, Najef Bey, and demanded the resignation of the Cabinet from the Grand Vizier. He held the form of the resignation and asked for their signature, which was meekly complied with by Kiamil Pasha and a few others. But Nazim Pasha got up in a rage and ordered his A.-D.-C. to get these intruders arrested by the gendarme. Shots were exchanged in which Nazim Pasha, his A.-D.-C. Najef Bey and two other were killed, but the remaining Ministers were kept under guard. Enver Bey then processed to the Sultan's palace and got the Imperial *iradeh* appointing Mahmood Shevket Pasha as the Prime Minister and entrusting him with the formation of a new Cabinet. The crowd was waiting for the arrival of Enver Bey, Talat Bey and Mahmoud Shevket Pasha was the signal for a tremendous outburst from the crowd outside Bab-i-Aalee. Enver Bey was the hero of the moment, and the crowd carried him shoulder high to the Bab-i-Aalee. He was embraced and kissed until he was nearly smothered. Then the Grand Vizier, according to the ancient custom, made a short speech to the crowd in which he expressed the hope that he would receive their cooperation and help in the difficult task of government at such a critical time. The crowd cheered him very heartily. The party then entered the Bab-i-Aalee, followed by the great crowd in which some of the members of the Mission were also included. They entered every room and also saw the chair in which Nazim Pasha had been killed. Very soon after the streets were quiet, and no external sign of such a great revolution was obvious even in the streets round the Bab-i-Aalee.

It struck an outsider as a very extraordinary thing that events of such great moment should be enacted in such a quiet manner without any obvious change in the daily life of the Turks. Is it possible that the Turks have got inured to these vicissitudes and take them with a philosophical calm, unthinkable by us Indians to whom such events are extraordinary and unusual? Or, is it they have grown indifferent and callous and take any sudden change in their government with the indifference of an absolutely lifeless and spiritless people?

I think probably the former is the truer explanation; for on the opposite side of the Bab-i-Aalee, inside the editorial office of Sheikh Abdul Aziz Chawish, were gathered a good number of people quite hidden from the passers-by, discussing with obvious jubilation the great triumph of the only patriotic party in Turkey. I am told that every moment an emissary would enter this place with news of what was going on inside the Bab-i-Aalee to the intense joy of the people gathered in this house.

At about half past nine, just as we had finished our dinner in the Kadirgah Hospital, a telephone message was received from the Bab-i-Aalee to send ambulance bearers and doctors at once. The director of the Hospital, with six of my ambulance bearers, and a few others from the Hospital, reached the Sublime Porte immediately, but the men were returned after a long wait, the staff of the Hospital, however, being asked to remain. I was informed the next morning that they had quietly buried the dead during the night, with the exception of Nazim Pasha whose funeral took place the next day, most of the members of the new Cabinet being present.

Next day the State Entry of the Grand Vizier and the new Shaikh-al-Islam (Ziyauddin Efendi) took place in a very quiet manner. I cabled to you on the night of the 23rd the names of the chief ministers in the new Cabinet; but there have been some changes since then the principal one being Prince Said Halim Pasha, who has been appointed Minister for Foreign Affairs. Every day the Grand Vizier first visits the War Office, where things are made to move. Already a great many changes have been made in the army and every day one sees troops being moved from one place to another. To-day six mountain batteries were seen going in the direction of the harbour.

There is a great change in the attitude of certain European Powers, the Triple Alliance openly giving assurance of help to Turkey. The Deutsche Orient Bank has made an advance of half a million Turkish pounds, and has promised 2 1/2 million by the end of January. The attitude of Russia has changed from a threat to an assurance of neutrality. Only England and France are still reticent. It is obvious that the Young Turks have saved the prestige of Turkey and mean to die honourably, if death must come.

Appendix

It is impossible even for an adversary to abstain from admiring their pluck, although it still remains to be seen whether this pluck is going to save Turkey. The new Ministers have come to power on condition that they would not cede Adrianople or give up the Aegean Island, even if it comes to a re-declaration of war. I am sure that the Balkan Confederacy is exhausted and will not be able to proceed with the campaign. We wish to God that Turkey would declare war again, and regain a moral and territorial victory over her toes.

My previous letters must have made plain to you what impression I had of Kiamil's Cabinet. It was the Hamidian regime, only in a more obviously constitutional garb hence the manner in which all the business was transacted. We think Indian Moslems have now no desire to 'harass' the Minister with frantic resolutions and telegraphic appeals.

M. A. Ansari

22 February 1913

On the 20th of January I wrote to you just before my departure to Ömerli. I arrived there with Dr. Fyzee, Dr. Abdur Rahman, Mr. Khaliquzzaman and Mr. Hussain Raza Bey, Abdul Waheed and Haji Abdullah our dragomen, having arrived there the day before. The first thing we did was to make a little bridge over the little strain between the railway line and the valley where our tents were to be pitched, some of the soldiers stationed in Ömerli helping us in this work. We then started pitching the first tent. As none of us had any experience in tent pitching, it took us quite a long time, with a great deal of discussion to put up this tent. By the end of the evening we succeeded only in pitching up one double-tent and a bill tent. Next day we succeeded in putting up three double-tents, one single tent, the operation tent and the remaining two bill tents: a mixed shower of rain and sleet prevented us from putting up the last tent. It would have done your heart a lot of good if you had seen the members of your Mission working in the teeth of a most bitterly cold wind and the mud almost knee-deep. Here at least there was no distinction between the doctor and the dresser, everyone hammering the pegs, fixing the poles or spreading the canvas and doing the work like real enthusiasts. The next morning there was a heavy downpour of rain, and, although one hundred soldiers arrived from Handemkoi for our aid, we could not avail ourselves of their services owing to the wretched weather. I left the next day for İstanbul in order to send all our equipment to Ömerli and proceed there with the utmost dispatch possible in this country.

I must mention that bitter experience has taught me never to rely in matters of provision on anybody but ourselves. My men and myself having been driven to eating nothing but cheese and bread for three days, owing to the box containing our provision having been stolen by someone on the line. I have now arranged for a bi-weekly supply of stores from İstanbul, at least one of my men always accompanying the stores.

[Here we have omitted Dr. Ansari's account of the coup d'etat which we published in the last issue—Ed. Comrade.]

I have been waiting ever since my return from Ömerli to make enquiries regarding the issue of the Turkish Treasury Bonds. I visited Talat Bey who promised to make enquiries about it. But not being satisfied with this indefinite promise I went and saw the Minister of Interior who understood English, made notes of all I had told him and promised to give me definite information this afternoon. He could not fulfill his promise owing to an important meeting of the Cabinet. Tomorrow I am going to visit the Grand Vizier with the Drafts you have sent for him and a translation of both your letters in Turkish. I am hoping to get information about the Treasury Bonds, which I intend cabling to you at once. I am sure a loan of three or four million Turkish pounds would be of immense help to Turkey. To write to you for hastening this matter on my part is obviously superfluous, as you are already too keen on the matter and besides it would be impossible for you to hurry up the matter without the receipt of Treasury Bonds from Turkey.

I must end my letter with a brief account of the Mission. I have sent out two wagons full of the baggage, mostly those things which had arrived from London. Half of another wagon has also been loaded and the other half will be loaded tomorrow. This wagon contains a portion of the articles which have been bought for us here in İstanbul. These things are mostly for kitchens and other general stores, a complete list of which is being prepared for your perusal. These articles have not been paid for as yet, as the Red Crescent have not sent the bill yet. I may mention that this list was carefully prepared on comparing our invoice with the authorized list of articles supplied to the Field Hospitals worked under the auspices of the Ottoman Red Crescent. I will send you the bill as soon as it is presented after I have carefully scrutinised the same.

There is one thing which is notably inadequate for our equipment and that is, the tents. They have sent us four double-tents, 30 by 16, and two single tents, 30 by 16. These tents would hold with utmost difficulty not more than 16 beds each, that is, altogether 96 beds for patients. Besides these there is one tent for operations and three bill tents, which are very small and would not hold more than three attendants. You would see that we have no tents for the doctors and dressers, nor any tent for dispensary kitchen, store or the office. We have been fortunate in being able to borrow two tents from the Bombay Mission but we still require at least four to six tents more. It is impossible to get tents in İstanbul for love or money, and I am afraid we will have to rely on the kindness of the Bombay Mission for tents. Absolutely it is impracticable to cable for tents to England or India, as it could take a mouth before we get them.

I have sent you a cable after getting the answer from the Minister of Interior but I wish I had not done so, as two days after during my interview with Rifaat Bey, the Minister of Finance proved that the Minister of Interior had given me absolutely wrong information on the subject of the Bonds. I explained to Rifaat Bey who was naturally very grateful to you for all that you are doing to raise money in India by the sale of the Turkish Treasury Bonds, but after explaining to me all the details of the manner of issuing the Bonds, he expressed his utter inability to issue these Bonds to less than three months' time. He was very sorry at this delay, but he suggested that I should cable to you do you to arrange with the Banks if it was possible to receive money from the people for these Treasury Bonds and give them receipts for their money to be changed for these bonds when they were ready. He would like to know if such an arrangement was possible, and also the names of the Banks, and the conditions on which they were willing to sell the Bonds. I had been waiting for your reply to my first telegram before cabling to you the above instructions received from the Minister of Finance.

I went to Bab-i-Ali on the 30th of January with your first letter to the Grand Vizier, enclosing a cheque of hundred and twenty odd pounds and your second letter enclosing two cheques of 1000 pound each. I had your letters translated in Turkish, as previous experience had taught me that this was the best way in order to facilitate matters. I also took your telegram along with two others, one from Rangoon and the other from Bombay, with their Turkish translation. I found Sheikh Abdul Aziz Shawish also waiting in Bab-i-Ali, and as we were both called in together he acted as my interpreter. Mahmoud Shevkat Pasha received me most courteously, and shook hands with me in a most cordial manner. I explained to him the feelings of the Muslims of India at the great crisis which Turkey was going through and the hopes they now centred in him and his Cabinet for saving Turkey and the whole Islamic world from disgrace and utter loss of prestige. He was very brief in his reply, but his words were pregnant and sincere. He said, among other things, that the Muslims of India had been very generous in their help towards the relief of the wounded and the sick, and that the Turks would never forget their kindness and help at such a time. After reading the Turkish translation of your letters and cable he was very pleased, and made enquiries about you and all that you have done in organizing the All-India Medical Mission and the Red Crescent Fund for the relief of the wounded soldiers and the refugees. He promised to send your telegram to his Imperial Majesty the Sultan, and said that I will have the receipt sent to me in due course of time for the three drafts I had given him from you. I asked him about the war to which he replied that they were ready for it, but he was not sure of the Balkan Confederacy. As regards Adrianople, he said that the garrison had enough provision for two months. In the end, he promised a private presentation of all the Members of the All-India Medical Mission to His Majesty the Sultan, and expressed a desire to see them himself.

I had sent all the Members of the Mission previously to Ömerli where they had all the tents ready. Our stores, provisions and equipment had all reached Ömerli also and were being stored in one of the tents which we were compelled to use exclusively for this purpose. This tent is single and very dilapidated. The snow and sometimes rain gets through inside it and hence it could not be used for wards for which it had been designed. I regret to say that in the choice of the tents both the quality and number have put as to a lot of trouble and expenditure. I have been compelled to buy tents from a local English firm, luckily at a very moderate cost. I have already bought ten small double tents for the staff and the office at thirteen pounds (£13) each, each tent accommodates three persons. I have also ordered three large tents at £20 each for holding 8 patients in each. It is absolutely necessary to have these tents double, as the winter here is terribly severe, and living in single tents would be absolutely impossible. The British Red Crescent Mission has been compelled for the same reason to give up its tents and erect wooden barracks at a cost of more than twice the price of a tent.

We have all been working terribly hard and have got our camp ready to receive soldiers from Çatalca day after tomorrow, as the war is going to begin tomorrow, Monday, at 7 P.M. I may tell you that our field hospital, if not the best, is second to none in Turkey. Not only are our wards, dispensary, operating theatre and general provision most excellent, but every member of the Mission has got the zeal and energy of ten persons, and a most excellent expert de corps exists among them, of which I feel naturally very proud.

Dr. Barry has been invalided due to rheumatism and would soon be returning home.... Husain Raza Beg has also got some lungs trouble and I am thinking of sending him back to India. I have secured the service of Dr. Fouad at £8 mensem. He will act both as a doctor and interpreter.

P.S.—I am afraid Unicode cables would not be allowed. They even cen-sored my last cable to you about the revolution. Five names and several words were removed from the cablegram. But rest assured I will keep you posted with all important news.

M. A. Ansari

Comrade, 1 March 1913

I am afraid my weekly note is impossible this time, I have had to divide the Mission into two units: one remains in Ömerli—under Dr. Naim, and the other is going under me to an unknown destination with Enver Bey's attacking army. This news ought to immensely please you, as ours in the only Mission out of the seven which had applied which has been given this great honour and distinction of accompanying Enver Bey. The British Red Crescent and the Egyptian Missions were all refused on the score of insuf-ficient equipment, I may also tell you that I have personally gained much favour with the party of Union and Progress and the Red Crescent Ottoman. They consult me in all their affairs connected with Hospital organization. As regards the Bonds, I have seen the Minister of Finance and have given him the fullest possible details about them. He promised to send the Bank of Bengal and the Alliance Bank of Simla and yourself official cables with full details. That is the reason I have not cabled to you myself with a view to economy.

Yesterday I saw Talat Bey, who promised to urge the party not to waste valuable time. He has also promised to send you news free through the Agence Ottoman. I have received the official receipt of the money you sent to the Grand Vizier through me, but as it is not with me just now I will send it next week. I have to buy a lot of things for the Mission. I spent £T.50 for tents, although the Bombay Mission had very generously given us six tents. I have to buy a lot of drugs and stores. These, by the way, can be had in İstanbul from an English firm at a slightly higher cost than in England, but one can save time and a lot of annoyance by buying here, and one can personally satisfy oneself about the articles. That is the reason why I have requested you to send me £2,000. We have also got to supply provisions for the Mission, which is the most costly item. The Ottoman army has driven the Bulgars all along the line so far. They are near Adrianople now, and the relief of the fortress is expected daily. I will cable all important news. Abdur Rehman will remain in future in İstanbul for keeping the accounts of the Mission and arranging for the food supply. He will in future send you the weekly letter, as I don't think I would be able to do so owing to our march with the advancing army.

After learning that a unit of the All-India Mission has gone with Enver Bey's attacking column, we would all of us be naturally eager to hear from Dr. Ansari about his experiences. He says, however, that he would be unable to send his weekly letter. We are sure the Manager's letters will be equally interesting and will give us full information about the doings of both the units of the Mission. The landing of the expeditionary column of 60 thousands of all arms under the command of Enver Bey was reported by Reuter long ago and later on the expedition was declared to have failed. We cannot, however, believe that a column of 60 thousands, after effecting a successful landing, would 'fail' without fighting a battle and even encountering the enemy. The movements of Enver Bey have for some time past been shrouded in mystery, but we are confident soon to hear of him and his column and that in a way which may not perhaps be a pleasant theme for a 'Reuter's Message'.

M. A. Ansari

Chanak Kila, Dardanelles, 3 March 1918
[From 4th to 11th February]

It is nearly a month that I have not been able to write to you at any length. My reason has been simply that I have been unsettled and never certain as to where I would be tomorrow. The urgent telegram from Bassim Ömer Pasha called me to İstanbul early in February, just when my hospital in Ömerli had started working and ever since I have been kept in hope and despair by the authorities in the War Office. At last I am glad to say that I have been able, by sheer dint of dogged perseverance, to secure a beautiful place for our hospital which, I hope in a day or two, will be full of patients, numbering some 125 to 150.

The object of my hasty summons to İstanbul was (1) the desire of War Minister to see me regarding the Treasury Bonds and (2) to send a portion of our hospital with Enver Bey's army which was trying to effect a landing at Charkhui [22] (on the coast of Marmara). As regards the Treasury Bonds I interviewed the Finance Minister and his Chief Secretary at least a dozen times and explained to them all the matter especially the points you had cabled to me regarding the interest, its payment, the capital, the security, and the urgent need of issuing the Bonds at the earliest possible moment. I fully explained that the present time was the most suitable for the sale of these Bonds in India, and that free and regular supply of news was essential for its success. I saw Talat Bey who may be said to be the moving spirit of the Party of Union and Progress, and arranged all these matters with him as well. I have already cabled you the essential points in this connection and I hope that this matter is now receiving your fullest support, and the Bonds are being well patronized by the Muslims of India. One cannot help feeling that the Turks have got absolutely no business capacity, and in arranging the issue of Bonds on such favourable terms they are not as prompt as they might be. That money is most urgently needed by them at present is most obvious to all, and at such a critical state in the life of their country they should be lacking in energy and zeal to expedite the issue of Bonds shows a great weakness and explains a great deal why they have failed so miserably.

The National Defence Association, which may be called an unofficial body of the Party of Union and Progress, has recently shown a great deal of activity at various meetings held in İstanbul and the provinces. It has collected funds which are devoted to the purposes of the Army and the Navy, and has done especially good work in connection with the Commissariat arrangements of the Army. It is due to the activity of this body that the food for the soldiers and the fodder for the horses and the animals regularly reach the armies in the field. It is not generally known by the people that it is this body which supplied to the Navy a good many of the troopships and a few armoured cruisers, which form part of the Turkish Navy. I have had several interviews with Dr. Col. Ali Darwesh Bey, who is one of the leading lights of this Association. He told me that the greater portion of the Navy and much of the improvements in the Army were effected by the financial help of this Association.

The Navy League is another similar body which has done much for the Turkish Navy. Two of the armoured cruisers, at present in the Turkish Navy, were presented to the nation by this League, and the 'Dreadnought', which is being built for Turkey in England and has been wholly subscribed for by this Navy league.

Anyone who has seen the soldiers which compose the present Turkish army, as I have had several occasions of seeing in the hospitals, would not doubt that the Anatolian soldiers are about the only soldiers whose spirit would remain undaunted in spite of the severest winter and the greatest hardships that any army could be exposed to. They had not only to fight against the soldiers of the Balkan Confederacy and the resources of the whole of Europe, but the forces of Nature seem to be working against them. Mere words can hardly express the bitter cold and the severe, icy wind and snow which at present the Turkish Army has to face. The snowstorm, which has been prevailing recently, has been the severest I have ever seen—and I have seen some of the worst in the Peak districts of Derbyshire. Here the wind seems to blow from every direction all at once, and the flakes of snow pour down so thick that it is impossible to see more than few yards ahead. It seems like a mixture of snow, fog and cyclone. In a few minutes' exposure the hands, feet, nose and ears become numb and lifeless. What would it be to those who are lying exposed to this inclement weather in their trenches I was told by English resident of İstanbul that he had actually seen an unboiled egg frozen inside: It sounds a bit tall but he seems a respectable sort of man.

After the re-commencement of the war the Turks have had several successes and advanced several kilometres specially along Çatalca, but the weather prevents them from taking any offensive at present.

As regards the division of our Mission, it was early in January that at your suggestion I had divided it into two units, intending to keep one on Ömerli and the other somewhere in Asis Minor. The present units are essentially the same as submitted to you except that Dr. Naim is now in charge of the Ömerli mission instead of Dr. Fyzee, who, as you are aware, has been sent to the Bombay Mission and is at present their Director. I had some troubles regarding tents. You are aware of the fact that we had been supplied with very few tents from London. Those sent to us being insufficient for our needs, I had been obliged to buy tents from an English firm in İstanbul, and now; that I had to divide all the provisions, stores, appliances and the other articles of the mission it was impossible to proceed without securing some more tents, especially as I had decided to increase the total number of beds, leaving 75 beds in Ömerli and taking 75 with the other section. I have to thank the Director and the members of the Bombay Poor Muslim's Medical Mission, as well as to Sir Adamjee Peerbhoy, for the loan of eight tents without which we could not have proceeded. I was also fortunate in buying three tents from a military provision-supplier at a very cheap price. I have had necessarily to spend large sums in buying kitchen canteens, provisions and stores for this section. Fortunately, we have been able to find a very good firm of chemists in İstanbul who had supplied as with medicines at London prices. I have had to buy food-stuff to last us for several weeks, as we were uncertain of our destination. The Ottoman Red Crescent gave us provisions for 75 patients, but they were quite insufficient even for a dozen people, besides they consisted of rice, bread and sugar. It is obvious we have to make provisions for the food of the patients coming to our hospital.

I have to thank the Red Crescent for the services of Dr. Fuad Bey and Dr. Ali Hasan Bey who are Egyptian gentlemen, graduates of the Turkish, Faculty of Medicine, and are of invaluable help to us, as they can speak Turkish and English perfectly besides being very good medical men. I have also added one more to the list of our dressers in the person of

Mr. Aaley-Imran from Balliol College, Oxford, who had been working in a hospital in İstanbul as a volunteer. You would see that the loss of Dr. Barry has been more than made up.

I was very glad to get a draft for £11,000 as in order to make the necessary purchases I had not only spent all the money at our disposal but have had to borrow £100 from the Red Crescent.

I have also received the registers you sent.

M. A. Ansari

[11th to 20th February 1913]

The week's stay in İstanbul was very tedious and trying. We were asked by the war office to have all our things ready to depart at a moment's notice. We were told to remain at the Kadirgah Hospital and not to leave the premises without informing the Central Office of our whereabouts. I had to call at the War Office and the Central Office of the Red Crescent for orders, morning, noon and night. Fortunately these days of tedium were spent usefully owing to the large number of wounded received in the Kadirgah Hospital. The Greek doctors on the staff of this hospital were absolutely callous and indifferent in attending to the wounded, and were it not for the hard work I had put in on the request of Dr. Sobami, the Director of the Khasta Khana and Baroness Rosen, the matron, good many lives would have been lost. We worked often until 3 and 4 in the morning, dressing the wounds and doing the needful for the patients. I cannot help expressing my greatest esteem and admiration for the zeal, care and the great sympathy shown by the Baroness to all her patients. She is untiring in her work for the relief of suffering, and, although brought up in the lap of luxury and ease, she does not hesitate in doing the meanest kind of work. I have seen her scrubbing the floor, bathing patients and even lifting them up to their beds. It is good to see persons like her who do the work of charity and love for the Turks in spite of their being of a different religion from her own.

I visited Ömerli twice during my stay and found the hospital working splendidly. I would have loved you to see the work done by our men whose behaviour would be called nothing short of heroic in the bitterly cold weather, with mud, and snow in places coming up to the calf, when their hands and feet were becoming powerless owing to the cold. I must specially mention here the work done by Abdul Waheed Khan and Dr. Mirza Riza Khan (of Edinburgh). These two have proved themselves incomparable; Abdul Waheed unfortunately caught a bad chill and had to be removed to

İstanbul as he developed Bronchitis, Pneumonia and Pleurisy. In spite of all care he did not improve and had to be returned home. I hope mild winter in Egypt and the Arabian Sea and the sea voyage would cure him by the time he lands in India. I was exceedingly sorry to lose him.

The National Defence Association consulted me regarding some telegrams which they were sending to the ruling Moslem chiefs of India in aid of the Turkish Treasury Bounds. I had asked them to send you a copy for publication in the *Comrade*.

I hope you are receiving telegraphic news regularly from the Ottoman Agency. I had arranged with Talat Bey for the regular supply of news free of charge to be sent to India and had specially deputed Abdur Rahman Siddiqi to collaborate with them. As regards Uzun Kieupuri[23] the mistake arose owing to there being two places of the same name, one being on the line of Midia in the Black Sea, the other being near Adrianople.

On the 17th of February, we were ordered to proceed at once, but it proved a false alarm, the boat Cambridge not being able to leave until next day. We embarked with all our baggage, hospital equipment, provisions and stores, the packages numbering about three hundred, and sailed on the night of the 18th Gallipoli on the evening of the 19th. I landed at once in company with Dr. Fuad Bey and Colonel Khalil, Enver Bey's uncle. Khalil Bey is gallant soldier and has been doing invaluable service to the Turkish Army with his band of volunteers from Crete, Arabia and Anatolia. Often he has fought with his three hundred men against several Bulgar Regiments with such bravery and pluck that the Bulgars thinking them to be backed by a large army have vacated places, leaving a quantity of guns and provision behind.

Enver Bey advised me to take my hospital to Çanakkale (the town of Dardanelles) as the weather was too severe for the patients to remain in tents. At my special request for giving us his best advice he assured me that Çanakkale being the centre where all the patients going to İstanbul have to embark on the hospital ship I would have the best chance of taking as many patients as I wanted in my hospital. He also gave orders for converting the troopship Rechid Pasha[24] into a hospital boat under our management but that idea was abandoned owing to the movement of Enver Bey's Army towards Çatalca. My intention of giving up the Ömerli Hospital was also abandoned due to the same cause. Enver Bey was especially nice to me and sent Dr. Zia Nuri Bey, the medical Inspector of this portion of the army, and Dr. Ibrahim Bey, the Army Medical Officer in Gallipoli, to help me in establishing my hospital at Çanakkale.

I was introduced by him to Prince Abdul Halim, the nephew of the present Sultan and the brother of Enver Bey's fiancée. The Prince was very warm in his appreciation of the Moslems of India sending money and the Mission in aid of the Turkish wounded soldiers and said that it would be impossible for Turkey to repay this debt of gratitude. He showed me the badge worn by the Bulgarian soldiers on their caps. It was a lion rampant prodding over the Crescent and carrying a cross on its head.

M. A. Ansari

March 1913

5 April 1913

To the members of the Bombay Poor Moslems Medical Mission:

Dear Sirs,

Your repeated requests to help you in your troubles and the obvious dissentions and quarrels in your Mission had obliged me as an Indian and a Muslim to try and smooth your differences and to help you in your mission of peace and mercy by lending you the services of Dr. A. H. Fyzee, as Director of your Mission. But it has pained me beyond expression to find that my efforts have been in vain. You have neither succeeded in settling your disputes nor have you refrained from constant intrigues and quarrel amongst yourselves. I am compelled to recall Dr. Fyzee to resume his duties as Assistant Director of my Mission. I am afraid nobody can help you as long as you remain divided amongst yourselves and as long as you do not have the good sense to see that by your constant differences you are not only dissipating your energies in a wrong direction but spoiling the good name of the community which you represent and country you hail from.

At the very longest only a few weeks remain for our stay in Turkey and I pray you even now to work with a united effort in the best interest of the cause entrusted to you by the poor Moslems of Bombay.

Dr. Fyzee must, however, return to the All-India Medical Mission as I cannot allow him in fairness to himself to remain any longer with you.

Yours Ever Sincerely,
M. A. Ansari

1 April 1913

The news of the fall of Adrianople must have caused deep grief to the Muslims of India; but Shukri Pasha [25] and his garrison have convinced the whole world of the bravery of the Turkish soldiers. The Bulgars only got one great smouldering ruin when they got there. For the last two days Enver Bey has been pressing the enemy hard at Çatalca. Yesterday he advanced to Silivri and captured two batteries of the Bulgars and killed between three to five thousands of the enemy. The spirit of the army is splendid, and if God will help them they would do some considerable damage to the enemy. Last night the Powers presented their note for peace: the Midia-Enos[26] line was proposed and the fate of the islands was to be decided by the Powers later on. It is most likely in three to four days peace would be concluded. Mr. Zafar Ali Khan is here; but, owing to the great preoccupation of the Cabinet, has not been able to see many ministers. In my next letter I will write to you at length. To-day I have only time to write a brief note. I arrived here yesterday from Çanakkale, as, owing to Dr. Naim's departure, I found it necessary to personally conduct the Ömerli section. Most of the fighting is, as you know, at present on this side.

M. A. Ansari

Ömerli, 7 April 1913

My letter last week was very brief owing to lack of time. You must have by now received the details of the fall of Adrianople.[27] Ghazi Shukri Pasha's noble defence has at least added to the military prestige of the Turkish army and has elicited appreciation from almost every European country. Adrianople would have gone to the Bulgars in any case, but now besides adding to the honour of the Turkish soldiers it has cost the Bulgars and the Serbs several thousands of lives. In well informed circles in İstanbul the fall of Adrianople was known to be imminent a week or two days before the actual occurrence. But the general public was very profoundly affected by the news. It was only after the recent Turkish victory at Boyuk Chekmedje[28] that people are again feeling hopeful and re-assured.

On the 31st of March, about eight O'clock in the evening, the sound of cannonade lured out two members of my Mission and they began to climb over the range of hills beyond the village of Ömerli until they were in sight of the Sea of Marmora and the Büyük Çekmece lake. They could see the searchlights from the Turkish fleet in the Sea of Marmora thrown over the hills beyond where the Bulgarians lay entrenched. The searchlight from the Black Sea was also thrown over the higher range of the hills, and the Turkish and the artillery on land directed their fire on to the hills occupied by the Bulgarian forces. The Bulgars did not make much resistance. Their firing was feeble and ineffective. As the night was very dark and wet our members in spite of their enthusiasm returned to their camp after two or three hours. In the morning the Bulgarian main column stationed beyond the bridge of Çatalca made a desperate and deadly attempt under the screen of a thick fog to cut off the Turkish left wing from the main body. But fortune favoured the Turks for once, fog lifted and the Turkish batteries opened fire with such disastrous results that the Bulgars were utterly routed. They fled back towards the hills many of them leaving even their rifles and caps behind. It is estimated that their losses were between six to eight thousand. The spirit of the Turkish soldiers has been raised by this victory, and they are determined to fight to death should the Bulgars try to force the Çatalca lines.

Moulvi Zafar Ali Khan, who is our guest at present in Ömerli, went with me two days ago to Hadımköy. We called on Abuk Pasha and Izzet Pasha. The latter received us very warmly in his saloon in the railway carriage. It surpasses description—the deep emotion his manner showed when he received us. For a few minutes the great Turkish Generalissimo was speechless, his eyes full of tears and downcast and his whole bearing showing how bitterly he felt about the present situation and how deeply he was moved by the sympathy shown by his brethren of India. We were both naturally moved by what we saw and could hardly express in words what was passing in our minds. When we took leave of His Excellency Izzet Pasha, he invited us to lunch with him next day and promised to send us in his motor-car to see all the fortifications. The lunch proved to be a much more sumptuous meal than we had been prepared for, and during the course of the meal H. E. made a thousand and one enquiries about the condition of the Indian Muslims—their social, educational and political condition, their trade and industries—and was agreeably surprised to find so much advancement among them. He expressed his desire to visit India and see the flourishing condition of his co-religionists there.

We started in two motor-cars and first went to Mahmad Pasha then to Büyük Çekmeceside and afterwards to Terkoz[29] side. We saw the magnificent fortifications and the previous soldiers—the Anatolian, the Kurd, the Arab and the Turk—all fresh and in high spirits and keenly awaiting to see some good fighting. The transport arrangements were ideal. They have thrown a narrow light railway by means of which they carry provision and stone with great expedition and speed. There is also a regular motor-car service between Hadımköy and the different sections of the army.

How different the picture is now from what it was during the time of the last Cabinet. Our return to Ömerli was on horseback.

This was a day of incidents. Just when we were starting, my mare started backing. My neck got caught in the branches of a tree and I came down, fortunately without receiving any injury. On our return journey from Hadımköy the great editor of *Zamindar* rode the most vicious horse, as he was voted to be the best horseman in the company. We had just climbed over the Mohae hills and were all riding side by side enjoying the beautiful scenery of the Sea of Marmara[30] on one side and the green valleys on the other when suddenly we saw two horses standing on their hind legs each trying to push the other down. But as it turned out afterwards it was only a ruse to rub the nose of their riders in the mud. One of these turned out to be no less a person than the indomitable editor of the *Zamindar* lying full length measuring the ground. I must say that it was only for a few minutes that we were treated to this never-to-be-forgotten picture.

A moment later and Zafar Ali Khan remounted his horse this time to punish the beast for playing him such a nasty trick. The horse and rider disappeared downhill in a short time, and when we reached our tents we found our friend sitting in the tent and philosophizing over the incident of the day with a big haematoma (in vulgar language black eye) on the left-side. We sympathised with him and had the privilege of adding his name to the list of our distinguished patients. I have just received from Çanakkale the returns for the month of March. There were 171 in-patients and 101 out-patients treated in this month. I have also received the returns of the Ömerli Field Hospital for the months of February and March. Their total number of in-patients for the two months was 177 and out-patients 140. The mortality at Çanakkale was nine and the cured 78. The percentage of mortality works out to be 3.3, a figure which speaks for itself and indicates the infinite attention and work which it must have involved to all the staff. And when it would be known that more than half the patients sent to the hospital were in the extreme stage of exhaustion due to exposure to cold and disease, some of them dying a few minutes after their arrival in the hospital, I am confident that all credit should be given to the staff of the Çanakkale Hospital for their splendid work.

But the Ömerli sections of our Mission have beaten all records. Their heroic adherence to their duties, in spite of the bitterest, and the severest winter when their tents were often completely snowed up and their camp was one mass of snow and mud, when the Turk's themselves would not venture out of their houses, has been rewarded with the splendid record of one single death out of a total of 310 patients, which works out to 3 per cent. No amount of words can adequately express their real work and worth. It is by their constant striving to keep up the high ideal that they have secured a reputation which induces the relations of many of the wounded soldiers to take them straight from Hadımköy and place them in their charge. Such a tribute from the patients and their relations to the honest and good work rendered by the Ömerli Hospital speaks for itself.

You will be very glad to hear that your earnest labours are already about to bear fruits. The presence of the two Indian Missions and the continual intercourse of the members of our Mission with the Turkish people of all shades and grades have brought home to the people of Turkey the intense sympathy felt for them by the Muslims of India. Many Turks hardly know of the existence of such a country as India, and they had no idea that the Muslims there would render them help at such a critical time in their national life. The generous financial help given by the Muslims of India to the Ottoman Red Crescent is deeply appreciated by them, and they have invited me to their meeting in İstanbul to discuss about the advisability of sending a few representatives of the Red Crescent to India to thank the Muslims of India for their help and sympathy. I am sure you would welcome this as the beginning of closer relations between the Muslims of India and Turkey. I may justly claim this to be the direct result of sending missions consisting of Indian Muslims to Turkey which no amount of money alone could have been able to do. I hope you would do all in your power to arrange for the suitable reception of this Turkish Mission by the Muslims of India in the different Provinces of India. I will let you know the details of their program after I have seen the members of the Council of Red Crescent. I am sending you accounts up to 4th April.

All the members of the Mission join me in sending you their love and regards. The Turkish authorities have named this village Hindia Köy, which is a great compliment to the Indian Muslims.

M. A. Ansari

April 1913

Hindia (Formerly Ömerli), 14 April 1913

Your Letter came after ages and gave me untold pleasures. I feel very much concerned about your health. Do take care of yourself....

As regards the Bonds, I have already spoken to Talat Bey who told me that they were being printed and would be ready in at least a month's time.

I have explained to him how absolutely necessary it was to send them to India at the earliest possible moment, but to-morrow I am returning to İstanbul and will see the Finance Minister and, if necessary, the Sadrazam about these bonds and ask them to cable you official instructions as well as to the banks.

As regards news, there has been none to send you. The Turkish Cabinet has expressed its readiness to accept as basis for peace the Enes-Midia line, no war indemnity and the settlement of the islands to be left in the hands of the Powers. It is rumoured to-day that a week's armistice will be arranged from to-morrow as a preliminary to peace.

As soon as the work of the Mission is over I am going to make a tour in Anatolia and Smyrna with Zafar Ali Khan, as a representative of Ottoman Red Crescent and probably a leading member of the Union and Progress to select a suitable place for the colonisation of the refugees. After forming a reliable organisation in which I may be able to induce some half a dozen members of my Mission to take practical part by staying for some time in Turkey and other reliable men in Turkey, I will request you to help the work with all the money that would be left with you after paying up all the dues of the Mission.

Owing to the rumours of peace there has been no fighting of late and hence we have only 57 patients in Ömerli and 100 in Çanakkale. As soon as peace is declared, I will transfer them all to İstanbul and will close the hospital, handing over all the things to the Ottoman Red Crescent with the exception of the painters and a few other things which I wish to bring to India for the permanent Indian Red Crescent Society.

To-day we have had a number of very distinguished visitors here—Izzet Pasha with staff, Talat Bey and Besim Ömer Pasha, Vice-President of the Ottoman Red Crescent. They had their lunch and tea with us and were very much pleased with their inspection of the camp. They have written very flattering remarks in our Visitor's Book.

I am getting your message to Enver Bey translated by Madam Halide Edip and will take it to Enver Bey myself as well as have it published in the Tanin.

All the members of the Mission join me in their affectionate regards.

Ghulam Ahmad's letter to you this week would take away some of your reproach from the members of the Mission. I think you would find it full of interest, as they have been exceptionally lucky in seeing what he has described in the letter.

M. A. Ansari

Comrade, 3 May 1913

The letter of Mr. Ghulam Ahmad to which Dr. Ansari refers in his letter runs as follows:

The reason why I have not written to you was the knowledge that you received weekly letters from the Director which gave you all the important particulars. My only excuse for venturing to write to you this letter is the fact that the experiences which Dr. Fyzee, Hafiz Muhammad Yusuf Ansari and myself have gone through has been unique. In fact we were told by the officers whose courtesy has enabled us to see all that I am about to describe, that we were the only persons who had during the course of this war been shown round their trenches and the actual working of the Turkish artillery. Twice before this we wanted to get permission from Zia Pasha to go to Boyuk Çatalca, but he very politely refused our request. The newspaper correspondents are only allowed bird's-eye view of the Çatalca fortification from a distance of some twelve or fifteen miles. The experience of our members has been that the unofficial source is the best when you happen to know one or two officers in the army. We all feel it that we owe so much to you that the best we could do is to write and give you a detailed description of our fortunate trip.

After the day's work was over, on Friday, April 11th, Dr. Fyzee, Hafiz Muhammad Yusuf Ansari and myself left our camp at Hindia (Ömerli) for a constitutional. As it was a beautiful sunny afternoon, we started with the intention of taking a long walk and took one of our soldiers with us. We walked over the hills beyond the village and then through the valley of the Moha range and over to the hills behind the Moha in continuation of the second line of defences. Here a clear view of the whole of Çatalca lines of defenses right up to Büyük Çekmeceon on the left and Nakash Kui on the right could be obtained. The plain of the Karasu river where the battle of the 17th November was fought was under our view, and we could not resist taking a photograph of this beautiful panorama. This gave Haflzji a little rest as he had strained his tendons in climbing up the hill. Our Doctor made straight for the milk bottle and had more than a lion's share of it. Not having started with any definite plan in our head we had a little discussion whether Bakhshaish or Büyük Çekmece should be our good. Büyük Çekmece appeared to us to be nearer, the longest estimation of distances in our mind to reach this place being two miles and a half. Once we got started the strained tendon and all were forgotten, and we were absorbed in admiring the beauties of nature which lay at our feet. There were fields of wild flowers as far as the eyes could reach and the undulating plains were yellow with daisies and in places purple with hyacinths or pink with tulips. Soon we reached towards the lake (Boyuk Chekmedje) where the soldiers were digging up fresh trenches under the supervision of some officers. As we reached the side of the lake which lay to our right, the sea was in front of us, and we could see the fortifications on the high hills to our left. The slanting rays of the sun and the beautiful evening breeze made the view so picturesque and absorbing that we walked on for some distance regardless of the muddy damp ground until we found our feet growing heavy and our boots increasing in size with all the need and grass sticking to the soles. Our attention was here diverted by the cannonade from behind the hills to our right on the other side of the lake. It gave us an idea of our destination which seemed just as far away as when we started. Hakki Pasha passed us here with an escort going in the direction of Bakhshaish. As we reached the banks of the lake the soil grew even more tenacious and sticky and in trying to finish the curve of the lake which seemed interminable to our P.M.O., we got the first specimens of his unparliamentary language which, I suspect, shocked Hafizji a little. But the sunset was so glorious that the 'interminable curve' was forgotten for the moment and we went on bravely fighting the mud—until we reached some old ruins of castles and turrets speaking eloquently of the ages gone by. We were thinking of the past glories of Islam and what mighty power those old fortresses must have seen when we were brought down to the realities by the chanting chorus of some Christian boys. It seemed like the singing of some Indian villagers giving expression to some pathetic and touching sentiments essentially Oriental. Was it really the wailing of the spirit of the East at the sight of such a great nation so suddenly bereft of all its greatness, or was it the subdued joy of the Christian people voicing their victory in the land that still remained under the sway of Islam?

We were at the outskirts of the town of Büyük Çekmecenow, and it suddenly struck us that we would have to arrange for the night's rest as it was already dark. We searched our pockets and the richest man amongst us produced less than two piasters (about three and a half annas). But Hafizji's resourcefulness came to our rescue, and the soldier who accompanied us became our banker and advanced us the large sum of one Mejideh (two and-a-half rupees). Greatly reassured by the advance we at once started a lively discussion at the bifurcation of the road as to the nearest way to the 'Hotel Cecil' in the village. Our P.M.O. is an easy-going man, and he selected the shortest route which brought us to a noble gateway by which we made our 'State Entry'. A short distance brought us to a house where we enquired from a soldier if there was any Zabit (officer) near about.

Imagine our joy when we discovered that there was not only a Zabit living in that very house but he bore the name of the great Fethi Bey, the hero of Tripoli. In spite of our trampy appearance the prompt production of a neatly printed card by our P.M.O. had the desired effect on the soldier and convinced him that we were people of some importance. He took our card at once and came with an invitation from his master to enter the house. But when we looked at our boots which were not exactly as they wear them in Bond Street, you can imagine our hesitation in entering an immaculately clean house with a polished wooden floor. As we walked through the hall we left big lumps of mud behind us which the servant swept away, only to do it over again when anyone of us passed the hall again. Our host showed us great hospitality and that essentially Turkish courtesy which has earned the Turks the deserving epithet of 'the gentleman of Europe'. We vaguely hinted about some hotel where we could spend the night, but our host would not hear of it, although the poor man possessed only two beds in the house and searched all over the village to procure some more beddings in which he did not succeed. Nevertheless he was rather suspicious of us and made enquiries about us and wrote profuse notes and dispatched them, I think, to the authorities. The conversation was conducted through the medium of Arabic, Persian, Turkish, French, English and German with a good backing of Urdu where words failed us, and we succeeded to make ourselves generally understood. Captain Remzi Bey and another officer joined the party, the latter being specially invited owing to his knowledge of Arabic. The dinner was a sumptuous affair consisting of seven courses, all of us eating from the same plate in the good old Turkish fashion, the only incongruous element being the use of knives and forks. We were afforded a beautiful view of the lake in the moonlight through the powerful field glasses which these officers gave us. As bed time approached Hafizji began to wonder whether his highly scented stockings might not have the effect of an emetic and spoil the evening's dinner. My own fears and tribulations were not small when I thought of the hundreds of thousands of my pet 'colonists' whom I had nourished on my own life-blood, and now that they were fattened and sleek the agony of losing them in this house was great, indeed. There was a regular tug-of-war at bed time, the host wasting to give us the beds and sleeping himself on the Ottoman; but we were three to one and at last prevailed on him to sleep in one of the beds.

Next morning we had an early tea and our host who had received a telegram on the previous evening was making preparations to start. He was still suspicious, but the production of a small packet containing the dust from the graves of the Shuhada who had died in the battle of the 17th November which Hafizji carried with him, cleared his suspicion and changed his attitude entirely. He gave us a letter to the Markaz commandant, Mahmud Bey, and we started to the office of that dignitary. We were waiting outside the house for the reply of the letter, but the soldier who accompanied us returned soon with a disappointing message that the Commandant was not at home. We were thinking of returning when we saw someone looking at us from the window and scrutinizing our appearance. I believe our dark colour proved a positive advantage here, as a man was forth with sent to us with a pass to go further to Enver Bey's headquarters. The first soldier was sent away, and we accompanied our new guide. We had to cross a bridge, a very old construction which was strictly guarded by sentries all along, no one being allowed to cross it without a pass. Even the military officers had to show a pass to get over the bridge. The view from the bridge was very extensive, the sea on one side with a flotilla of transport ships anchored in the port and one of the cruisers painted invisible grey ready with its guns for action and the Büyük Çekmecelake on the other side with the hills sloping down to its shores. There were two pontoon bridges also recently constructed there. On reaching the village of Kale Karası, where Enver Bey had his headquarters, we passed British Red Crescent Hospital and two Ottoman Red Crescent Hospitals and met Tevfik Bey, the Russian aviator, who has got a wonderful invention by means of which an aeroplane can be stopped in mid-air for two minutes. He was here to present his plan to Enver Bey and place this new invention exclusively at the service of the Ottoman Government. If this invention proves to be what he claims for it, it would revolutionize aviation and prove a formidable weapon for military purposes.

We went to Aziz Bey, the commandant, who spoke Persian fluently and hence understood us perfectly. He spoke to us about Langar Shah, an Afghan volunteer, who had fought with Enver Bey in Tripoli and had recently shown marvellous courage and bravery in fighting against the Bulgars at Yalor. He was killed on the 3rd of April in engagement where he rushed with a small number of soldiers in the Bulgar ranks which numbered some six thousand. Aziz Bey is one of the famous officers who had distinguished themselves in Tripoli with Enver Bey's army. We expressed to him our desire to see Enver Bey to whom he took our message. Enver Bey sent for us at once and on seeing us and saying 'Biliyorum' (I know them) the whole aspect of all the officers and men changed towards us like the magic words of Ali Baba, and all the mysteries and secrets were to be shown to us without any further suspicion or questioning. We told Enver Bey how the whole Islamic world looked to him to retrieve its lost honour and save the sinking ship of Turkey from utter destruction.

We expressed a desire to kiss his hands for all the Muslims of India and Hafizji had a regular tussle with him before he succeeded in kissing the tips of his fingers, which the returned by kissing him on his cheek. Enver Bey spoke also very highly of Langar Shah's courage and bravery. He forestalled our request and asked us if we should like to see the newly won position, which they had captured on the 31st March with such heavy losses to the Bulgars. We took a photograph of Enver Bey just before we left him. This place was simply a beehive of activity, every soldier and officer moving with alacrity and determination. We returned to Aziz Bey again who was to provide us with soldiers and guide for the most interesting part of the trip. Here we met Nishat Bey, a young member of a Pasha's family working as common soldier, and two Pathan volunteers from Afghanistan— Abdul Hakim Chaush of Kandhar in a picturesque Kurdish dress and Syed Ismail Kabuli. We took their photographs. We met Capt. Mümtaz Bey, a cavary officer who had distinguished himself in Tripoli, and Ehsan Bey, a very brave artillery officer.

In our anxiety not to waste any further time we even refused the offer of a lunch by Aziz Bey and started on our horses, the Doctor of course getting the best mount. We had not proceeded a mile mostly spent in trying to save our P.M.O. from an ignominious fall from his horse when a brisk shower of rain caught us and gave us a drenching which proved rather refreshing. Our P.M.O. burst forth into a full throated chorus 'By the side of the Zuyder Zee' apropos of our ride along the sea shore. The view was very beautiful here. The green undulating plain and the hills beyond and the sea on the left side made one of those fascinating landscapes which are found in such abundance in Turkey. Half an hour's ride brought us to the position at Monastic Tepe were we met Salahud-din Bey, Reis Arkan Harbia[31] in his camp. We left our horses here and accompanied him. Fortunately for us he spoke Arabic and Hafizji was able to carry on a conversation with him.

Ghulam Ahmad

Dardanelles, 20 April 1913

I went to see the Minister of Finance on the 15th of this month immediately on the receipt of your cable. As Rifat Bey was indisposed I could only speak to him for some 15 minutes, but I had a long interview with his Chief Secretary and the Financial Advisor to the Ministry. After three hours' conversation I got the following information from them:

1. The Bonds could not be sent out to India in less than two months. They were at present being printed in Vienna (Liepzia) and as their printing involved a great deal of care that would be the least time in which they could be got ready.

2. Each Bond was divided into five separate portions by perforation—one for each year; and these yearly slips had two portions each, one for the principal and the other for the interest. Every year one of these slips would be presented, and one-fifth of the principal would be paid up by the Turkish Government. Persons desirous of taking interest would present the slip containing both the portions for the principal and the interest: but those who wanted only the principal but no interest could tear off the portion denoting the interest and present only the portion denoting the principal. The Turkish Government will thus pay up on every 30th of November one-fifth of the principal, and interest to those who desire it. The sketch given below would clearly explain the shape of the Bonds. The entire principal will be paid up in five years.

10/- Sterling.				
Interest. 1	2	3	4	5
Principal. 1	2	3	4	5
2/-	2/-	2/-	2/-	2/-

3. Printed circulars in English and Persian containing the *Irade* for issuing the loan and all the rules regarding the payment of the principal and the interest have been sent out to the Consul-General in Bombay some three weeks ago. Several thousand copies of these have been sent with the intention of circulating them freely in India. Please ask Jafar Bey to circulate them freely. I am sending you a dozen copies in English and Persian: in case the Consul-General does not circulate these, you could have similar ones printed for circulation.

4. The Turkish Finance Ministry has printed several hundred thousand provisional receipts to be given to the buyers in India till the Bonds are sent out. These receipts are ready and are being sent out by this mail to the different Banks in India that are willing through your efforts to act as Agents for the Turkish Government. I bought one of these receipts for 10 shillings and I am sending it to you as a sample.

5. I explained to these gentlemen in the Finance Ministry the urgent necessity of sending out cables to the Banks in India advising them to forward the money received at once by cable at the expense of the Turkish Government. I was promised that this would be done the following day.

After spending a fortnight at Ömerli and a week in İstanbul I returned the day before yesterday to Dardanelles. I have already reported to you about the Ömerli section. Here in Çanakkale they are working exceedingly well under the energetic and able guidance of Dr. Abdur Rahman. The total number of patients up-to-date has reached 292, the number of patients at this moment in the hospital being 108. The number of out-patients since my last letter has reached 102. I enclose the latest report written in our Visitors' Book by Emin Pasha, the head of the Army Medical Service. Now that the armistice has been arranged and peace would most likely he signed by the end of this month, I must naturally think of the time when we will have to close our hospitals. I think by the middle of May at the very latest both of our hospitals would be closed. At first I was thinking of handing over all our tents and equipments to the Ottoman Red Crescent, but I have changed my mind now. I mean to bring back to India everything that would be necessary to look after fifty patients. This would from the nucleus of the permanent Red Crescent Society at Delhi. Considering the innumerable claims on the generosity of the poor Muslims of India this is hardly a fit time to expect a great deal of support from them for establishing a permanent Red Crescent Society. But if we possess the necessary equipment a great deal of useful and humane work could be done in India with the help of only a small sum. For instance, a very small unit of two doctors, one compounder and three or four dressers, with equipment for twenty-five beds, could be sent out to combat dreadful epidemics like cholera, plague etc., which break out in India and carry off so many thousands of people every year. This Red Crescent Mission could also undertake with greater success than Government officials inoculation against plague, typhoid, etc. It could do a great deal of ambulance work and treatment of accidents, etc., by sending out units during big fairs like the Nauchandi in Meerut, the Numaiha at Aligarh, the Magh Mela in Allahabad, or the Sonepur fair in Behar. But the most useful service of the permanent Red Crescent would be when it would go out with the Hajis to Mecca. The rest of the things I intend keeping stored until after my tour in Anatolia where, as I have already told you, I wish to start immediately the work of colonization for the Muhajirs. I do not yet know what amount of money there would still be at your disposal to spend on this great work of mercy. If you could manage to collect twenty to thirty thousand pounds, a model village of 100 to 150 houses containing as many families should be built with this capital. It would relieve 1,000 to 1,500 emigrants only, which, as you very well know, would be a very small number considering the vast number of these homeless, wretched victims of the War. My rough estimate is one hundred pounds for each family consisting of about five individuals.

The cost would include a cottage with the necessary furniture, the implements of agriculture and cattle and seed for one year. To begin with the immigrants would be kept in the tents now used for patients and fed and clothed. They would provide all the labour necessary for building the houses with the exception of skilled labour such as masons, cabinet makers, joiners, etc. I think I would be able to induce some half a dozen members of my Mission to stay in Anatolia and conduct the construction of the houses and the supervision of the general work, etc., on a very moderate monthly pay. But this would be a most important essential as my experience has convinced me that the presence of our Indian compatriots here for supervising the work capably and honestly is indispensable.

I know you have got far too many things on your hands, but please remember and give me definite instructions by cable as to the amount of money that could be spent on this scheme and any other matter you may consider it necessary to advise me upon. It is necessary that I should know this, so that I may try and induce my men before our work is closed and they disperse. Think carefully about this scheme of colonization. It would sow the seed of greater things in future should Indian Muslims be disposed to invest their money which they are lending to the Turkish Government in developing some kind of industry in the very village which their own efforts would be able to bring into existence. Mr. Zafar Ali Khan has suggested an International Moslem Co-Operative League to be started on a capital of one million pounds. There would be one million shares of £1 each sold to the Moslems of Turkey, India, Egypt, Morocco, Persia, etc. The object of this Society would be to faster Moslem industries and to encourage industrial development in Turkey. The Mudafaa-i-Milliye where he discussed his scheme has appointed a committee for this Society, and I have been asked to be present in its meeting on Tuesday. I shall be going to İstanbul to-morrow for this purpose. I will probably start for my tour in Anatolia in the second week of May, after waiting for your instructions.

M. A. Ansari

May 1913

İstanbul, 6 May 1913

I forgot to tell you last week about the Annual Congress of the Ottoman Red Crescent Society. It was held in the great hall of the Dar-ul-Funoon.

There were about 150 members present. Mr. Zafar Ali Khan. Dr. Muhammad Hussian and I were also invited to attend.

The proceedings began with the election of the Chairman and two vice-chairmen in a very methodical manner. Two scrutinisers and two tellers were elected to count the votes. Hazrat Essad Effendi, a very venerable and universally respected hodja, was elected to the chair. This proceeding appeared to us a bit tedious, but later on when we witnessed the parliamentary way in which all the discussions of the Congress were carried on, it appeared quite consistent.

The Secretary was then asked by the Chairman to read the printed annual report which unfortunately we could not follow in all its details. But it was very extensive and exhaustive. I am sending it on to you although it is written in Turkish. You would see from the figures what a vast amount of work has been done by the Society. It has given substantial existence to almost all the foreign missions that were sent to Turkey in some cases furnishing everything, even the uniforms of the doctors and nurses. Besides the Turkish Red Crescent Hospitals, it has rendered help to the Military Hospitals and those under the Board of Sanitation. The vast organization for the relief of the refugees, who have been given shelter, food, clothing and bedding, has saved thousands of lives and enabled innumerable families to escape from perishing on account of starvation and other hardships.

Besim Ömer Pasha, who is the soul of this great organization, has been ceaseless in his efforts in this noble cause, and no less praiseworthy are the efforts of the devoted band of works associated with him. Colonel Mehmet Ali Bey, in spite of his old age, has shown such a remarkable energy as Inspector-General of the Society that it has earned the respect and devotion of every one of the staff of the various hospitals working under the auspices of the society. Dr. Akil Mukhtar, the Rais Sani, by his activity has added a good deal towards that smooth working of this useful organization. But the most useful member of the Central Committee, who is always ready to help wherever help is needed, is Kemal Ömer Bey, the younger brother of Besim Ömer Pasha.

In this connection the enormous work done by the Ladies' Committee presided over the Princess Nimet Hanum is worthy of note. It consists of 120 members, who have got under them a number of bands of workers distributed in the metropolis and the suburbs. The hundreds of thousands of clothes for the use of patients and Muhadjirn had been turned out week after week without the expenditure of a single penny for their sewing. They have also knitted the warm socks and night-caps, and prepared sheets, pillow-cases, aprons, caps and over-alls.

When the Secretary had finished his report it was put before the assembly for criticism. After a good deal of very animated discussion a committee was appointed to audit the accounts and to report in the next meeting of the Congress for their final adoption.

I had never seen Turks looking so interested and keen as I saw on this occasion. It would have convinced anyone who had seen this debate that the quiet and impassive Turk is at times quite capable of getting wound up into an impassioned denunciation or rejoinder. And after all he is not altogether incapable of discussing affairs in a representative assembly as many would have us believe.

Kemal Ömer Bey read a list of donations received up to date from different countries. It would gladden the generous Indian Muslims to learn that they stand first in the aid rendered to the Ottoman Red Crescent. This is the most convincing proof that the Indian Muslim has the largest heart although he has the shortest purse. I am sending you a copy of the list.

A meeting of the Indo-Ottoman Colonisation Society was held under the Presidency of Dr. Esad Pasha on May 2nd in which all the Members were present. Discussion took place regarding the Government Scheme for colonisation and the advisability of the Ottoman and Indian Committees working together, having a common advisory council, but separate executives. It was also decided that Dr. Esat Pasha should ascertain from the Government the various tracts of land at its disposal, their irrigation facilities, their proximity to railways and the sea, the condition of labour, the nature of soil, etc., and that after this a select committee with an agricultural expert should be sent out to Anatolia on a tour of inspection. The final scheme with the plans of the village and cottages is to be submitted to the Government after the return of the committee.

As regards the two hospitals, there are only 25 patients left in Ömerli. I have been considering whether it would not be advisable to close this hospital and send the members on the Kala-i-Saltanieh (Çanakkale), as the prospects of peace seem to be very great. But I have been advised not to do so until peace has been definitely signed. Two members of this section who have shown conspicuous good work are Dr. Mahmudullah and Mr. Hamid Rasul. Hafiz Muhammad Yusuf Ansari, who will always be remembered for his incomparable toasts and excellent cuisine, has exalted cooking to a fine art. But he is even more indispensable in the wards for performing night duty, and occasionally as an interpreter when an Arabic-speaking Pasha visits the hospital.

The Kala-i-Sultanieh hospital is working in full swing and has more than made up in number, although it started a month later. It has at present 110 in-patients and the average daily number of out-patients is between

40 and 50.We are also feeding daily 70 women and children refugees at Kala-i-Sultanieh and 30 at Hindia (Ömerli).

M. A. Ansari

Comrade, 31 May 1913

The unexpected sometimes happens even in Turkey. The scheme of a Moslem Bank and Co-operative Society is taking a definite shape and the deliberations of the committee are resulting in bringing the scheme to a head. The National Defence Association, which at present is doing considerable work in the matter of the commissariat arrangements of the Turkish Army and is showing its activities in many other directions, is about to place £25,000 in this Moslem Bank for the purchase of shares. This generous offer turns the co-operative society at once into a practical concern. Only £25,000 more have to be subscribed to start the society. The Iradeh would be issued as soon as the regulations are ready, and prospectuses would be prepared and sent out for the sale of shares to the different Moslem countries. You can well imagine how far-reaching the effect of the Bank and co-operative society would prove in developing the decaying industries of Turkey and other Moslem countries. Another important matter is the question of the University of Medina. A meeting of the Central Committee was held this week in which several Ministers and other leading men of Turkey were also present, showing what keen interest is being taken in this matter. The Minister of Evkaf showed great zeal, and wished the University to be started with as much expedition and dispatch as possible. The Nizam-nameh (copy of which I am sending) was discussed and sanctioned. Members of the Constitution Committee were appointed, including Mr. Zafar Ali Khan and myself. Shaikh Abdul Aziz Shaweesh, who is the soul of this movement, would probably be appointed Principal of the University. We have sent you a cable and hope you will not spare any pains in preparing the Constitution and Curriculum for the University of Medina on the lines of the Aligarh University, special regard being paid to the local requirements and the fact that Arabic would be the medium of instruction. Please consult Maulana Shibli No'mani, Dr. Iqbal, Major Syed Hasan Bilgrami, Maulvi Hamiduddin and any other persons that you may consider desirable. The Shaikh Saheb has also requested some friends in London and Egypt to prepare draft constitutions and on the receipt of the three drafts, the Constitution Committee will draw up the Constitution, taking the best and most suitable draft as its basis. Two more meetings of the Indo-Ottoman Colonisation Society have been held, and a Constitution has been drawn up for presentation to the Minister of the interior for approval. Hadji A'dil Bey has given us a list of lands in Anatolia which the Government has got at its disposal and would grant us for colonisation purposes. In Ankara 65,000 acres near the railway are available. There are also available in Adana 45,000 acres in a very well irrigated tract, but the climate here is warmer than would suit the emigrants from Macedonia. From 20,000 to 25,000 acres of land could also be got near Bursa and Konya. We are only awaiting the approval of the Minister of the Interior of the rules of our Society before we start on a tour in Anatolia. I hope we will not be delayed more than a week. I have already given you the names of members of our mission who are willing to stay up to the middle of September to look after the work, but you must be on the lookout for suitable men to reach here by the beginning of August, so that they may not be new to the work when the time comes for the old members to leave. Besim Ömer Pasha has got an expert to prepare a general plan of the villages and one for the cottages. Each village would contain 100 cottages, a mosque, a school, a dispensary, a washing house and a school for teaching practical farming. Each cottage is two storied. The ground floor will have a kitchen, a dining room, and a few small store-rooms, a bath and a lavatory. On the first floor there will be two bed rooms and a sitting room. In the compound there would be a shed for cattle and a place for keeping the harvest. I would send you the plans later on as soon as they have been approved after taking estimates from different contractors.

As there are only 30 patients left in Hindia, and the prospects of peace are very great, I have decided to close the hospital, sending to India materials for 50 beds and placing the remainder in the Hilal-i-Ahmar Stores. The members would be sent over to Çanakkale as there is still a considerable number of patients in the hospital there, and a daily growing out-patient department. Owing to a great deal of work in hand in connection with the Colonisation scheme, the Medina University and the Moslem Bank and Cooperative Society, I am not able to answer the letter of Mr. Kasim Hussain published in the *Comrade* received last week.

M. A. Ansari

İstanbul, 20 May 1913

Thanks to the efforts of Talat Bey and Dr. Esad Pasha the 'Society for the colonization of the Macedonian Refugees' has been officially recognized by the Government and a Committee of four persons, including Mr. Zafar Ali Khan and myself, are leaving next Friday for Anatolia where we would choose the site for the colonization of the village with due regard to sanitary, agricultural and economic conditions. We are awaiting the draft constitution from India, Egypt and England for the drawing up of the final Constitution of the Medina University. In the meantime, the constitution committee has been busy in doing a lot of spade work and have drawn up a provisional syllabus for the two faculties of Divinity and Science. The most difficult question would be the finding of suitable professors and assistant professors who would be able to teach the sciences in Arabic. Once the university has started on the career even in a modest way, it is sure to pave its way to success. I have no doubt that every Muslim would hail this University as the beginning of the great renaissance in the Islamic world. I am getting letters from private individuals requesting me to bring some Turkish orphans to India for them. I have no doubt these people are actuated by the most human desire to help in bringing up these poor, homeless, fatherless, children; but it is impossible to accede to their wishes, as these orphans are at once sent to the Government orphanages and cannot be secured. I have decided to close both the Mission Hospitals by the end of May and sail for India by the middle of June with all the members of the Mission except such as will remain here for colonization work.

M. A. Ansari

Istanbul, 27 May 1913

Both the Hospitals have now been closed; the one is Hindia on the 22nd and the Çanakkale Hospital on the 24th May. The scenes of leave-taking as Hindia, and Sanjak Tepe, from General Izzet Pasha and Abdus Salam Pasha, were most touching and will ever remain in our memory. I will have to postpone their full description until next week; probably Shuaib or Hafiz Muhammad Yusuf will write to you about it. We have had several meetings of the Colonisation Society, and a definite plan of work has been decided upon. To-morrow a committee consisting of five persons is going to Anatolia to see the tracts of the land the Government is willing to place at the disposal of the Society for the Colonisation of the Macedonian refugees. This committee consists of Mr. Zafar Ali Khan; Agah Bey, representing the Ottoman Red Crescent; Saleh Bey, an Agricultural expect; Dr. Ahmed Fuad, Joint Secretary; and Mukhtar Ahmad Ansari, Secretary. The committee has been given every facility by the Government to inspect these tracts. The members are going first to Ankara to see 65,000 acres of land in Qurai Ilias, then to Konya and Ulukışla by train, and from there by carriage to Adana, where 45,000 acres of land near Jabali-Barakat are available. The exact location of the two villages would be decided upon after the completion of the tour. Mr. Zafar Ali khan and I had the good fortune of meeting Enver Bey again. I talked to him about your letter, but he said he did not deserve all the things mentioned in it. He believed in working loyally for his God and country. He was sure Turkey would rise soon to its full glory and power, but a great deal of sincere and hard work was needed to achieve it. He hoped one day to come to India, but at present he could not possibly say when that could be. Don't give credence to the irresponsible talk in some of the papers. Recently he has had a narrow escape from death by drowning; but he is destined to perform greater work for his nation, and God saved him. It must be a source of satisfaction to learn that England and Turkey are now about to arrange all their differences and establish an Entente. But I am assured by a high authority that the talk of Lord Kitchener or Lord Milner being appointed as Inspector-General, is without any foundation. On return from Anatolia, it is decided we would start on our return journey to India about the middle of June, so as to catch the Italian steamer on the 24th June at Suez.

M. A. Ansari

[Mohammad Ali introduced the following letter by Abdur Rahman Siddiqui as follows—Author]

Two days later Mr. Abdur Rahman Siddiqi, General Manager of the Mission, wrote as follows. The letter has a pathetic interest attaching to it, for little did Mr. Abdur Rahman dream at the time that in less than a fortnight he would have to announce the death of one so great whom he had the good fortune to meet.

Dr. Ansari started for Ankara yesterday morning. When going he gave me your letter to the Grand Vizier and the Bank draft. I took it to the Grand Vizier and thus had an opportunity of seeing the great Mahmoud Shevket Pasha. You will be interested to learn that he is exactly as we used to find him in his published photographs except that he is a bit more pulled down perhaps because of the heavy work at the War Office and at the Grand Vizierate.

Abdur Rahman Siddiqui

[Here the sequence of Dr Ansari's letter is altered in order to reflect his account of the Indian Medical Mission's tenure in Turkey in historical order. This is because Dr Ansari described his tour of Anatolia in his letters which he wrote aboard the ship during his return to India.—Author]

Comrade, 12 July 1913

In my last letter, I had time only to describe the tragic murder of the greatest Ottoman soldier and statesman, Field Marshal Mahmoud Shevket Pasha. But so many things had been crowded together during the few days between my return from the Anatolian tour and our departure that I will have to give you the whole to three different letters.

On my return from Anatolia on the 14th of June, I found that there was so little time left and so much to do that I decided to leave Abdur Rahman behind to complete the work. He will spend a week or two on his own account in seeing İstanbul, as he never got any chance of doing so owing to pressure of work.

I wound up all my accounts after paying all our dues to the Hilal-i-Ahmar and obtained a receipt to that effect. The only accounts still to be settled are those for the articles purchased for your Turkish exhibition and a few minor ones.

Kamal Ömer Bey, by his Kindness, courtesy and ever-ready assistance has, indeed, placed us under an everlasting debt of obligation to him. He compiled a complete list of all the Moslem industries and manufactures of the different vilayets of Turkey, and with Abdur Rahman spent three or four days from morning till evening in purchasing these articles and labelling them with full statements of their wholesale and retail prices.

I have been forced for want of time to leave the question of the orphans half-finished in the hands of our Manager. I have seen and selected ten children (six boys and four girls), their ages varying from six to nine years; but owing to the necessity of getting the final permission of Cemil Pasha, Chief of the Municipality, I was unable to bring them with me. But these children will follow in a week or two together with two Turkish ladies, the widow and the daughter of a Turkish officer, who have been left destitute and absolutely unprovided for. Those ladies come from a respectable family and know French, Arabic and Turkish perfectly and are expert on needle work. As arranged with you, the ladies services will be utilized as teachers in your family or in a girl's school. I have left Haji Abdullah, an Indian, who worked as interpreter in our Çanakkale Hospital, to accompany them to India.

The visit of our Mission to Topkapı Serai, the ancient palace of the Byzantine Emperors and all the Sultans up to the time of Sultan Abdul Aziz, is worth recording. This is the palace which meets the eye of a traveller when the boat enters the Boğaziçi and rounds the Seraglio Point. Its palatial marble buildings with domes and minarets, its ancient towers and modern kiosks seen in the half light of the early morning makes İstanbul look like an enchanted place, leaving an everlasting impression on the minds of those who are fortunate to see it. We entered the central court, which was guarded by soldiers, after passing the buildings containing the Imperial Museum of Antiquities, the School of Fine Arts, the Mint and the famous court of Janissaries, with its historical plain tree where in olden days and where good many plots and revolts were hatched by the Janissaries. This courtyard which is beautifully green and leafy, with an avenue of fire majestic tress, led us to a square marble building of the period of Mohamed the Conqueror. The throne-room, where the monarchs used to give audience to the foreign Ambassadors and where the Council of Ministers used to meet, has a small fountain in it, which flowed noise-lessly but produced such a loud, roaring sound outside that no one could hear the conversation going on inside the room. Next to the throne room is the Library of Sultan Ahmed. It is built with white marble, with beauti-ful pillars of green marble. It contains most valuable Arabic and Persian books and manuscripts. The next building which is built in pure Saracenic style is the Khirka-i Shariff tomb. In this shrine are placed the Prophet's mantle, the javelin and the sword. The Sanjak Sheriff, the sacred standard of the Prophet, is also kept here closely guarded. The place where those holy relies are deposited is a square hall with a central place shut from public gaze by beautifully worked green curtains. The marble screens sur-rounding this hall gave us a glimpse of the central shrine. In this buildings are also kept a carpet of Syyedena Abu Bakr and four copies of the origi-nal Quran arranged by Syyedena Osman. The Quran of Syyedena Osman when he was murdered is also presented here, with blood stains on its pages. Syyedena Ömer's arms and turban are also deposited here. This shrine is opened only once a year on the 15th of Ramazan for the proces-sion of the Khirka-i-Shariff. In the lobbies surrounding this central hall are kept some historical aims. The sword of Sultan Mohamed the Conqueror and the guns used in his time are to be seen here. A beautiful specimen of calligraphy executed by Sultan Mahmud II is hung to the lobby. Baghdad Kiosk built by Sultan Murad IV in true imitation of a Kiosk he had seen in Baghdad, is a wonderful piece of pure Saracenic white architecture. Built of spotless white marble, it commands an extensive view of the beauti-ful blue Boğaziçi and the limpid, mobile waters of the Sea of Marmara. Here the Sultan retires when he visits the Khirka-i- Shariff Jame on the 15th of Ramazan. On the entrance to the central hall is executed following couplet in mother-o- pearl:

Let the door of happiness be open for you always in this Dargah
Because I am witness that there is no other God but Allah

The walls of the kiosk are artistically decorated with blue tile, and the interior of the dome is covered with deer-skins wrought with most artistic floral designs and perfect tughras. The doors, dewans and sofas are inlaid with mother-o'-pearl and are of the rarest and choicest kind, and give an idea of the life of the period of Khalifa Haroon-ul-Rashid. There is a historical clock, which curiously enough, still keeps time, presented by Napoleon to Sultan.

Numerous other buildings built by a succession of Sultans carried one back in imagination to those glorious times when the Ottoman power was irresistible and ever on the increase. We were shown Sultan Murad's latest hall where he read out the granting of the Constitution, and the room where the janissaries attacked him. We were shown the golden corridor and the staircase leading to the Harem where, after the murder of Sultan Murad, the janissaries rushed to kill all the royal princes, but they were turned back by the coolness and presence of mind of the Sultan's wife, who threw buckets of glowing charcoal on their faces. The window through which the Sultan made Sultan Mahmud jump out is adjoining this staircase, also the room where he was proclaimed Sultan in the very teeth of the revolt of the Janissaries. There were secret ladders, hidden passages leading from one building to another. In fact all those contrivances which were necessary in those days when the palace intrigues and plots were the rule of the day. In passing out of the Harem we were shown the place where the chief of the eunuchs used to punish the offenders. On the gate could be seen the dried scalp of one of the eunuchs hung by Sultan Mahmud. A secret balcony which we entered from the Harem overlooked the hall, where the discussions of Vozara and Vokals used to take place. In this balcony the Sultan used to sit and over hear all the discussions without being seen.

The building on the extreme right with yellow domes is the remains of the Byzantine palace, used as the sweet kitchen in the time of Sultan Selim, where he had hidden himself from the Janissaries.

The Military Museum, which is the ancient church of St. Irene, contains the most complete collection of the armaments, standards and other trophies from the time of Osman I to the present day, the latest addition being some guns, standards, uniforms and other articles captured, during the Turco-Balkan War.

The greatest event of our stay in Turkey—the presentation of the All-India Medical Mission to His Imperial Majesty the Sultan—took place on Tuesday afternoon, the 17th of June 1913. Besim Ömer Pasha accompanied us to the Yıldız Palace, wither we drove in carriage. We were received by Khalil Khourshed Pasha, the 2nd Chamberlain of His Majesty, and

Dr. Kheri Bey, Chief Physician to the sultan. We had only to wait for twenty minutes in the saloon, where we were treated to some refreshments. Then we were ushered into the audience hall where Besim Ömer Pasha presented me to His Majesty, and I in turn presented the members of the Mission individually. His Majesty bowing graciously as every member was presented. His Majesty then stepped forward and expressed his appreciation of our assistance to the Outman soldiers during the Turco-Balkan War. His Majesty was visibly touched as he spoke these words; he invoked God's blessing on the members of the Mission for their work of mercy so asked us to convey to the Muslims of India the eternal gratitude of His Majesty and the Ottoman nation. The cable which I dispatched to you on our return from Yıldız palace would have reached you by now.

On the evening of the 18th an official dinner was given to us by the Ottoman Red Crescent Society, His Excellency Bassim Ömer Pasha, the vice-President, Dr. Akil Muktar Bey, the 2nd vice-president, Dr. Mohamed Ali Bey, the Inspector General, Dr. Adosan Bey, Kamal Ömer Bey, Dr. Ali Derwesh Bey, members of the Central Committee of the Ottoman Red Crescent and many other notable persons were present. Our valued and esteemed friend Mr. Zafar Ali Khan was also invited. After a most sumptuous meal Besim Ömer Pasha and several other members of the Ottoman Red Crescent Society made speeches, praising the work of the All-India Medical Mission and thanking the Muslims of India for the generous help they had given to the Ottoman nation in their trial and distress and expressing fervent hopes for a closer and more constant relations between the Muslims of India and Turkey. A suitable reply was made to these speeches by Mr. Zafar Ali Khan and myself. An album containing photographs of the All-India Medical Mission from the time of its departure to the present moment, containing different views of the Hindia Field Hospital and the Hospital at Çanakkale, was presented to Besim Ömer Pasha as a souvenir, and a watch to which Mr. Zafar Ali Khan added a gold chain was given to Dr. Ahmad Firad as a remembrance for the most valuable assistance he had given to the Mission.

On the morning of the 19th, His Excellency Talat Bey, Minister of Interior, paid as a visit at the Kadirgah Hospitals on behalf of the Turkish Government. A group of the members to the Mission was taken with His Excellency.

But the most overwhelming and touching expressions of fraternal regard and brotherly feelings were exhibited when our Ottoman brothers came out to strong numbers to bid us farewell at the docks. His Excellency Talat Bey come down again on behalf of his colleagues, the members of the Government, His Excellency Ameen Pasha, the Head of the Army Medical

Department, was sent as a Vakil by General Izzet Pasha. Minister of War and ex-Commander-in-Chief His Excellency Bassim Ömer Pasha with all the members of the Central Committee of the Ottoman Red Crescent, His Excellency Dr. Essed Pasha, President of the Sanitary Department of İstanbul and President of the Indo-Ottoman Colonization Society and representation from the Madala-i-Milliys, and many other Anjumans and Societies were present. Maulana Sheikh Abdul Aaiz Chawish, Principal of the Medina University, and many other Egyptian and ottoman gentleman were present. His Excellency Talat Bey made a short and touching speech bidding as farewell and expressing gratitude on behalf of the Ottoman Government and the Ottoman People. He said that the last war had caused them much sorrow and entailed great sufferings, but the sympathy and the great help of the Muslims of India and the presence of the Indian Mission had consoled the nation and had made them forget their great trouble. They will never forget this brotherly help rendered by the Modems of India. He then kissed and embraced every member of the Mission and said that he was leaving them to the care of God. All present followed Talat Bey's example, and we departed with tearful eyes and sorrowful hearts, feeling that we were learning our home and family in Turkey only to go to another home and family in India.

I must not forget mentioning our visit to Hamidiyeh yesterday morning. We had heard that the Hamidiyeh was cruising in the Red Sea, but never in our wildest dream did we think it possible that we would actually be able to visit her and meet her gallant and indomitable commander, Husain Rauf Bey; but by merest good luck that was what exactly happened. We found just enough time to spend half an hour on board the Hamidiyeh before out boat sailed.

Rauf Bey, who is a young, most handsome and frank Turkish gentleman, received us with that genuine and sincere cordiality which the Ottomans have shown us all along. He told us he was feeling very much depressed as he had just then received newspapers from home; our visit had made him happy and enabled him to forget the troubles at home. He was exceedingly kind and he thought that nothing he did to entertain us was sufficient or good enough. He related to us some of the most thrilling incidents of bombarding Greek ships, of chasing torpedo boats, how he found the troopship Lyrgs and sank her, how he needed to smuggle coal and articles of provision. He praised his officers' pluck and bravery and specially felt proud of his gunner Husain, who never sent a shot without severely damaging of or sinking a boat. He has sunk altogether ten Greek boats and damaged a good many. He worked and showed us the mechanism of the big guns on Hamidiyeh, and told us that more than two hundred shots had been fired only by front gun. On the covering of the gun in a prominent place was written in bold letters the Ayetul Karimah:

In the Name of Allah, the Most Beneficent, the most Merciful
Verily We have granted thee a manifest victory.

He also showed us his mottos written in very large Arabic characters on the bridge of the boat, which were:

The Heaven is under the swords' shadow
Help from Allah and an imminent victory

He thought that this motto was infinitely superior to that of the English Navy: 'England expects every man to do his duty'. As to his men, death had no fear but a welcome means to transport them to heaven. He gave some interesting photographs of the Hamidiyeh in actual action and the sinking of the boat Lyres with his autograph on them. We also took some photographs with him and then departed among the loud and lusty cheers of his sailors, the band playing the 'National Anthem'.

M. A. Ansari

SS. 'Sicilia', 26 June 1913

The Indo-Ottoman Colonisation Society had in their meeting decided to send a commission as a tour of inspection in the different vilayets of Anatolia, in order to inspect the lands which the government had placed at their disposal for the colonisation of the muhadjirin from Macedonia. The Commission consisted of an agricultural expert (Saleh Bey), an expert on town planning (Aagha Bey), a medical man with intimate knowledge of sanitations and hygiene (Dr. Ahmed Fuad) and two representatives of India (Mr. Zafar Ali Khan and Dr. Ansari). It was aimed that this Commission would inspect the land and make necessary investigation on the spot regarding the fertility of the land, its mining resources, its proximity to the railway and the sea, its water supply, its sanitation, the question of labour and the most suitable and cheapest material at hand for the construction of house in the colony. On the basis of these facts a correct estimated of the cost of construction of a model colony of one hundred houses with a mosque, a school, a dispensary and an experimental farm would be formed.

The commission left İstanbul on the 28th of May, by the morning train from Haider Pasha.

The railway line runs along the sea coast through the most beautiful suburb of Kazi Keni and Moda. Here the villas of the well-to-do Ottomans are situated along the sea shore and one can truly call it a garden city. The deep blue sea of Marmora here dips towards Islands forming the gulf of that name and the Principo islands with their red soil and modern red tiled villas make a contrast picture worthy of sight. Hereke was passed soon, and we saw the great factory from the train. Here fazes, silk cloths, rugs, carpets and many other goods are manufactured and worked by purely Turkish capital. Unfortunately the output is not sufficient for the demand; otherwise the quality and the finish of the materials would enable them to compete with any other manufacturer. Tutun Chiftlik, which was once the favourite hunting ground of Sultan Abdul Aziz and one a very thick forest, is most used as the name implies mainly for the cultivation of tobacco for the Regie Factory. All that remains is the kiosk of sultan Abdul Aziz situated on a foot hill commanding the most glorious land and sea view. It is here that the best Turkish tobacco is grown. The original line from Haider Pasha was constructed as far as Tutun Chiflik by Sultan Abdul Aziz for use during his hunting expeditions. The most striking was the fact that only women were seen working in the fields: probably the male population was all drained by the army.

Ismidt[32] was soon reached. It is situated on a hill overlooking the bay: the town consists of mostly two-storeyed homes with latticed balconies made of wood in a purely Turkish style. The population consists of Armenians and Turks, numbering some 45,000 of which the Turks are a little over fifty per cent. Beyond Ismidt the foot-hills gradually rise to about a thousand feet, the scenery becomes most varied and picturesque. The mountain tops, the valleys and the plains are all covered with groves of olive trees. Cultivation is done everywhere as far as the eye could reach. Neat little houses and villas could be seen here and there peeping through the green foliage. Nature is seen here in its greatest profusion and makes it an ideal spot of beauty. The railway line now runs along the shores of Sapanja Lake which is enclosed on every side by green hills and extends in length to some fifteen miles. There are several little villages of the Caucasian refugees along the shores of the lake; they could be seen working is the fields in their picturesque costumes. To those who have seen the Swiss mountains, this part of the Turkish dominions would appear equally enchanting if not superior. There are beautiful fruit gardens and orchards all along the shores the lake and some of the best grapes are grown in this district.

The journey to Boyuk Derbind and Beledjek is achieved through the most difficult ravines and gorges the railway going through numerous tunnels, over-bridges with roaring mountain torrents running under and galleries cut along the most precipitous mountain. The town itself is of a fairly good size, is purely Muhammadan, and nestling among green smiling hills, looks happy and contented with its white houses and tall slender minarets. We had our midday meal here which the care and thoughtfulness of our friend Ageyah Bey had provided for us. He had brought a variety of viands which we did full justice to. Ageyah Bey is a typical Turk and his natural kindness and solicitude for the comfort of other makes him a most agreeable and loveable companion. He has most beaming, smiling and jovial countenance and simply adores little children and animals. At times he behaves like an overgrown boy amusing himself as he did here by trivial things such as throwing pepper and salt in the nose of dogs while feeding them or putting a stone in a morsel of meat and roaring with laughter when the dogs were slugging hard to bite at the tough morsel. We arrived at Eski Shahar at 6 pm and stayed at Hotel Tadia as the trains do not run expect in the daytime.

Eski (old) Shahar as the name implies is a very old town. It was in the vicinity of this town that the Saljuks had granted a free land to Toghral for his services in helping their army which was about to be defeated by the hosts of Tamerlane. The little village of Qarajah Hissar where Osman, the founder of the present dynasty, raised the flag of independence first is nearby and a monument marks the place where Osman made his declaration. The town has grown owing to its being the chief emporium and headquarters of the Anatolian line and the Baghdad Railway. It has a natural hot spring which supplies the whole town with beautiful clear and chalybeate water. The population is almost entirely Moslem and numbers 80,000. There is a first class secondary school, three primary schools, one girls' school, an agricultural school and an agricultural bank with a capital of £T 50.000. It belongs to the vilayet of Bursa. The Mutasarrif, Faredun Bey, is a very able and sympathetic official. We learnt some interesting facts about litigations and criminal cases. The average number of litigations yearly does not exceed 125, and the number of criminal cases was only 37 during the previous year. This gives us a fair idea of the law-abiding and peaceful character of the Ottoman subjects. In the vicinity of Eski Shahar we inspected same colonies of the Muhadjirin from Crimea and Roumelia, and also some land which we found rather arid, of poor productive capacity, there being only one crop of serials every year. Another industry is Meerchum mines which are let by the Government to private individuals who work the mines and make rosaries, mouth-pieces and such articles.

Our journey to Ankara lasted seven hours. We passed through absolutely barren and rocky plain devoid of any herbage or trees as far as the eye could reach. There were some small hamlets to be seen and a few herds of cattle and sheep. Indeed this part of the country presented the most desolate and depressing view. Here and there were some low-lying marshy plains, but even in these parts nothing but rank grass and reeds grow. Ankara or A-kara (meaning black) receives its name from the peculiar slate-grey colour of the rocks on which the town is built. It is situated on the southern side of a hill and dates back to the time of the Romans. In the times of the Seljuks this city was besieged by the conquering hosts of Tamerlane and would have been lost if it had not been for the timely help of Toghral and his well-trained horsemen. At present the town consists of narrow winding streets made of cobble stones without any regard to sanitation or drainage. The shops are generally low-roofed, showing their wares in the most primitive fashion. The farmers and people seen in the market places and streets look very poor. The population of over 60,000 consists mainly of Muslim, there being less than 5 per cent Armenians, yet all the industries and the banks are in their hands, and the Muslim Turks are being heavily dealt with by the usurious Armenian money-lenders. The chief industry of the place consists in sheep farming, the wool we got from them is of the very finest quality. There are woollen factories belonging to wealthy Armenians, but all the handwork such as knitting of shawls, stockings etc., is done by the Muslim women.

We stopped at an Armenian hotel which was anything but clean; the ravages of the millions of little dwellers in our beds made the faces and bodies of our companions a beautiful purple and blue. But we had no other alternative but to remain there, as there was no other hotel in the town. The Vali Ibrahim Sousa, a very handsome and imposing person, very fussy and talkative was a Greek. He gave us the services of the head of the Agricultural Department, Haider Bey, from whom we got all the necessary information about the land in Serrie Hissar, which the Ministry of Interior had given us reference to. This land which was 50,000 acres in area was situated in a low marshy locality, its productive capacity being not more than 1 to 20. Seven previous colonies had been settled here with most disastrous results, not one of the families surviving to the present day. The climate is damp, malarious and most unhealthy, and unless the swamp is drained it could not possibly be habitable. The crops of serials produced only once a year did not bring much prosperity to the tillers of the soil and hence they had to take to sheep-farming which is not a very paying occupation either. These facts made us decide against planting our colony here.

In spite of the depressing general appearance of the town signs are not wanting of sincere efforts on the part of the unionist Government to improve the conditions of the people. Directly after the Consultation the Government opened primary schools, one girls' school, one higher primary school and one secondary school where free education is given.

Recently the efforts of Nishat Bey, the delegate for the Party of Union and Progress, have brought into existence an up-to-date primary school on the latest model. There is a secondary school where all the modern sciences are taught and a Darul-Moallimin preparing teachers for primary schools. Under the able guidance of Maulana Hussain and his staff, this school is doing splendid work. A visit to the different classes in the school convinced us that the teaching here is very sound and practical. We were agreeably surprised to see how fluently the student to the 'Wanah ya sanat' (i.e. first form) could speak, read and write Arabic and Persian. In another form most lively discussion took place in our presence on Taleem Akhlaq.[33]

The most characteristic feature of every school that we visited was the mosque room and the offering of the prayers rigidly and regularly. Our visit to the school of industry and the agricultural college proved highly satisfactory. The latter institution has been working for the last three and a half, years and consists of a staff of eight teachers. There are forty boarders who are fed, clothed and taught free of any charges (thirty-five Muslims and five Christians). The class-room, library, scientific laboratory, zoological and geological museums were up to date and most complete. We saw here the rearing of silk-worms and the preparation of butter, cheese, etc., in the cow-shed attached to the college.

This dairy-farm was kept most scrupulously clean, the diet, the quantity of milk, the amount of butter, etc., being all noted on a chart in each shed. Attached to this institution was also a shed where six fine Arab stallions were kept for covering mares. Sabah was the most perfect specimen of an Arab horse it had been my lot to set eyes on. The experimental farm attached to the college covers an area of 1,000 acres, where all the modern, up-to-date agricultural implements and methods were being used. A very large poultry-farm is also attached to this institution. We had a very splendid lunch given us here by the Director of the College.

On our return to the hotel after spending a very pleasant half day we had several calls from the notables of the town. Ibrahim Sousa, the Vali, came to return our call, and then Nishat Bey, the delegate of the Party of Union Progress with Cemal Bey, the Chief of the Police, a red-hot Unionist and a most delightful person. The Commander of the town with his Chief Medical Officer also paid us a visit. He was an İhtilafi[34] and spoke many bitter things against the Unionist Government, though he granted that they were honest and sincere. We visited the hospital Gaziya-yı Muslimeen[35] and went round the wards. The special feature of this institution was a separate wing for the treatment of syphilis, which seems to be very prevalent here. The explanation given by Dr. Faiq Bey was that the people here were very simple and ignorant, and the disease which was contracted by the soldiers in İstanbul was given to their wives and inherited by the children: but curiously, it is twice as common amongst the Christians and Jews as amongst the Muslims, which does not seem to support the theory of the able doctor, as it is only within the last few years that these races have been allowed to enroll for the military service. We visited the ancient mosque of Sultan Alauddin Seljuki which was built by Abu Nasar Nasood ibn Hilij Arsalan in the month of Safar, 475 Hijri. The canopy where the ancient throne was kept until the time of Sultan Abdul Hamid, when it was removed to the Kazeena-i-Khassa and theminbar[36] (both worked in ebony by Ibrahim Abubakar) are the finest, rarest specimens of Turkish workmanship and artistic carving. We paid a visit to the ruins of the ancient Roman tower and castle of the time of Augustus, and a well-fortified place now used as a khan which was once the citadel of the Seljuk kings.

In the evening an open air dinner was given to us by the notables of Ankara which proved a most enjoyable and entertaining function. After the dinner speeches were made by Zafar AliKhan: Haji Atıf, member of Majlis-i-Idara: Haji Mustafa Alam, ex- Deputy; Ali Bey, ex-President of the Municipality, and myself, and it was decided that a branch Association of the Khuddam-i-Islam Society should he formed with Mufti Rafaat Effendi as its President, Nishat Bey as its Secretary, and twenty notables of Ankara as its members. The object of the Society was briefly the industrial, agricultural, economic end religious revival of the Muslims of the Vilayet. This Association was to work in harmony with similar associations in other Vilayets and the Central society in İstanbul. We left Ankara on the 31st May and reached Eski Shahar the same evening. Hotel Tadia now looked a heaven compared to our hotel in Ankara, the clean beds and the good wholesome cuisine was a blearing form heaven, which only those who have stayed in the Armenian hotel in Ankara can fully appreciate.

We had just time to drive with Feridun Bey, the Mutasarrif to the village of Muttalib, where the oldest Ottoman Turks consisting of 200 families have settled down and who still live in their pristine simplicity. Their law-abiding sober, truthful, industrious and quiet life is an example to all the people in the district. The Mutasarrif told us that theft or crime of any kind or litigation is unknown to the inhabitants of that village, their little difference being settled by the elders of the village. Their honesty is so proverbial that the villages from the district deposit all their little savings with the elders of this village. These people are quite well-to-do as they are hardworking and industrious. No one is allowed to beg. In the evening a meeting of the notables was arranged in the hotel, and a branch Association of Khuddam-i Islam was formed with the Mufti as President.

We left next morning by a very early train for our long journey to Konya. Our journey up to Alyund was through a country similar in character as that in the vicinity of Eski Shahar. At Alyund we saw green fields and fruit gardens with white walled and red-roofed little cottages and villages dotting the plains, and altogether showing every sign of prosperity. There were some beautiful China-ware sold here from Kütahya china works. A branch line runs from here to Kotahia which is an important *mutasarrifiyat* of the vilayet of Bursa. Kotahia is a historical place where a treaty was signed between the conquering Egyptian General Ibrahim Pasha and the Sublime Porte appointing Mohamed Ali, the ruler of Egypt and Ibrahim Pasha the Governor of Syria and Adana. At Afyon Karahisar halt was made for lunch. This is a very thriving little town and is an important place, being the junction between the Anatolian Railway and the Smyrna-Kassava Railway. As the name of the town implies it is the chief centre for the cultivation of poppy, besides being famous for its green jungles and plums. Aak Shahar, the ancient Philadelphia, is a town dating its antiquity to the Grecian times. Near it are the ruins of an ancient town with an amphitheater, forum, baths, marble chariots and everything complete. Here also Nasiruddin Khoja was born and buried. He is the Turkish counterpart of our own Mulla Do Peyaza and many a humorous and witty anecdote attributed to his great wit brightens the winter evening in a Turkish home.

Gazli-Gul-Hammam which we reached late in the afternoon is noted for its hot sulphur springs where patients suffering from gout and skin diseases flock for a cure.

Konya, the ancient Iconium, was reached at 7 P. M. Here we were met by many of the notables of the town at the station as they were informed by their friends at Eski Shahar of our arrival. After a long and tiresome journey we felt only fit to retire to our beds after the evening meal. Early next morning we called at the Hukumet and saw the Vali, Ali Rıza Bey, who was very courteous and ready to assist as in every way possible. We talked with him of our scheme of colonization, and he expressed fervent hope that it would be in his Vilayet that we would select the site for the colony. He introduced us to Dr. Besim Bey, Chief of the Sanitary Department and Nadir Bey, the Chief Engineer of the Irrigation Department of Konya. I must mention here that the Ottoman Government has canalized and completed the irrigation of half a million acres of land in Konya. It was arranged that we should go next day with Nadir Bey and Dr. Bassim Bey to inspect this canalised land. The Vali asked us if we belonged to the same society which Colonel Surtis represented. On being informed in the negative he spoke to us of the utter distrust shown by the colonel in the Turkish people by distributing aid to the refugees in Konya through a foreign missionary institution in preference to the Ottoman peoples. We then visited the Government depot where a large number of modern agricultural implements were exhibited and sold to the farmers on hire-purchase system. There was also a German mart for agricultural implements. But the thing which delighted us most was our visit to a large magazine started by the Maulvis where every kind of article from finest silk down to ordinary broom was sold by these Maulvis themselves. The next most pleasing visit was to the 'Moslem' Bank which has been started for the last two years with a capital of £T 70,000. The Manager, Ahmed Haznee Bey, told us that the last year's net profits were £T 8,000, a tidy little sum which speaks volumes for the management of the Bank. This year they were going to undertake the electric installation in the town and an electric tramway which the Manager of the Bank hoped would bring larger profits to the shareholders. Their new building situated in the principal street of the town was almost complete, and they hoped to transfer the Bank there within a month. These signs of commercial and economic activities amongst the Musalmans of Konya gave us great heart and hopes for the real consolidation of the Ottoman Empire. It must be mentioned that all this is the result of the activity of the Party of Union and Progress in Konya.

M. A. Ansari

July 1913

26 July 1913

Visit to the Tomb of Maulana Jalaluddin Rumi

The great saint, *muhaddis*, philosopher and poet, Maulana Jalaluddin Rumi, whose interpretations of Al-Quran in his immortal and classical *Masnavi*, is read everywhere Islam has spread, is buried here in Konya. His shrine has been always held in highest veneration by the Sultans, noblemen, ulama and the common people. It is a place of pilgrimage from all parts of Turkey and indeed all the Islamic world. Here the great Maulana Jami made a pilgrimage and wrote in his own hand the couplets which are hung up in a frame at the gate of shrine.

This house has become the Kaaba of Lovers
Anyone who came here incomplete left as complete

The visit of Hazrat Shams-i-Tabraz and his preachings in the Madrassah and his subsequent murder by the suspicious students, who took him to be a Shia, and the throwing of his body into the well over which to the present day a tomb marks the place, was related to us by one of the Maulavis of the shrine. The shrine itself is a beautiful building with a green dome over the grave of the Maulana. The tomb is cornered with richly embroidered green silk cloth enclosed with a beautiful silver railing which is a precious work of art. The huge candles outside the railing and the antique lamps have stands studded with most costly gems, being the devotion offerings from the different Sultans and emirs.

We also visited several modern mosques in the town, that of Sultan Salim being the most magnificent. There are numerous objects of historical interest in Konya, the chief being Sultan Alauddin's Jame and his tomb. The mosque is of little interest except the forty-two pillars on which the roof and the dome are supported. The mihrab and mimber are of exquisite workmanship and of the best Ottoman period. The tomb of Alauddin Saljuki, the last of that dynasty, is a plain one with a simple inscription bearing the name and date of the monarch:

Alauddünya veddin Ebul-Feth Keykubat ibnus-Sultan sa'idush-shahid Keyhusrev bin Kılıçarslan bin Mesud. Year 617 Hijra.

There are some objects of great antiquity and interest deposited in this shrine: (1) a green banner, on each corner of which are embroidered the names of the four Khalifas and the Prophet's name in the centre, and (2) a very ancient copy of the Quran in Khatt-i-Kufi and one in Khatt-i-Suls.

Alauddin's kiosk is nearby, commanding a beautiful view of the surrounding country. It is fast crumbling down.

Two beautiful mosques, one built by Fakhruddin Saheb-i-Ata in 682 Hijri, and another by Karatagh-i-Kabeer, one of the viziers, contain the most beautiful and rarest China that could be found. The mosaics on the roof are the finest specimens of their kind. The carving on the wooden gates and the raised stone carvings round these gates are most wonderful.

There are six schools, five for primary and one for secondary education and a girls' school. There is a school of law and a very fine industrial school which turns out furniture and cabinets of newest designs and ploughs, water pumps and other industrial implements, besides doing a considerable amount of repairing work.

There is a very old church half of which is used by the Armenians and other half by the Greeks.

Next morning we started with Nadir Bey and Dr. Bassim Bey to Chomra where the staff of irrigation engineers have their headquarters. The source of the water is a very large like in the Karadağ Mountains some ten miles distant. The water is diverted into a river, the Çarsamba Çayı, from which by means of dams and sluice-gates the flow of water is maintained into the primary canals and thence into the secondary and tertiary systems. The irrigation scheme, which was started more than four years ago, has now been completed and supplies an area of half a million acres. We inspected nearly the whole of this area and selected an artificial hillock, the sight of an ancient town, for our village, should we select this track for our colonization scheme. This hillock is situated about four miles from the railway line and would be the most suitable place for building a village. Nearby we saw the remains of an old Roman village, Binbir Kalissa, where there are also remains of many old churches and monasteries. We returned to Chomra late in the afternoon and did full justice to the lunch provided by Shauket Bey, the Chief Engineer. Mr. and Mrs. Her Kener gave us a very fine tea in the afternoon. Our host was the wife of the German expert, who is employed by the Ottoman Government. She is a young lady of great culture and refinement and charmed our friend Aageyah Bey very much by her brilliant conversation. Mr. Zafar Ali Khan was also a privileged person owing to the supposition that he was a parson (due to his long black frock coat).

We returned to Konya in the evening and were given an invitation to dinner by Chalaki Effendi, the Sajjadanashin of Maulana Rum's shrine; dinner was simple and wholesome as befits the life of a hermit. After the meal, we were introduced to all the notables of Konya, and Mr. Zafar Ali Khan made a stirring speech asking them to be up and doing, working for the regeneration of their motherland by means of commercial and industrial regeneration. Noori Effendi, the Deputy for Konya, made a reply and showed the work of industrial progress which they in Konya had been carrying on for some time and which he hoped would gradually bring about the consolidation of the vilayat. A branch Association of the Khuddam-i-Islam was also formed here with the Rayes-i-Baladia as its President, and Huznee Bey, the Manager of the Bank, as the Secretary of the Association. The Chairman of the Municipality then presented us with an album containing photographs of all the antique and historical buildings and monuments in Konya. For the valuable souvenir of their brotherly goodwill and friendship, I thanked them in suitable and cordial terms.

Our journey to Bozanti next day was a gradual ascent along a tableland, the highest point of which was Eregli 2,500 feet above the sea level. Beyond this, as far as Bulgarloo, a height of 5,400 feet, the train passed through the Tarsus system of mountains, its highest peaks being snow covered. We had to pass over numerous bridges and through no less than

21 tunnels, on numerous embankments and galleries, the wild and rugged mountains all around us full of grandeur and majesty seemed to be an unceasing chain until we reached Bulgarloo, its highest point. Here the rarified air and the low-atmospheric pressure caused some respiratory embarrassment to one or two of our companions, notably Dr. Ahmed Fuad. But an amyl nitrite capsule, which I fortunately had in my bag, relieved the symptom instantly. The descent to Bozanti which lies in the hollow between the two peaks of the Taurus was steep and difficult. The German engineers have expended considerable skill and ingenuity in achieving this great feat. Bozanti, which is situated in the vale of that name, is the last station on the Baghdad Railway. From here the line goes a few miles and there stops owing to the long tunnel they are boring through the Taurus to reach the Cilician plains.

We made a halt here for the night and had to stay in a *khan* infected with fleas and vermins of all sorts. This is a very historical place and though it have passed the armies of Darius and Alaxander, the hosts of Cyrus and the conquering armies of the Egyptian General Ibrahim Pasha. What vicissitudes, what changes this green, smiling valley must have seen. Many empires have risen, reached their zenith, decayed and disappeared, before the very eyes of these unchanging mountains and rocks. It makes one wonder what fate awaits the only remaining Moslem State which now holds this historical place under its away.

A very touching and pleasing little incident happened here. I was taking some snapshots of the snow-covered Taurus and the green valleys when I was accosted by a farmer who was returning from his field. He asked me where I came from and, on learning my country and my religion, he looked so immensely pleased that he kissed my hands and invited me to a cup of tea in his cottage. Here was as example of that true fraternity which is only practiced in Islam though preached by many other religions. As he was from the borders of Persia, we could talk with each other in Persian. His hospitality was real and genuine. I will never forget the happiness that cup of tea gave me and my host. It was the best cup I ever had in my life. In the evening we visited some refugees from Tchorlu who were on their way to Adana and who had run short of food and provision. They were 70 in number, men, women and children, and we offered a small help of five piastres a head. We passed the night in the infested khan, but we did not get a wink of sleep owing in the irritating attention of our friends the vermins.

We started at 3 in the morning on our journey to Adana. Our carriages, which were four-wheelers, were a cross between a brougham and a Victoria. They had to take all our baggage and two of us in each.

They were drawn by a pair of strong horses. As we went along the Roman road which goes winding—uphill and downhill, often in a zig-zag fashion to make the climb less steep, we passed through most gorgeous and enchanting scenery. And were it not for the rough and continuous jolting the journey would have been ideal. I do not believe that the roads have been repaired since the Byzantine period when they were constructed. It is only the Turkish horses and the strong spring of the carriages which could have stood the rough roads. We passed a very old fort which at first sight could not be distinguished from the rocky mountain and which it stood. Its date is lost in distant ages. Some say it dates from the time of the Assyrians, others gives it a much later date in the Roman period. It was obvious from the condition of the walls and the moat surrounding the castle that it must be very ancient as time and exposure to weather had absolutely worn out all traces of inscriptions on the walls. A few miles beyond we came across two modern fortresses on hills commanding the road and of great strategic position. These were constructed by Ibrahim Pasha, the conqueror of Egypt, about the year 1845. It was a beautiful morning and we decided to walk along the road in order to enjoy better the magnificent scenery just as much as to escape the increased bumping and jolting inside the carriages. We came across few low roofed cottages along the road with one or two solitary occupants selling cigarettes and coffee to the way-farers. We met long caravans of camels loaded with packages of all sorts this being the chief means of transport between Bozanti and Adana. A halt was made at midday at a wayside inn give rest to the animals and to take some refreshment. Our friend Aageyah Bey, who was the master of ceremonies, is always very thoughtful in matters relating to food. The fare he provided us here was worthy of any first class restaurant in İstanbul. His memory never deceives him in such matters, even in such details, as chocolates, peppermint drops and delicacies like pat de fois gras, although he may forget such unimportant details as the letter of introduction to the Vali of Adana or many other such foolish unnecessary things. And even if the latter omission caused a little inconvenience, his bearing countenance and smiling eyes made up for it. After our meal we were lounging about and some of the party had gone up to reconnoitre the adjoining hill, when the sharp eyes of our dear friend Mr. Zafar Ali Khan perceived engraved on a steep rock on the opposite band of the river, the bearded face and the crowned head of an ancient Assyrian King, facing another image presumably that of the Queen. He could see the sceptre, the flowing robe and every detail complete. We at once decided to cross the mountain torrent, and after a laborious and steep climb, at times on all fours, reached the summit panting and perspiring only to find that our visions had played us false, and that was nothing but an optical illusion, the images probably conjured up by the highly imaginative brain of our friend Zafar Ali Khan, the classical ground and the romantic surroundings probably taking a great share in it.

The second half of our journey, though every bit as interesting as the first half, was marred by the extreme roughness of the road, and the tropical heat of the sun. In one place our road passed through a perpendicular gorge rising up to some 3,000 feet, the steep rocky wall on one side and the deep dark ravine on the other, in which a foaming, roaring river pursued its course. In the middle of this stream stood a rock on which an inscription was carved by the order of Marcus Aurelius, the great Roman philosopher and the tutor of Emperor Nero. The name 'Kibir Sanduk'[37] is aptly given to this place owing to its shape like a box. About 4 o'clock we reached the summit of a hill from which we could see the plain of Cilicia, which for its fertility and richness has always been the coveted possession from the time of Egyptians and Assyrians, Darius and Alexander the Great, the Greeks and the Romans, to the present day. This plain stretches as far as the sea and on its south-eastern and north-eastern sides is limited by the Karadagh Mountains and the Taurus system which we had just traversed. Three rivers flow from the mountains and irrigate these plains, the Saihan, the Jaihan and the Bardan. The great Egyptian Queen Cleopatra used to come up the river Saihan in her galleys dressed as a Greek goddess to meet her Roman lover Antony at Tarsus. We reached the railway station Gulen Bughaz just in time to catch the train to Adana, where we reached in one hour. This section of the Baghdad Railway runs between Mersina and Osmanieh with a branch line to Alexandretta. It is expected that the tunnel in the Taurus Mountain would join the second section of the Baghdad Railway with this, the third section somewhere near the station of Gulen Bughaz.

At Adana we were met at the station by a large number of the notables of the town. Sukhi Pasha, the Chairman of the Municipality, and Mufti Haji Ali being amongst them. These gentlemen had been informed of our arrival by our friends from Konya. After a good Turkish bath and supper, we retired to our beds in our hotel.

Early on the morning of the 7th June we called on the Vali, Amin Bey, who was very prompt in arranging our journey to Erzine, where the land (more than 40, 000 acres) we wished to inspect was situated. He told us that it was the most fertile district and the productive capacity of the land was very high: wheat, maize, but-root, cotton, fruits and almost anything could be grown on this land with equal success. He told us that manure was never used in Adana, and in fact it was unnecessary and no irrigation was required unless fruit trees were grown, the annual rainfall being quite sufficient for the crops.

The population of this vilayet is 450,000, out of which there are 80,000 Armenians. But the curious fact was that in spite of the richness and fertility of the land and the wealth of the farmers the revenue derived by the Government was only half a million pounds. The chief cultivation in the vilayet was wheat and other serials, but recently cotton growing is being carried on an extensive scale although the quality of the cotton is inferior to that produced in Egypt and India. Fruits of all kinds are grown here in abundance and are shipped at Mercina to Europe. Some of the finest apricots and plums I have ever tasted in my life were given to us by Dr. Rafiq Bey, Chief of the Sanitary Department here. We visited the secondary school, which has 180 boarders and is one of the finest institutions of the kind. The school of industry here is a very extensive institution with a large carpentry department, a smithy with an iron forge attached to it. I saw several engines being repaired here and a large number of ploughs, sheaving machines and other agricultural implements. They have a printing press where every description of printing was being taught to the students and the local bi-weekly paper, *Ceyhan*, was printed here. The agricultural college is the most up-to-date institution, has a staff of twenty teachers and over 200 students and has been doing splendid work for the fast five years. Some very important experiments on cotton growing are at present being carried on in this institution, the results of which are expected to be of greatest economic importance to the vilayet. The orphanage which is constructed to accommodate 300 inmates is very well governed and looked after. Most of the children there, numbering 140 altogether, were Armenians.

We caught the train for Erzine at 4 pm, our train passing through the fertile valley of Ceyhan, where as far as the eyes could reach nothing but cultivated fields could be seen. This was the reaping season for the wheat crop. The reaping was done by means of the modern machinery driven by a horse, which cuts the corn and collects it in sheaves at the rate of 20 acres a day. In another place one saw grain being cropped and separated from straw and husk by engine-driven machinery. Indeed all the agricultural operation here are carried on in the most modern and up-to-date manner with the least amount of labour. It makes one wonder could some of the Indian journals have the audacity to call Turkey the most backward country, when they must know that in India agriculture is still being carried on in the most primitive condition without the least improvement in the methods of agriculture for the last 150 years. I assure you, Adana, could give many lessons to most up-to-date agricultural districts in India.

We passed the village of Hamidieh, which belongs to ex-Sultan Abdul Hamid and which he has rented to a French baron for 30 years. The ancient town of Annivers, which is a most magnificent Roman ruin with its citadels, its forum, amphitheatre and marble baths complete in every detail, is situated near here. Ilan Kale (Ilan—serpent), which was built by the Persians in time of Darius, still stands. There was a myth that the Persian army astrologer invoked the aid of the deity, and his prayer was answered in the shape of a serpent who guarded the fortress against any enemy, and hence the name Ilan Kale. The fortress is still infested by poisonous snakes and visitors are forbidden entrance into it.

We arrived at Toprak Kale Station from where we had to take carriages to Erzine but the vehicles which were to have come from Osmanieh had not reached and we took advantage of this delay to explore the ancient fortress built in the time of Alexander the Great and commanding the road to Alexandretta. Although the sun was setting, we thought we would be able to return before it was dark. We started with a gendarme at a brisk pace and had to wade through two streams and many fields full of prickly bushes before we reached the base of the fortress. Some of the party had gone halfway up the hill, others had reached the gate of the fortress, when we heard a groan and our gendarme guide was not be found any more. We searched in the darkness, slipped, fell down, tore our clothing and got bruised all over in our attempt to find the gendarme, but we found it impossible to trace him. We had almost given up hopes when in response to one of the many shouts from Aageyah Bey the man replied and came down saying that he had been inside the fortress searching after us. I really believe that he had hid himself behind a bush to be spared the trouble of climbing up the steep hill. Our exertions had quite exhausted us and our friend Aageyah Bey who is by nature an easy going man insisted that we should wait there along the road and let the carriages pick us up here, this being our route to Erzine. We remonstrated against this, but he insisted on the point and gave a hundred and one reasons why we should remain where we were, the strongest reason was that if the shepherd's dogs barked we will be shot at being taken for a burglar. After three hours of patient waiting we had to face the shepherd's dogs and made through streams, losing our way in the darkness and reaching the railway station at about midnight. I do not believe this strength of character (as Ageyah Bey would call it, but which we thought was stubbornness) is a common Turkish trait.

After three hours' journey in the country cart (I do not think the vehicles could be called by any more dignified name) we reached the village of Erzine and were taken to a house where beds were provided for us for the night, but we found that five gendarme soldiers had occupied our beds after making a sumptuous repast which had been provided for us. The soldiers were not a little discomfited when their chief rudely rowed them from their slumbers. This officer of the gendarme was very apologetic to us for the inconvenience caused by the thoughtlessness of his subordinates but we passed it off good humouredly and after a cup of tea started off on horses to see the domain. A couple of hours' ride brought us to this tract of land which lives along the shores of the Bay of Alexandretta in a most ideal locality. On its northern side is situated the village of Bashlania at the foot of a bill of that name. There is a plentiful supply of water by means of three fair sized springs situated in this mountain. One of them runs to very near the centre of this land and then turns towards the west to irrigate the fields and the fruit gardens in the village of Ersine. The second is about forty times the volume of the first and runs to a low-lying tract of ground on the south eastern side and ends into a sort of marsh. The third is partially utilized by the villagers of Bashlamia and then allowed to run into the sea. Anyone or all of them can be utilized for irrigating the domain in view at a very modest cost. The soil in this domain is very rich, of dark-brown colour and is virgin, not having been under cultivation for centuries. Judging from the adjoining Armenian Village of Dartiol, it will very soon be a flourishing place owing to the proximity to sea and to the railway line running to Alexandretta. Our agricultural expert, Saleh Bey, was entirely satisfied and inquiries about the cost of labour and material make it most likely that the cost of the houses would be 20 per cent less than our original estimates. As regards sanitation it is a most healthy locality and combines the benefits of mountain and sea air. The little swamp could be drained off once the stream which runs into it is diverted to irrigate our domain, and then ten or fifteen thousand acres of marshland would be worth its value in gold. After thoroughly investigating everything we returned to Erzine highly satisfied and determined to take this domain for planting our first colony there. What with our previous night's adventure at Toprak Kale and what with want of sleep and the six hours' ride on horses, we were so tired that we dropped off to sleep immediately after our food and did not wake up until 5 P.M. an hour before our return to Osmanieh.[38]

We had a very comfortable hotel in Osmanieh, and after a good night's rest left for Adana in the morning and reached there at 10 A.M. We thanked His Excellency the Vali for all his kindness and he promised to communicate the choice of this land to the Minister of Interior and make all necessary arrangements for the official transference of this domain for the colonization of the muhadjirin to Indo-Ottoman Colonization Society. At a meeting held in the Primary School of Union and Progress we met all the notables of Adana. Mr. Zafar Ali Khan and myself made speeches explaining the necessity of economic and industrial co-operation, the formation of a Muslim bank and the Khuddam-i-Islam Society. Sukhi Pasha was elected President, and the Principal of the school as secretary of the Association. A little school boy often recited a patriotic poem in Turkish in such a perfect manner that it moved the assembly to tears. The last words of this poem meant something to this effect. 'Our great and mighty ancestors—rest yourselves in peace in your graves; we your descendants, in whose veins is still running your blood, will not tarnish your fame. We will live for revenge.'

We left for Tarsus the same afternoon, where we were met by Sadi Pasha, ex-Deputy of Adana, Shakir Bey, Rais-e-Baladia,[39] Besim Bey and the Mufti of the town and many other notables. We visited the tomb of Khalifa Mamun-ul-Rashid, that elegant, cultured Abbasside monarch, who died in this vicinity where he had come on a political mission, and was buried at Tarsus. The Tomb of one of the greatest of the Arabian Monarch, the grandeur of whose court is still recounted in many an Arabic poem, is simple to the extreme and devoid of any of those paraphernalia which mark the last resting place of the great monarchs. It was his express will that this should be so, as simplicity was the key-note of the private life of this monarch and that of his father, the great Harun-ul-Rashid. The following 'ketebehu'[40] is the only engraving found on the headstone of the tomb:

La Illah-il Fatiha
You will see the shrine of Mamoon and Ameen tomorrow. among the greatest evil people of Khalil
You will not see his grave as bright; he is not the son of Badar (full moon) though with all the brightness
Haroon Rashid was the best personality in the Bani Abbas era

There were several banners and standards which unfortunately we could not see as it was very dark.

In the same premises are two other tombs said to be those of Hazret-I Şit Aleyhi and Lokman Hekim, Ashab-i Kehf. Not very far from here is a place where Ashab-i Kehf and their dog were buried.

Sadiq Pasha gave us a very fine dinner in the town gardens, where many other guests were also invited. At a meeting held after the dinner we met with an unexpected success, as not only the Khuddam-i-Ka'ba Association but a Muslim Bank was decided to be formed. Early next morning we visited Sadiq Pasha's flour mills, Rassim Bey's extensive cotton mills, the famous Burdan waterfalls and the electric power house which lights the town. We left for Mersina[41] hoping to catch a boat in the afternoon, but

Appendix

on arrival there we were told that there was no boat until the 12th June reaching İstanbul on the 17th. As I had decided to sail for Egypt on the 19th it would have given me hardly any time had I waited for the boat at Mersina. I was obliged to return by the same route by which we had come. And thanks to the kindness of Shatir Bey, Rais-e-Baladia of Tarsus, who responded to my telegram and sent coaches to meet our party at Gulan Bughaz station the same afternoon, and travelling all night we were able to catch the train at Bozanti[42] on Wednesday morning, 11th June. I was thus able to reach İstanbul on Friday afternoon.

M. A. Ansari

June 1913

İstanbul, 17 June 1913

The Colonization Commission was on its way back to İstanbul when the news of the assassination of Marshal Mahmoud Shevket Pasha came to us like a thunderbolt from the blue. This news for a moment paralysed us. It was inconceivable that the Grand Vizier should be assassinated so brutally just on the morrow of the signing of the Peace. Yet this was exactly what had taken place. With one fiendish blow the greatest soldier and statesman of Turkey was snatched from the nation at a time when he was most needed by it. On our arrival in İstanbul we gathered further details of the dastardly deed. The funeral of Marshal Mahmoud Sherket Pasha and Ibrahim Bey, his heroic A.-D.-C., who lost his life in defending his master, took place on Tuesday, the 12th June. The prayers were offered in St. Sophia in which ten thousand people were present, but the crowd outside the mosque and in the streets was so thick that it was difficult to walk without discomfort. Everywhere along the route of the funeral the deepest sorrow was evinced by the populace and the cries and sobbing of the women and children were heard from the balconies and terraces all along the route. The two coffins of the 'Shohada-i-Moazzam' were carried in the strictest Islamic manner on the shoulders of the bearers. They were covered with blood-red silk richly embroidered with gold, the cap being placed over the coffin indicating the head. At Sirkedji landing stage the two coffins were placed on a steam launch and carried to Dolme Bagche, the mourners following in three large troopships. As the procession passed the different cruisers, belonging to the European powers, had their soldiers standing in files on the deck with their flags flying half-mast. On the landing at Dolma Bagche, the representatives of the different Embassies and the commanders of the different cruisers were present. Here the procession was greatly increased by the sailors of the different foreign cruisers as well as by the Ottoman soldiers and officers and became a full military funeral with artillery infantry, etc. All the members of the two Missions also took part in the procession. The remains were interred in the enclosure at Hurriyet Tepe where the Column of Liberty indicates the site where the remains of the martyrs for the cause of liberty are buried. A meeting of all the Indians resident in İstanbul and members of the Indian Red Crescent took place on Saturday and passed the following resolutions which were duly submitted to the Grand Vizier, Prince Said Halim Pasha. His Excellency expressed his thanks on behalf of the Ottoman Government and the Ottoman nation and wished us to convey his sentiments to the Muslims of India. The resolutions were the following:

1. That this meeting of the Muslims of India, representing 75 million compatriots, places on record its intense loathing and horror at the dastardly deed which has cut short the career of one of the greatest Moslem statesmen whose services to Islam can never be sufficiently acknowledged.
2. That this meeting on behalf of Moslem India joins the Ottoman nation in mourning the untimely loss of the martyrs to the cause of constitutional progress and Moslem advancement.
3. That this meeting fervently prays that Allah will confer His eternal peace on the martyred remains of Mahmoud Sherket and will vouchsafe patience and strength to the widow and family of the 'Shahid-i-Moazzam' in this great bereavement.
4. That copies of the above resolution be submitted to (a) His Imperial Majesty the Caliph's Government, (b) the widow of the late lamented Marshal Mahmound Sherket Pasha, (c) the leading papers for publication.

It is obvious from the investigations which the police have been carrying out that it has been a deep-laid plot by men of high station in life, some members of the Liberal Union Party and men of the Hamidian regime. The Turkish papers have been publishing accounts showing the complicity of the Kiamilian clique. It is also said that some of the foreign subjects are also suspected of having played a part in this plot. Shariff Pasha had predicted the fall of Young Turk Cabinet a week before the assassination and Raschid Bey, the Minister of Interior during the last Government, had also indicated something similar. The Government is going to publish a full account of the plot after they have been finished that investigation. At present five hundred persons have been arrested, including Topal Towfiq, the first assassin, Djawad, Koramun, and Zia. Cemal Bey, the Commandant of İstanbul, had given information the day before the murder to Mahmoud Sherket Pasha of the suspicion of a plot against Mahmoud Sharvet Pasha, Enver Bey, Talat Bey and himself. He had warned him to change the route which he usually took to go from the War office to the Sublime Porte, but Mahmoud Sherket Pasha made little of the matter and took no precautions. On Wednesday morning he left as usual the War office at 11-30, and proceeded in his motor car towards the Sublime Porte. At one end of Beyazid Square the tram lines were under repairs and the road was so narrowed for the traffic that the passing of a mock funeral obliged him to stop. Immediately his car stopped. Topal Tewfik fired at him the bullet passing into the brain from his right temple. His A.-D.-C. Ibrahim Bey, threw himself in front of the Grand Vizier to shield him from the firing which at this moment was begun by all the assassins. Ibrahim Bey was shot dead. The other A.-D.-C., Ashrif Bey and Kazim Agha, the attendant, began firing at the assassins having dismounted from the car, but Kazim soon fell down wounded and Ashraf Bey ran after one of the assassins who was retreating in the direction of War Ministry. All this took place in about two minutes, and after firing 35 shots the assassins got inside a motor car which was waiting for them near the fountain of Fatima Sultan and drove as fast as was possible, leaving Topal Tewfiq behind. They rode via Aak Serai, Tash Kassab, Top Kapon and then to Amphiajee and out of the city wall to Sishbe. Topal Tewfiq was seen by Ismail Haqqi of the police force who ordered him to stop, but the murderer ran firing his revolver all the time towards Assheratkhan (aserai in the neighbour-hood). Reaching the staircase he threw away a revolver and dagger there, hid himself in the water-closet, where he was caught by the police with a revolver and some cartridges. Kamila Khanun of Scutari had seen the trag-edy and had noticed Topal Tewfik firing the revolver. The police who were sent after the motor car discovered it in Shishla and found its owner to be no less a person than Abdur Rahman, the son of the Chief of the spies in Abdul Hamid's time. His cousin Djavid was the chauffeur. The police also captured Qoramneen, one of the assassins, and found in his posses-sion a paper from Damad Saleh Pasha for one thousand pounds to be paid to him on accomplishing certain works entrusted to him. The proprietor of Alsidar Hakki Bey, was followed by the police and was seen to enter a suspected house in Pera Muhammad street. He was also arrested and from him a clue was obtained as to the inmates of the house. The owner of this house is a certain Nichola Villich, an English subject. The police was refused admission unless someone from the Consulate accompanied them. They surrounded the house and two police officers in plain clothes got admission into the house. One of them was Hilmi Bey, a very gallant and brave officer as A.-D.-C. of Cemal Bey, the Commandant of İstanbul.

Both these were fired at and wounded in the house. Then the gendarme surrounded, and about one thousand shots were exchanged between the police and the inmates, one of the assassins Muhammad Ali being wounded in the hand. The fire brigade men climbed the house and made a hole in the roof through which the police entered the building, and after a desperate and terrible fighting the inmates were all captured. The house proved to be a regular magazine; for they found in it boxes of Mauzer revolvers of ammunitions, two hand grenade shrapnel's large stores of food and drink and dressings for the wounds. The four assassins Muhammad Ali, Kasim and two others were arrested in the house on Friday. The remaining assassin Ziya was also arrested on Sunday at Besiktas. Of the five hundred arrested most of the people had been found with bombs, rifles, and a number of documents relating to the plot and proving that they were simply tools in the hands of the members of the Liberal Union Party. Prince Salahuddin, it is said, has been living for the last two months in a cruiser belonging to one of the foreign powers anchored in the Boğaziçi. A gloom has been cast over İstanbul by this great tragedy, and the consequent stringent measures started by the police have altered the social aspect of the capital. I have been very much pressed for time since my return from Anatolia. We have had the meeting of our Colonization Society, the complete report of which would have been sent to you this week under ordinary circumstances, but I found it impossible for reasons stated above. I will, however, publish it on my return and explain everything in the minutest details.

The All-India Medical Mission is going today for audience of His Imperial Majesty the Sultan, and I am dictating this letter whilst awaiting for the members to get ready. This is a distinction which we are naturally proud of, for a Muslim it is a great honour to kiss the robes of the Khalifat-ul-Muslimeen. We will by the Romanian boat, leaving İstanbul on the 19th, and would catch the Italian boat from Suez on the 29th. You will of courses, get a cable long before this letter reaches there. I am enclosing an account of the tragedy written by a friend of Abdur Rahman, Kasim Bey, which you can utilize in the most suitable manner. My next letter will be delivered to the Editor of the *Comrade* personally.

M. A. Ansari

Notes

1. Greetings!
2. Tip.

Appendix

3. Serbians.

4. Çanakkale Boğazı (Çanakkale Strait).

5. Mecidiye.

6. Üsküdar, on the Asian side of İstanbul.

7. Çanakkale.

8. Boğaziçi. The second of the Turkish Straits between the Black Sea and the Aegean Sea.

9. Kadırga Hastanesi.

10. Besim Ömer Akalın.

11. Beyoğlu.

12. Hadımköy.

13. Çatalca.

14. Sancaktepe.

15. Halide Edip Adıvar.

16. Ömerli.

17. Mahmud Şevket Paşa.

18. Dr. Esad Paşa.

19. Haydarpasa.

20. Yeşilköy.

21. Kamil Paşa.

22. Şarköy.

23. Uzun Köprü.

24. Reşit Paşa.

25. Şükrü Pasha.

26. Midye-Enez.

27. Edirne.

28. Büyükçekmece.

29. Durusu (Terkos).

30. Sea of Marmara.

31. Chief of Staff.

32. İzmit.

33. Ethics education.

34. Dissident.

35. Muslim daughters.

36. The pulpit.

37. The chest of conceit.

38. Osmaniye.

39. Belediye Reisi, namely Mayor.

40. Words.

41. Mersin.

42. Pozantı.

Select Bibliography

ABDÜLHAMİD. *Siyasi Hatıratım* (İstanbul: Dergah Yayınları, 1975).

ABRAHAM, Jose. 'A Discussion on the Possibility of a Subaltern Reading of Indian Muslim History', AMSS 35th Annual Conference 'Muslim Identities: Shifting Boundaries and Dialogues', co-sponsored by Hartford Seminary, Hartford, CT, 27–29 October 2006.

ADA, Hüsnü. 'The First Ottoman Civil Society Organization in the Service of the Ottoman State: The Case of the Ottoman Red Crescent' (Osmanlı Hilal-i Ahmer Cemiyeti), unpublished Master's Thesis, Sabancı University, September 2004.

ADEEB, Khaled. 'Pan-Islamism in Practice: The Rhetoric of Islamic Unity and Its Uses', in Elisabeth Özdalga, ed., *Late Ottoman Society: The Intellectual Legacy* (New York: Routledge Curzon, 2005), pp. 203–26.

ADIVAR, Halide Edip. *Inside India* (London: George Allen & Unwin, 1937).

AHMAD, Ishtiaq. 'From Pan-Islamism to Muslim Nationalism: The Indian Muslim Response to the Turkish War of Liberation', International Conference 'Turkish War of Liberation', 12–13 May 2005, National Institute of Cultural and Historical Research, Pakistan.

AKBAR, M. J. *The Shade of Swords: Jihad and the Conflict between Islam and Christianity* (New Delhi: Lotus Roli, 2006).

———. *India—The Siege Within: Challenges to a Nation's Unity* (Suffolk: Penguin Books, 1985).

ANSARI, Mukhtar Ahmad. 'Introduction' in Halide Edib, *Conflict of East and West in Turkey* (Delhi: Maktaba Jamia Millia Islamia, 1935).

ANSARI, K. H. 'Pan-Islam and the Making of the Early Muslim Socialists', *Modern Asian Studies*, vol. 20, no. 3 (1986), pp. 509–37.

AHMED, Feroz. 'The Late Ottoman Empire', in Marian Kent, ed., *The Great Powers and the End of the Ottoman Empire* (London: Frank Cass, 1996).

AYDIN, Cemil. 'Islamic Traditions of the Muslim World: The Legions of the Late 19th Century Intellectual History', AMSS 38th Annual Conference 'Islamic Traditions and Comparative Modernities', 25–26 September 2009.

———. *The Politics of Anti-Westernism in Asia: Visions of World Order in Pan-Islamic and Pan-Asian Thought* (New York: Columbia University Press, 2007).

BABUR, Zahiru'd-din Muhammad Padshah Ghazi. *The Babur-Nama in English (Memoirs of Babur)*, translation from the original Turki by Annette Susannah Beveridge, vol. 1 (London: Luzac and Co, 1922).

BALABANLILAR, Lisa. 'The Begims of the Mystic Feast: Turco-Mongol Tradition in the Mughal Harem', *The Journal of Asian Studies*, vol. 69, no. 1 (February 2010), pp. 123–47.

BERKES, Niyazi. *The Development of Secularism in Turkey* (Montreal: McGill University Press, 1964).

BHARASPATI, K. C. D. 'Muslim Influences on Venkatamakhi', in G. Kuppuswamy and M. Hariharan, eds, *Readings on Music and Dance* (Trivandarum: B. R. Publishing Corporation, 1979).

BİLKAN, Ali Fuat. 'Halide Edip Adıvar', ın Hindistan 'daki Konferansları', *Bilig*, Kış 2011, Sayı 56, pp. 33–44.

BLUMI, Isa. *Reinstating the Ottomans: Alternative Balkan Modernities 1800–1912* (New York: Palgrave Macmillan, 2011).

BURKE, Edmund. 'Pan-Islam and Moroccan Resistance to French Colonial Penetration, 1900–1912', *The Journal of African History*, vol. 13, no. 1 (1972), pp. 97–118.

CASALE, Giancarlo. *The Ottoman Age of Exploration* (Oxford: Oxford University Press, 2010).

CHAKRABARTY, Dipesh. *Provincializing Europe: Postcolonial Thought and Historical Difference* (Princeton: Princeton University Press, 2000).

CHOWDURY, Rashed. 'Pan-Islamism and Modernisation during the Reign of Sultan Abdülhamid II, 1876–1909', PhD dissertation, McGill University, 2011.

ÇETİNSAYA, Gökhan. 'The Ottoman View of British Presence in Iraq and the Gulf: The Era of Abdulhamid II', *Middle Eastern Studies*, vol. 39, no. 2 (April 2003), pp. 194–203.

DAMES, Longworth M. 'The Portuguese and Turks in the Indian Ocean in the Sixteenth Century', *Journal of the Royal Asiatic Society of Great Britain and Ireland*, no. 1 (January 1921), pp. 1–28.

DERİNGİL, Selim. *The Well-Protected Domain: Ideology and the Legitimation of Power in the Ottoman Empire, 1876–1909* (New York: IB Tauris, 2009).

————. 'Osmanlı İmparatorluğu'nda "Geleneğin İcadı", "Muhayyel Cemaat" ("Tasarımlanmış Topluluk") ve Panislamizm' (Invention of Tradition in the Ottoman Empire, Imagined Group and Panislamism), Toplum ve Bilim, Sayı 54–5, Yaz-Güz 1991, 47–64, pp. 53–4.

DURSUNOĞLU, Halit. 'Türkiye Türkçesindeki Farsça Kelimeler ve Kullanım Şekilleri', *Atatürk Üniversitesi Sosyal Bilimler Enstitüsü Dergisi*, vol. 13, no. 1 (2009), pp. 131–42.

ERARSLAN, Cezmi. *Abdülhamid II ve İslam Birliği* (İstanbul: Ötüken Neşriyat, 1992).

ESENBEL, Selçuk. 'Japan's Global Claim to Asia and the World of Islam: Transnational Nationalism and World Power, 1900–1945', *The American Historical Review*, vol. 109, no. 4 (October 2004), pp. 1140–70.

ESPOSITO, John, ed. *The Oxford Dictionary of Islam*, Oxford Islamic Studies Online, available at http://www.oxfordislamicstudies.com/article/opr/t125/e1819 (accessed on 17 January 2013).

FAROOQI, Naimur Rahman. *Mughal–Ottoman Relations: A Study of Political and Diplomatic Relations between Mughal India and the Ottoman Empire, 1556–1748* (Delhi: Idarah-i Adabiyat-I Delli, 2009).

————. 'Pan-Islam in the Nineteenth Century', *Islamic Culture* (October 1983), pp. 283–96.

FINDLEY, Carter Vaughn. *The Turks in World History* (Oxford: Oxford University Press, 2005).

————. 'An Ottoman Occidentalist in Europe: Ahmed Midhat Meets Madame Gulnar, 1889', *American Historical Review*, vol. 103, no. 1 (1998), pp. 15–49.

FRASER, Glenda. 'Enver Pasha's Bid for Turkestan: 1920–1922', *Canadian Journal of History*, vol. XXII (August 1988), pp. 197–211.

FROMKIN, David. *A Peace to End All Peace: The Fall of the Ottoman Empire and the Creation of the Modern Middle East* (New York: H. Holt, 2001).

GLADSTONE, William Ewart. *Bulgarian Horrors and the Question of the East* (London: J. Murray, 1876).

GREEN, Abigail and Vincent Viaene, eds. *Religious Internationals in the Modern World: Globalization and Faith Communities since 1750* (Houndmills: Palgrave, 2012).

GREENE, Molly. 'The Ottoman Experience', *Daedalus*, vol. 134, no. 2, On Imperialism (Spring, 2005), pp. 88–99.

GÜNALTAY, Şemseddin M. *Hurafattan Hakikate* (İstanbul: Tevsi-i Tıbaat Matbaası, 1916).

HAIDAR, Mansoura. *Turco-Indian Architecture* (İstanbul: Archaelogy and Art Publications, 2010).

HAIM, Sylvia G., ed. *Arab Nationalism: An Anthology* (Berkeley: University of California Press, 1962).

HALL, Richard C. *The Balkan Wars 1912–1913: Prelude to the First World War* (London: Routledge, 2000).

HASAN, Mushirul. *Between Modernity and Nationalism: Halide Edip's Encounter with Gandhi's India* (Oxford University Press, 2010).

———. *A Moral Reckoning: Muslim Intellectuals in Nineteenth Century Delhi* (Delhi: Oxford University Press, 2005).

———. *A Nationalist Conscience: M. A. Ansari, the Congress and the Raj* (Delhi: Manohar, 1987).

———. *MA Ansari: Gandhi's Infallible Guide* (New Delhi: Manohar, 1987).

———. 'Pan-Islamism versus Indian Nationalism? A Reappraisal', *Economic and Political Weekly*, vol. XXI, no. 24 (14 June 1986).

———. *Muslims and the Congress: Select Correspondence of Dr. M. A. Ansari, 1912–1935* (New Delhi: Manohar, 1979).

HUSAIN, S. M. Azizuddin, ed. *Calendar of Dr. M.A. Ansari's Correspondence* (New Delhi: Kanishka Publishers, 2007).

IQBAL, Afzal. *The Life and Times of Maulana Mohamed Ali* (Lahore: Institute of Islamic Culture, 1979).

KARA, İsmail. 'Turban and Fez: Ulema as Opposition', in Elisabeth Özdalga, ed., *Late Ottoman Society: The Intellectual Legacy* (New York: Routledge Curzon, 2005), pp. 163–202.

———. 'Ulema–siyaset ilişkilerine dair metinler-II, Ey Ulema! Bizim gibi konuş!', *Divan*, no. 7 (1991/92).

KARPAT, Kemal. *The Politicization of Islam: Reconstructing Identity, State, Faith, and Community in the Late Ottoman State* (Oxford: Oxford University Press, 2001).

———. *Türk Dış Politikasi Tarihi* (İstanbul: Timaş, 2012).

KAYALI, Hasan. *Arabs and Young Turks: Ottomanism, Arabism, and Islamism in the Ottoman Empire, 1908–1918* (Berkeley: University of California Press, 1997).

KEDDIE, Nikkie R. 'Pan-Islam as Proto-Nationalism', *Journal of Modern History*, vol. 41, no. 1 (March 1969), pp. 17–28.

KEDOURIE, Elie. 'The End of the Ottoman Empire', *Journal of Contemporary Society*, vol. 3, no. 4, 1918–19: From War to Peace (October 1968), pp. 19–28.

KHALIDI, Tarif. 'Islamic Views of the West in the Middle Ages', *Studies in Interreligious Dialogue*, vol. 5, no. 1 (1995), pp. 31–42.

KHALIQUZZAMAN, Chaudhry. *Pathway to Pakistan* (Lahore: Longmans Green and Co, 1961).

KIDWAI, Shaikh Mushir Hosain. *Pan-Islamism* (London: Lusac and Co.: 1908).

KINROSS, Lord. *The Ottoman Centuries: The Rise and Fall of the Turkish Empire* (New York: Perennial, 1979).

KINZER, Stephen. *Crescent and Star* (New York: Farrar, Straus & Giroux, 2001).

KURTZ, Stanley. 'Root Causes', *Policy Review*, no. 112 (April–May 2002).

LANDAU, Jacob M. *The Politics of Pan-Islam: Ideology and Organization* (Oxford: Clarendon Press, 1990).

LELYVELD, David. 'Three Aligarh Students: Aftab Ahmad Khan, Ziauddin Ahmad and Muhammad Ali', *Modern Asian Studies*, vol. 9, no. 2 (1975), pp. 227–40.

LEWIS, Bernard. *From Babel to Dragomans: Interpreting the Middle East* (Oxford: Oxford University Press, 2004).

———. *The Middle East: A Brief History of the Last 2,000 Years* (New York: Simon and Schuster, 1995).

———. *The Muslim Discovery of Europe* (New York: W. W. Norton, 1982).

MACFIE, A. L. 'British Intelligence and the Causes of Unrest in Mesopotamia, 1919–21', *Middle Eastern Studies*, vol. 35, no. 1 (January 1999), pp. 165–77.

MAHMUD, Syed. *The Khilafat and England* (Patna: Sidaqat Ashram, 1921).

MALCOLM, Noel. *Bosnia: A Short History* (New York: New York University Press, 1994).

MATAR, Nabil. *In the Lands of the Christians: Arabic Travel Writing in the Seventeenth Century* (London: Routledge, 2003).

———. *Turks, Moors and Englishmen in the Age of Discovery* (New York: Columbia University Press, 1999).

MAZOWER, Mark. *The Balkans* (London: Phoenix, 2001).

MINAULT, Gail. *The Khilafat Movement: Religious Symbolism and Political Mobilization in India* (New York: Columbia University Press, 1982).

MINAULT, Gail and David Lelyveld. 'The Campaign for a Muslim University, 1898–1920', *Modern Asian Studies*, vol. 8, no. 2 (1974), pp. 145–89.

MISHRA, Pankaj. *From the Ruins of Empire: The Revolt against the West and the Remaking of Asia* (London: Allen Lane, 2012).

NADVI, Sayyed Suleman. 'Khilafat Awr Hindustan', in Sayyed Sabah al Din, M. A., ed. *Maqalat-i-Nadvi*, vol. I (Karachi: National Book Foundation, 1989).

NECİPOĞLU, Gülru. 'Framing the Gaze in Ottoman, Safavid, and Mughal Palaces', *Ars Orientalis*, vol. 23, Pre-Modern Islamic Palaces (1993), pp. 303–42.

NEW YORK TIMES. 'Balkan War's Effect on India: British Viceroy Hastens to Reassure Both Moslems and Hindus', 19 October 1913.

NICHOLSON, James. *The Hejaz Railway* (London: Stacey International, 2005).

NIJENHUIS, Emmie Te. *Indian Music: History and Structure* (Leiden: Brill, 1974).

NOJEIM, Michael J. *Gandhi and the King: The Power of Non-Violent Resistance* (Westport: Greenwood, 2004).

OCHSENWALD, William. 'The Financing of the Hijaz Railroad', *Die Welt des Islams*, vol. 14, no. 1/4 (1973).

ÖZAYDIN, Zuhal. 'The Indian Muslims Red Crescent Society's Aid to the Ottoman State During the Balkan War in 1912', *Journal of the International Society for the History of Islamic Medicine*, vol. 2 (October 2003), pp. 2–18.

ÖZCAN, Azmi. *Pan-Islamism: Indian Muslims, the Ottomans and Britain, 1877–1924* (Leiden: E.J. Brill, 1997).

———. 'Büyük Hind Ayaklanması ve Osmanlı Devleti', in *İslam Tetkikleri Dergisi*, Cild IX (1995), pp. 269–80.

ÖZDALGA, Elizabeth, ed. *Late Ottoman Society: The Intellectual Legacy* (New York: Routledge Curzon, 2005).

PALMER, Alan. *The Decline and Fall of the Ottoman Empire* (New York: Barnes and Noble, 2005).

PEKESEN, Berna. 'Vertreibung und Abwanderung der Muslime vom Balkan', Europaische Geschichte Online (accessed on 2 April 2011).

PERICA, Vjekoslav. *Balkan Idols: Religion and Nationalism in Yugoslav States* (Oxford: Oxford University Press, 2002).

PERRY, John. 'The Historical Role of Turkish in Relation to Persian of Iran', *Iran & the Caucasus*, vol. 5 (2001), pp. 193–200.

PICK, Walter Pinhas. 'Meissner Pahsa and the Construction of Railways in Palestine and Neighboring Countries', in Gad G. Gilbar, ed., *Ottoman Palestine 1800–1914* (Leiden: E. J. Brill, 1990).

PRAKASH, Gyan. 'Postcolonial Criticism and Indian Historiography', *Social Text*, vols. 31/32 (1992), pp. 8–19.

QUATAERT, Donald. *The Ottoman Empire: 1700–1922* (New York: Cambridge University Press, 2005).

QURESHI, Naeem. *Pan-Islam in British India: The Politics of the Khilafat Movement 1918–1924* (Oxford: Oxford University Press, 2008).

RANGER, Terence. 'Connexions between "Primary Resistance" Movements and Modern Mass Nationalisms in East and Central Africa', *Journal of African History*, vol. 9, no. 3 (1968).

RAUF, Abdul. 'Pan-Islamism and the North West Frontier Province of British India (1897–1918)', *Perceptions*, Winter (2007), pp. 21–47.

REDHOUSE, J. W. *A Vindication of the Ottoman Sultan's Title of 'Caliph': Shewing Its Antiquity, Validity, and Universal Acceptance* (London: Beffingham Wilson Hoyal Exchange, 1877).

REMOND, Georges. *Bir Fransız Gazetecinin Balkan İzlenimleri: Mağluplarla Beraber* (İstanbul: Profil Yayıncılık, 2007).

REUBEN, Roxanne L. *Journeys to the Other Shore: Muslim and Western Travelers in Search of Knowledge* (Princeton: Princeton University Press, 2006).

SADIQ, Mohammad. *The Turkish Revolution and the Indian Freedom Movement* (New Delhi: Macmillan, 1983).

SAID, Edward. *Orientalism* (New York: Vintage, 1979).

SARI, Nur and Zühal Özaydın. 'Dr. Besim Ömer Paşa ve Kadın Hastabakıcı Eğitiminin Nedenleri (II)', *Sendrom*, Mayıs (1992), pp. 72–80.

SARKAR, Benoy Kumar. *The Futurism of Young Asia and Other Essays on the Relations between the East and the West* (Berlin: Julius Springer, 1922).

SCHIMMEL, Annemarie. *The Empire of the Great Mughals: History, Art and Culture* (London: Reaktion Books, 2004).

SHUKLA, Ram Lakhan. *Britain, India and the Turkish Empire: 1853–1882* (New Delhi: People's Publishing House, 1973).

SIDOROV, Dmitrii. 'Post-Imperial Third Romes: Resurrections of a Russian Orthodox Geopolitical Metaphor, Geopolitics', vol. 11 (2006), pp. 317–47.

SONYEL, Salahi. 'Mustafa Kemal and Enver in Conflict, 1919–22', *Middle Eastern Studies*, vol. 25, no. 4 (October 1989), pp. 506–15.

SOYLUER, Serdal. 'Balkan Savaşı Sırasında Hintlilerin Osmanlı'ya Yardım Kampanyalarının Osmanlı Basınına Yansımaları', *şarkiyat Mecmuası*, Sayı 13 (2008), pp. 91–118.

SWANSON, Glen W. 'Enver Pasha: The Formative Years', *Middle Eastern Studies*, vol. 16, no. 3 (October 1980), pp. 193–9.

TANGRI, Shanti S. 'Intellectuals and Society in Nineteenth-Century India', *Comparative Studies in Society and History*, vol. 3, no. 4 (July 1961), pp. 368–94.

TONER, Jerry P. *Homer's Turk: How Classics Shaped Ideas of the East* (Harvard University Press, 2013).

TOSUN, Hale. 'İstanbul'da Kurulan Cumhuriyetin İlk Milli Hemşirelik Okulu: Kızılay Hemşirelik Okulu', *Maltepe Üniversitesi Hemşirelik Bilim ve Sanat Dergisi*, Sempozyum Özel Sayısı, 2010, pp. 126–30.

TRIVEDI, Raj Kumar. *The Critical Triangle: India Britain and Turkey: 1908–1924* (Jaipur: Publication Scheme, 1994).

UYAR, Mesut and Edward J. Erickson. *A Military History of the Ottomans: From Osman to Atatürk* (Santa Barbara: Praeger, 2009).

ÜNAL, Hasan. 'Young Turk Assessments of International Politics, 1906–9', *Middle Eastern Studies*, vol. 32, no. 2 (April 1996), pp. 30–44.

VEHBİ, Ali. *Avant la debacle de la Turquie: Pensées et souvenirs de l'ex-Sultan Abdul Hamid* (Paris: Attinger, 1913).

WASTI, Syed Tanvir. 'The 1877 Ottoman Mission to Afghanistan', *Middle Eastern Studies*, vol. 30, no. 4 (October 1994), pp. 956–62.

———. 'Mushir Hosain Kidwai and the Ottoman Cause', *Middle Eastern Studies*, vol. 30, no. 2 (April 1994), pp. 252–61.

———. 'Two Muslim Travelogues: To and From Istanbul', *Middle Eastern Studies*, vol. 27, no. 3 (1991), pp. 457–76.

———. 'The 1912–13 Balkan Wars and the Siege of Edirne', *Middle Eastern Studies*, vol. 40, no. 4 (July 2004), pp. 59–78.

———. 'The Indian Red Crescent Mission to the Balkan Wars', *Middle Eastern Studies*, vol. 45, no. 3 (May 2009), pp. 393–406.

YILMAZ, Şuhnaz. 'An Ottoman Warrior Abroad: Enver Paşa as an Expatriate', *Middle Eastern Studies*, vol. 35, no. 4, Seventy-Five Years of the Turkish Republic (October 1999), pp. 40–69.

Index

Din-i Ilahi 61
Diu, Battle of 63
Dolmabahçe 207
Dr. Ali Azhar H. Fyzee 162
Dr. Esad Pasha 196, 286, 288
Dr. Fouad 163, 264
Dr. Mahmudullah 202, 286
Dr. Muhammad Husain 191, 253–5
Dr. Rahman 163–4, 174, 181, 184, 202, 215, 238, 254, 261, 270, 283, 290–1, 315–16
Dr. S. Muhammad Naim Ansari 162
Dr. Shamsul Barry 162–3
Dusan, Stephan 37
Dutch Empire in the Indian Ocean 64, 123–4
Dysentery 41, 214

East India Trading Company 77, 123, 125
Eastern Question 31, 36
Edirne 40, 42–6, 80, 185, 187–9, 207, 317, 325
Egypt 29, 31, 38, 49, 72–3, 91, 98, 106, 116, 121, 127, 130, 141–2, 148–9, 151, 169, 181, 191, 194, 196, 208–9, 212, 216, 220, 238, 241–2, 270, 274, 284, 287, 289, 302, 307, 309, 313
Egyptian Red Crescent 181, 253
Ekmecic, Milorad 37
Empire 1–2, 4–5, 7, 9–11, 15–16, 22–8, 30–8, 43, 46, 48–9, 51, 53–67, 69–70, 72–5, 77–81, 83, 85–6, 90–1, 93–9, 101–2, 104–6, 108–9, 111–18, 120–8, 130–2, 135–7, 142, 145–50, 160, 165–70, 172, 175, 177–8, 183, 199–200, 208, 210–11, 219–20, 227–9, 230–1, 245, 303, 306, 319–22, 324
Enver Pasha (also Enver Bey) 17, 44, 165, 185–7, 189, 203, 320, 325
Erarslan, Cezmi 135, 320
Erickson, Edward J. 39, 45, 52, 325

Ertuğrul frigate, tour of the Indian Ocean 117
Esenbel, Selçuk 135
Esposito, John 97, 134
Euro-Americans 91–3, 95–6, 105–6
Europe 25–7, 30–2, 35–6, 46–7, 49, 50, 60, 64, 73, 81, 89–90, 92, 94, 96, 102, 122, 124, 127–8, 130, 134, 142–3, 146–7, 150, 153–4, 160, 175, 180, 188, 212, 228, 239, 244, 252–3, 267, 279, 309, 319–20, 322
European Modernity 89, 146
European Union 21, 24, 32
Europeanness 9, 89

Faith Communities 135, 321
Farooqi, Naimur Rahman 11, 58, 67, 86, 100, 320
Farrukbsiyar 67
Feth Ali. *See* Tipu Sultan
Fethi Bey, the hero of the Turkish–Italian war of 1912 in Tripoli 154, 245, 279
Filofei 35
Findley, Carter Vaughn 85, 134, 136, 320
Firangi Mahal 128–9, 230
First War of Independence 9, 12, 76–9, 118, 123–4
First World War 4, 11, 32–4, 47, 51, 75, 81–2, 118, 121, 131–2, 157, 164–5, 167, 169, 173, 178, 180, 197, 202, 210, 217, 223, 321
Fleischauer, Jan 141
Fraser, Glenda 203, 320
French empire 4, 10, 31–2, 68–9, 72, 74, 150, 167–8, 170–1, 180, 186, 209, 252, 260
Fromkin, David 81, 87, 320

Gallipoli 44, 173, 177–8, 185, 187–9, 207, 245, 259, 270

Landau, Jacob M. 100, 116, 135, 322
Lawrence, T. E. 121
Lelyveld, David 18, 137, 322–3
Lewis, Bernard 143, 160, 322
London 3, 5–6, 11, 14, 17, 43–6, 51–2, 68, 70, 72, 75, 78–81, 85–6, 95, 105, 116, 125–7, 134, 136–7, 150, 160, 163, 169, 173–5, 180, 185, 216, 236–7, 252, 262, 268, 287, 318, 319, 321–4
London Conference 43–4, 185
London Peace Treaty, 30 May 1913 45–46
Lucknow 76, 80, 163, 175, 233
Lüleburgaz 41–5
Lytton, Lord 80–1, 119

Macedonia 21, 24, 29, 40, 43–8, 166–7, 171, 197, 207, 217, 288–9, 296
Macedonia, Republic of 21, 24
Madame Noureddin Bey 151, 242
Madrasatul Uloom Musalmanan-e-Hind 127
Mahmud al-Hasan 130
Mahmud I 67
Mahmud Muhtar Pasha 41
Mahmud of Ghazni 55
Malabar 68
Malcolm, Noel 51, 322
Mamluk Turks 63
Mansoor Ali Amethi 163
Marathas 68, 124
Marco Polo 122
Marmara Sea 42, 45
Matar, Nabil 160, 322
Maulana Hasrat Mohani 130
Maulana Mohamed Ali 14, 18, 175, 244, 294, 302, 321
May, Karl Friedrich 141–2
Mazower, Mark 49, 52, 322
McCarthy, Justin 48, 52

Mecca 61, 71, 97–8, 114, 123, 143, 193, 283
Mecidiye warship 178
Medina 97–8, 114, 120–1, 287
Medina University 202, 206, 216, 288–9, 295
Mehmed V 8
Meriç River 44, 46
Mevlana Celaleddin Rumi 157, 235
Mezar-i Sherif 119
Middle East 18, 22, 87, 123, 136–7, 161, 203, 229, 320, 322, 325
Millet system 30, 47
Minault, Gail 99, 137, 323
Mirza Abdul Qayyum 163–4
Mishra, Pankaj 134, 323
Missionaries 33, 76, 89, 92–4, 96, 116, 126
Modernities 29, 51, 134, 319
Modernity, the role of education 12, 89–90, 94, 96, 109–10, 113–14, 124–7, 149, 151, 152, 166, 172, 199, 209, 217, 229, 273, 299
Mohammad Inshaullah 121
Mohammad-Uddin 202
Mohammed Abdul Aziz Ansari 163
Moldova 21
Montagu, Edwin 125
Montenegro 21, 25, 29, 34, 37, 47, 80
Morocco 116, 169, 196, 284
Moscow 25, 35–6, 169
Moynier, Gustave 190
Mughal court, Turkish influence in 54–9
Mughals, Turkic roots 55–9
Muhammad Ali 11–12, 18, 31, 72, 149, 316, 322
Muhammad Shah 67
Muhammad Shah (Mughal Emperor, 1719–48) 67
Muhammed Qasim (1833–77) 80

About the Author

Burak Akçapar is a Turkish diplomat, author, and scholar.

As a career diplomat, Ambassador Akçapar has served as the Ambassador Plenipotentiary and Extraordinary of the Republic of Turkey to India, Nepal, and Maldives. His previous postings included Deputy Director General for Political Affairs with a focus on South Asia; twice the head of the Policy Planning Department at the Ministry of Foreign Affairs in Turkey; Deputy Head of Mission of the Turkish Embassy in Washington; international officer at NATO, where he received Award for Excellence; as well as other postings in Germany and Qatar.

As a scholar, Burak Akçapar has authored two international peer-reviewed books: *Turkey's New European Era* (2006) and *The International Law of Conventional Arms Control in Europe* (1996). He has also contributed to various edited books as well as numerous journals on international affairs, international security, and arms control.

Burak Akçapar lives in New Delhi and is married to Şebnem Köşer Akçapar, social anthropologist and former director of Eastern Mediterranean Center of Georgetown University. They have a son, Ziya Onat Akçapar.